Intelligent Systems Reference Library

Volume 140

Series editors

Janusz Kacprzyk, Polish Academy of Sciences, Warsaw, Poland
e-mail: kacprzyk@ibspan.waw.pl

Lakhmi C. Jain, University of Canberra, Canberra, Australia;
Bournemouth University, UK;
KES International, UK
e-mail: jainlc2002@yahoo.co.uk; jainlakhmi@gmail.com
URL: http://www.kesinternational.org/organisation.php

The aim of this series is to publish a Reference Library, including novel advances and developments in all aspects of Intelligent Systems in an easily accessible and well structured form. The series includes reference works, handbooks, compendia, textbooks, well-structured monographs, dictionaries, and encyclopedias. It contains well integrated knowledge and current information in the field of Intelligent Systems. The series covers the theory, applications, and design methods of Intelligent Systems. Virtually all disciplines such as engineering, computer science, avionics, business, e-commerce, environment, healthcare, physics and life science are included. The list of topics spans all the areas of modern intelligent systems such as: Ambient intelligence, Computational intelligence, Social intelligence, Computational neuroscience, Artificial life, Virtual society, Cognitive systems, DNA and immunity-based systems, e-Learning and teaching, Human-centred computing and Machine ethics, Intelligent control, Intelligent data analysis, Knowledge-based paradigms, Knowledge management, Intelligent agents, Intelligent decision making, Intelligent network security, Interactive entertainment, Learning paradigms, Recommender systems, Robotics and Mechatronics including human-machine teaming, Self-organizing and adaptive systems, Soft computing including Neural systems, Fuzzy systems, Evolutionary computing and the Fusion of these paradigms, Perception and Vision, Web intelligence and Multimedia.

More information about this series at http://www.springer.com/series/8578

Kenji Suzuki · Yisong Chen
Editors

Artificial Intelligence in Decision Support Systems for Diagnosis in Medical Imaging

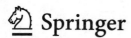 Springer

Editors
Kenji Suzuki
Medical Imaging Research Center
 and Department of Electrical and
 Computer Engineering
Illinois Institute of Technology
Chicago, IL
USA

and

World Research Hub Initiative (WRHI),
 Institute of Innovative Research (IIR)
Tokyo Institute of Technology
Yokohama, Kanagawa
Japan

Yisong Chen
Key Laboratory of Machine Perception
 (Ministry of Education), School of
 Electronics Engineering and Computer
 Science
Peking University
Beijing
China

ISSN 1868-4394   ISSN 1868-4408   (electronic)
Intelligent Systems Reference Library
ISBN 978-3-319-88666-4   ISBN 978-3-319-68843-5   (eBook)
https://doi.org/10.1007/978-3-319-68843-5

Printed on acid-free paper

This Springer imprint is published by Springer Nature
The registered company is Springer International Publishing AG
The registered company address is: Gewerbestrasse 11, 6330 Cham, Switzerland

I dedicate this book to my wife, Harumi Suzuki, for her support, encouragement, and love, and to my daughters, Mineru Suzuki and Juno Suzuki, for their love.

Kenji Suzuki

I dedicate this book to my wife, Hong Cui, for her unwavering support and love.

Yisong Chen

Foreword

Medical images of CT, MRI, PET, ultrasonography, etc., prevail in clinical diagnosis. Usually, it takes years of training for physicians to conduct the interpretation of medical images. Still, it may happen that interpretations may change from physician to physician. Computer-aided diagnosis (CAD) is a technology to help physicians efficiently ease the interpretation procedure. The first CAD product for detection of breast lesions in mammography was approved by the FDA about 20 years ago. Many CAD systems have been installed in hospitals or shipped with scanners and help improve the diagnostic performance of physicians. The need of healthcare organizations for CAD systems is ever growing. In addition to its success in clinics, CAD can also be used for education and for remote diagnose, among others.

CAD is an interdisciplinary field of traditional disciplines, such as statistics, mathematics, physics, medicine, computer and imaging technologies, and new disciplines, such as artificial intelligence, especially, pattern recognition and machine learning. It usually takes a long leaning curve to train sophisticated researcher and engineers for CAD. Many scientific discoveries and technological inventions have resulted during the interdisciplinary collaborations. This book demonstrates the picture of CAD by contributions from active groups and state-of-the-art techniques for CAD. Students may find his/her own path by reading this book if they are to pursue a career in CAD.

This book is a timely publication for CAD. It is only under the appreciated effort of the well-respected CAD researchers Drs. Suzuki and Chen that it is possible to bring together the state-of-the-art advances in CAD in one readily accessible source. This book demonstrates a number of CAD applications in a variety of diseases and body regions, and for different imaging modalities. This book covers also a number of machine-learning methods and their CAD applications. Researchers, engineers, and professionals may find this book a comprehensive reference on CAD.

With the performance of AlphaGo, a deep learning approach is becoming popular in CAD because it is able to learn from examples and prior knowledge. Several successful applications have been reported. A number of start-ups and big vendors are investing in this technology. Although most of current CAD systems are organ-specific, modality-tailored, and disease-specific, the diseases, organs, and imaging modalities covered within CAD systems are rapidly expanding. It is expected that CAD systems will evolve with the development of machine learning to cover whole-body and cross-modalities and to incorporate other patients' symptoms and clinical tests.

Will physicians lose their jobs with the development of CAD? Very unlikely in my opinion. Although machine learning is becoming ubiquitous, it is necessary to understand what the machines are doing to trust it. The problem with the deep learning is that knowledge is trained into a neural network of a huge number of parameters, rather than into us. It works like a black box at present. Moreover, successful examples of CAD are only for typical diseases, but not for rare diseases because of insufficient data to train the network. In such rare cases, the engagement of physicians is indispensable. There are, and will remain, debates if machine intelligence will perform over human beings and whether CAD will replace physicians in the future. This book is a valuable source for reads to envisage the future of CAD while reading the vivid stories in this book.

Beijing, China   Ming Jiang
                                                                Peking University

Preface

A decision support system for diagnosis is a crucial element in medicine and patients' healthcare, because diagnosis is a complex task that is often difficult for even experienced physicians. Medical imaging offers useful information on patients' medical conditions and clues to causes of their symptoms and diseases. Thus, medical imaging is indispensable for accurate medical decision making in modern medicine. Medical images, however, provide a large number of images, which physicians must interpret. That would lead to "information overload" for physicians, and it can complicate medical decision making further. Therefore, intelligent decision support systems are increasingly demanded to help physicians in their decision making in diagnosis and treatment through medical images. In the computer aids in medical decision making, computational intelligence plays very important roles to intelligently support physicians' decision making. The areas of research in this field include computer-aided diagnosis, computer-aided surgery and therapy, medical image analysis, automated organ/lesion segmentation, automated image fusion, automated image annotation, and content-based image retrieval.

As this field of intelligent decision support systems for diagnosis through medical images is one of the most promising, growing fields, the efforts are currently scattered, and a large number of researchers participated in the field and developed a number of intelligent diagnosis methods based on medical imaging. This book covers the state-of-the-art technologies and recent advances in the field of intelligent decision support systems for diagnosis through medical images. We expect that this book will be useful for professors, students, researchers, engineers, and professionals in their studies, research, development as well as daily work and practice.

Leading researchers in the field contributed 13 chapters to this book in which they describe their cutting-edge techniques and studies on intelligent decision support systems for diagnosis through medical images. The 13 chapters are organized in five parts that represent five major research areas in the field of intelligent decision support systems.

Part I contains three chapters provided by leading researchers in the research area of advanced machine learning in computer-aided systems.

In Chapter "Multi-modality Feature Learning in Diagnoses of Alzheimer's Disease," Dr. Daoqiang Zhang introduces a label-aligned multitask feature selection method that can fully explore the relationships across both modalities and subjects, and then, they propose a discriminative multitask feature selection method to select the most discriminative features for multimodality-based classification. The experimental results on magnetic resonance imaging (MRI), fluorodeoxyglucose positron emission tomography (FDG-PET), and cerebrospinal fluid (CSF) data of subjects from the Alzheimer's disease neuroimaging initiative (ADNI) database demonstrate the effectiveness of their proposed method.

In Chapter "A Comparative Study of Modern Machine Learning Approaches for Focal Lesion Detection and Classification in Medical Images: BoVW, CNN and MTANN," Drs. Nima Tajbakhsh and Kenji Suzuki review and compare two major end-to-end machine-learning models, massive-training artificial neural networks (MTANNs) and convolutional neural networks (CNNs), and a well-known non-end-to-end machine-learning model, a bag of visual words (BoVW) with Fisher vectors in detection and classification of focal lesions in medical images. They show that MTANNs outperform CNNs and BoVW in detection of lung nodules and colorectal polyps and classification of lung nodules in CT.

In Chapter "Introduction to Binary Coordinate Ascent: New Insights into Efficient Feature Subset Selection for Machine Learning," Drs. Amin Zarshenas and Kenji Suzuki describe a novel optimization technique based on their originally developed optimization algorithm, the coordinate descent algorithm. The algorithm is an iterative deterministic local optimization approach that can be coupled with wrapper, filter, or hybrid feature selection techniques. The algorithm searches throughout the space of binary-coded input variables by iteratively optimizing the objective function in each dimension at a time. With their new technique, the efficiency in terms of the number of subset evaluations was improved substantially.

Part II contains two chapters provided by two leading groups working in the area of computer-aided detection.

In Chapter "Automated Lung Nodule Detection Using Positron Emission Tomography/Computed Tomography," Drs. Atsushi Teramoto and Hiroshi Fujita highlight their recent contributions to a hybrid detection scheme of lung nodules in PET/CT images. The method detects lung nodules by using both the anatomical information obtained by CT and the functional information obtained with PET. Their results demonstrate that the proposed hybrid method would be useful for computer-aided detection of lung cancer in clinical practice.

In Chapter "Detecting Mammographic Masses via Image Retrieval and Discriminative Learning," Drs. Menglin Jiang, Shaoting Zhang, and Dimitris N. Metaxas introduce an automatic computer-aided diagnosis (CAD) approach that integrates content-based image retrieval (CBIR) and discriminative learning. Their approach achieves a high mass detection accuracy and retrieval precision, comparing favorably with traditional methods. Compared with CBIR-based CAD methods, their approach serves as a fully automated "double reading" aid without radiologists' labeling of suspicious regions.

Part III contains four chapters in the area of computer-aided diagnosis.

In Chapter "High-Order Statistics of Micro-Texton for HEp-2 Staining Pattern Classification," Drs. Xian-Hua Han and Yen-Wei Chen aim to achieve automatic recognition of six HEp-2 staining patterns in indirect immunofluorescence (IIF) images in an open HEp-2 dataset. They propose a local structure representation called Weber local descriptors (WLD) and develop a method for extracting not only low-order but also high-order statistics based on WLD, which has high discrimination power in classification. Their approach for classifying HEp-2 staining cells automatically indicates the presence of autoimmune diseases by finding antibodies in the patient serum by means of indirect immunofluorescence image analysis.

In Chapter "Intelligent Diagnosis of Breast Cancer Based on Quantitative B-mode and Elastography Features," Drs. Chung-Ming Lo and Ruey-Feng Chang introduce three CAD systems focusing on quantitative B-mode texture, elasticity analysis, and the combination of both B-mode and elasticity features. They show that the malignant tumor detection rate can be significantly improved with all three methodologies of (1) intensity-invariant transformed tumor textures analysis, (2) shear-wave elastography (SWE) features, and (3) quantified strain features combined with B-mode features.

In Chapter "Categorization of Lung Tumors into Benign/Malignant, Solid/GGo, and Typical Benign/Others," Dr. Yasushi Hirano describes various categorization methods for lung tumors in chest X-ray CT images, which include a method for classification between benign and malignant tumors and methods for classification between solid nodules and ground-glass nodules. Furthermore, extraction methods for lung tumors and lung blood vessels are also described as the fundamental techniques for the structural analysis in these categorization methods.

In Chapter "Fuzzy Object Growth Model for Neonatal Brain MR Understanding," Drs. Saadia Binte Alam, Syoji Kobashi, and Jayaram K Udupa describe a brain region segmentation method in newborn brain MR images. The method employs a four-dimensional fuzzy object growth model (FOGM) that gives a prior knowledge of brain shape and position at any growing time. Using the growth index, FOGM is constructed from the training dataset. To evaluate the method, they segment the parenchymal region of 16 subjects using synthesized FOGM.

Part IV contains two chapters written by two leading groups in the area of computer-aided prognosis.

In Chapter "Computer-Aided Prognosis: Accurate Prediction of Patients with Neurologic and Psychiatric Diseases via Multi-modal MRI Analysis," Dr. Huiguang He's research group introduces their work on computer-aided prognosis technology based on multimodal MRI to assist the clinical diagnosis of neurologic and psychiatric diseases, especially Alzheimer's disease. Their method employs support vector machine classifiers and multikernel learning with multimodal features. They show the advantages of their framework for neurologic and psychiatric diseases prediction.

In Chapter "Radiomics in Medical Imaging—Detection, Extraction and Segmentation," Dr. Jie Tian's research group provides comprehensive descriptions of radiomics and CAD in medical imaging. Radiomics and CAD have pipelines of data acquisition, lesion segmentation, feature extraction and selection, classification with machine learning including deep learning, and clinical results. They describe radiomics and CAD methods for CT, MRI, and PET imaging.

Part V contains two chapters provided by two leading groups in the area of computer-aided therapy and surgery.

In Chapter "Markerless Tumor Gating and Tracking for Lung Cancer Radiotherapy Based on Machine Learning Techniques," Drs. Tong Lin and Yucheng Lin demonstrate how machine-learning techniques can be used for tumor gating and tracking in radiation therapy for lung cancer. In tumor gating, five-dimensionality reduction techniques and two machine-learning classification approaches are investigated. In tumor tracking, a novel tracking algorithm without implanted fiducial markers is proposed. They show the usefulness of their methods in tumor gating and tracking in radiation therapy.

In Chapter "Image Guided and Robot Assisted Precision Surgery," Drs. Fang Chen, Jia Liu, and Hongen Liao present several related technologies and application examples about image guidance and surgical robots in computer-aided surgery (CAS). Three key technologies are introduced, including image processing-based guidance, 3D augmented reality-based image guidance, and various surgical robots that can be implemented precisely to complete complex tasks under the image guidance in difficult procedures.

In summary, this book covers a comprehensive overview of the state-of-the-art research and technologies in intelligent decision support systems for diagnosis based on medical images. This book discusses major technical advancements and research findings in the rapidly growing field of intelligent decision support systems. This book demonstrates that such technologies and studies reached the practical level already and that they are becoming available in clinical practices in hospitals rapidly. We hope that this book will also act as a useful reference for professors, students, researchers, engineers, and professionals who demand textbooks or handbooks in the interdisciplinary field between computational intelligence and medical imaging.

Chicago, USA/Yokohama, Japan   Kenji Suzuki
Beijing, China   Yisong Chen

Acknowledgements

This work would not have been possible without the help and support of countless people. The authors are grateful to the thirteen leading research groups in the field of artificial intelligence in decision support systems for medical image diagnosis for valuable contributions to this publication, to all members in the Suzuki laboratory, i.e., postdoctoral scholars, computer scientists, visiting scholars/professors, medical students, graduate/undergraduate students, research technicians, research volunteers, and support staff, at Illinois Institute of Technology, at University of Chicago, and at Tokyo Institute of Technology for their invaluable assistance in the studies, and to colleagues and collaborators for their valuable suggestions. Many of the authors of chapters in this book served as reviewers of manuscripts submitted by their peers. The authors are grateful to all reviewers for their time and effort. The authors are grateful to their mentors in the past decades for their guidance in their career. One of the authors, Kenji Suzuki, is also grateful to his wife, Harumi Suzuki, for her support, encouragement, understanding, patience, and love, and her parents and brothers for their understanding and support; his daughters, Mineru Suzuki and Juno Suzuki, for cheering him up, and the joys that they have brought to his life; and his parents, Souichiro Suzuki and Mitsuru Suzuki, and his brothers, Eiji Suzuki and Junji Suzuki, for their support, encouragement, and inspiration.

Contents

Fuzzy Object Growth Model for Neonatal Brain MR Understanding 209

Saadia Binte Alam, Syoji Kobashi and Jayaram K Udupa

Part IV   Computer-Aided Prognosis

Computer-Aided Prognosis: Accurate Prediction of Patients with Neurologic and Psychiatric Diseases via Multi-modal MRI Analysis 225

Huiguang He, Hongwei Wen, Dai Dai and Jieqiong Wang

Part I
Advanced Machine Learning
in Computer-Aided Systems

Multi-modality Feature Learning in Diagnoses of Alzheimer's Disease

Daoqiang Zhang, Chen Zu, Biao Jie and Tingting Ye

Abstract Many machine learning and pattern classification methods have been applied to the diagnosis of Alzheimer's disease (AD) and its prodromal stage, which is mild cognitive impairment (MCI). Recently, multi-task feature selection methods are typically used for joint selection of common features across multiple modalities. In this chapter, we review several latest multi-modality feature learning works in diagnoses of AD. Specifically, multi-task feature selection (MTFS) is proposed to jointly select the common subset of relevant features for multiple variables from each modality. Based on MTFS, a manifold regularized multi-task feature learning method (M2TFS) is used to preserve both the intrinsic relatedness among multiple modalities of data and the data distribution information in each modality. However, most existing methods focus on mining the relationship across multiple modalities of the same subjects, while ignoring the potentially useful relationship across different subjects. In order to overcome this issue, label-aligned multi-task feature selection (LAMTFS) which can fully explore the realtionships across both modalities and subjects is proposed. Then a discriminative multi-task feature selection method is proposed to select the most discriminative features for multi-modality based classification. The experimental results on the baseline magnetic resonance image (MRI), fluorodeoxyglucose positron emission tomography (FDG-PET), and cerebrospinal fluid (CSF) data of subjects from AD neuroimaging initiative (ADNI) data base demonstrate the effectiveness of those above proposed methods.

D. Zhang (✉) · C. Zu · T. Ye
Nanjing University of Aeronautics and Astronautics, 29 Jiangjun Road, Nanjing 211106, People's Republic of China
e-mail: dqzhang@nuaa.edu.cn

C. Zu
e-mail: chenzu@nuaa.edu.cn

T. Ye
e-mail: yetingting@nuaa.edu.cn

B. Jie
Anhui Normal University, 1 Beijingdong Road, Wuhu 241000, People's Republic of China
e-mail: jbiao@nuaa.edu.cn

© Springer International Publishing AG 2018
K. Suzuki and Y. Chen (eds.), *Artificial Intelligence in Decision Support Systems for Diagnosis in Medical Imaging*, Intelligent Systems Reference Library 140, https://doi.org/10.1007/978-3-319-68843-5_1

1   Introduction

Alzheimers disease (AD) is the most common type of dementia, accounting for 60–80% of age-related dementia cases [36]. It is predicted that the number of affected people will double in the next 20 years, and 1 in 85 people will be affected by 2050 [3]. As AD-specific brain changes begin years before the patient becomes symptomatic, early clinical diagnosis of AD becomes a challenging task. Therefore, many studies focus on possible identification of such changes at the early stage, that is, mild cognitive impairment (MCI), by leveraging neuroimaging data [29, 36].

Neuroimaging is a powerful tool for disease diagnosis and also evaluation of therapeutic efficacy in neurodegenerative diseases, such as AD and MCI. Neuroimaging research offers great potential to discover features that can identify individuals early in the course of dementing illness. Recently, a number of machine learning and pattern classification methods have been widely used in neuroimaging analysis of AD and MCI, including both group comparison (i.e., between clinically different groups) and individual classification [23, 36]. Early studies mainly focus on extracting features (e.g., based on regions of interest (ROIs) or voxels) from single imaging modality such as structural magnetic resonance imaging (MRI) [6, 10, 18, 22, 34] and fluorodeoxyglucose positron emission tomography (FDG-PET) [9, 11–13], and so forth. More recently, researchers have begun to integrate multiple imaging modalities to further improve the accuracy of disease diagnosis [14, 40].

In many clinical and research studies, it is common to acquire multiple imaging modalities for a more accurate and rigorous assessment of disease status and progression. In fact, different imaging modalities provide different views of brain function or structure. For example, structural MRI provides information about the tissue type of brain, while FDG-PET measures the cerebral metabolic rate for glucose. It is reported that MRI and FDG-PET measures provide different sensitivity to memory between disease and health [31]. Intuitively, integration of multiple modalities may uncover the previously hidden information that cannot be found using any single modality. In the literature, a number of studies have exploited the fusion of multiple modalities to improve AD or MCI classification performance [1, 8, 11, 15, 17]. For example, Hinrichs et al. [14] and Liu et al. [18] proposed to combine MRI and FDG-PET for AD classification. Zhang et al. [40] combined three modalities, that is, MRI, FDG-PET, and cerebrospinal fluid (CSF), to discriminate AD/MCI and normal controls (NCs). Existing studies have indicated that different imaging modalities can provide essential complementary information that can improve accuracy in disease diagnosis when used together.

For imaging modalities, even after feature extraction (usually from brain regions), there may still exist redundant or irrelevant features. So, feature selection, which can be considered as the biomarker identification for AD and MCI, is commonly used to remove these redundant or irrelevant features. However, due to the complexity of brain and the disease, it is challenging to detect all relevant disease-related features (i.e., regional features) from a single modality, especially in the early stage of the disease. Different imaging modalities may provide essential complementary information that can help identify these dysfunctional regions implicated by the same underlying pathology. In addition, recent studies also show that there is overlap between the disease-related brain regions detected by MRI and FDG-PET, respectively, such as regions in the hippocampus and the mesia temporal lobe [15]. Some feature selection techniques (e.g., t-test) have been used for identifying the disease-related regions from each single modality data [40]. However, an obvious disadvantage of these techniques is that they do not consider the intrinsic relatedness between features across different modalities. Recently, a few studies have exploited to jointly select features from multi-modality neuroimaging data for AD/MCI classification. For example, [15] proposed to jointly identify disease related brain features from multi-modality data, using sparse composite linear discrimination analysis method. Liu et al. [18] embedded intermodality constraint into multi-task learning framework for AD/MCI classification. However, a disadvantage of those methods is that the distribution information of each modality data is ignored, which may affect the final classification performance.

In this chapter, we review several latest multi-modality feature learning works in diagnoses of AD. Specifically, multi-task feature selection (MTFS) [39] is proposed to jointly select the common subset of relevant features for multiple variables from each modality. Based on MTFS, a manifold regularized multi-task feature learning method (M2TFS) [16] is used to preserve both the intrinsic relatedness among multiple modalities for data and the data distribution information in each modality. However, most existing methods foucus on mining the relationship across multiple modalities of the same subjects, while ignoring the potentially useful relationship across different subjects. In order to overcome this issue, label-aligned multi-task feature selection (LAMTFS) [42] which can fully explore the realtionships across both modalities and subjects is proposed. Then a discriminative multi-task feature selection (DMTFS) [37] method is proposed to select the most discriminative features for multi-modality based classification.

2 Subjects

The data used in the preparation of this chapter were obtained from the Alzheimers Disease Neuroimaging Initiative (ADNI) database (https://www.loni.ucla.edu/ADNI). The ADNI was launched in 2003 by the National Institute on Aging (NIA), the National Institute of Biomedical Imaging and Bioengineering (NIBIB), the Food and Drug Administration (FDA), private pharmaceutical companies and non-profit organizations, as a 60 million, 5-year public-private partnership. The primary goal of ADNI has been to test whether serial MRI, PET, other biological markers, and clinical and neuropsychological assessment can be combined to measure the progression of MCI and early AD. Determination of sensitive and specific markers of very early AD progression is intended to aid researchers and clinicians to develop new treatments and monitor their effectiveness, as well as lessen the time and cost of clinical trials.

ADNI is the result of efforts of many coinvestigators from a broad range of academic institutions and private corporations, and subjects have been recruited from over 50 sites across the U.S. and Canada. The initial goal of ADNI was to recruit 800 adults, ages 55 to 90, to participate in the research approximately 200 cognitively normal older individuals to be followed for 3 years, 400 people with MCI to be followed for 3 years, and 200 people with early AD to be followed for 2 years (see https://www.adni-info.org for up-to-date information). The research protocol was approved by each local institutional review board and written informed consent is obtained from each participant.

The ADNI general eligibility criteria are described at https://www.adni-info.org. Briefly, subjects are between 55–90 years of age, having a study partner able to provide an independent evaluation of functioning. Specific psychoactive medications will be excluded. General inclusion/exclusion criteria are as follows: (1) healthy subjects: Mini-Mental State Examination (MMSE) scores between 24–30, a Clinical Dementia Rating (CDR) of 0, non-depressed, non MCI, and nondemented; (2) MCI subjects: MMSE scores between 24–30, a memory complaint, having objective memory loss measured by education adjusted scores on Wechsler Memory Scale Logical Memory II, a CDR of 0.5, absence of significant levels of impairment in other cognitive domains, essentially preserved activities of daily living, and an absence of dementia; and (3) Mild AD: MMSE scores between 20–26, CDR of 0.5 or 1.0, and meets the National Institute of Neurological and Communicative Disorders and Stroke and the Alzheimers Disease and Related Disorders Association (NINCDS/ADRDA) criteria for probable AD.

In this chapter, only ADNI subjects with all corresponding MRI, CSF and PET baseline data are included. This yields a total of 202 subjects including 51 AD patients, 99 MCI patients (43 MCI converters who had converted to AD within 18 months and 56 MCI non-converters who had not converted to AD within 18 months), and 52 normal controls. Table 1 lists the demographics of all these subjects.

Table 1 Subject Information

	AD (n = 51; 18F/33M)			MCI (n = 99; 32F/67M)			NC (n = 52; 18F/34M)		
	Mean	SD	Range	Mean	SD	Range	Mean	SD	Range
Age	75.2	7.4	59–88	75.3	7.0	55–89	75.3	5.2	62–85
Education	14.7	3.6	4–20	15.9	2.9	8–20	15.8	3.2	8–20
MMSE	23.8	2.0	20–26	27.1	1.7	24–30	29	1.2	25–30
CDR	0.7	0.3	0.5–1	0.5	0.0	0.5–0.5	0	0.0	0–0

The numbers refer to baseline data. AD = Alzheimer's Disease, MCI = Mild Cognitive Impairment, NC = Normal Control, MMSE = Mini-Mental State Examination, CDR = Clinical Dementia Rating.

2.1 Data Acquisition

All structural MR scans used in this chapter were acquired from 1.5 T scanners. Data were collected across a variety of scanners with protocols individualized for each scanner, as defined at https://www.loni.ucla.edu/ADNI/Research/Cores/index. shtml. Briefly, raw Digital Imaging and Communications in Medicine (DICOM) MRI scans were downloaded from the public ADNI site (https://www.loni.ucla.edu/ ADNI), reviewed for quality, and automatically corrected for spatial distortion caused by gradient nonlinearity and B1 field inhomogeneity.

We downloaded the baseline PET data from the ADNI web site[1] in December 2009. A detailed description of PET protocols and acquisition can be found at https://www.adni-info.org. Briefly, PET images were acquired 30–60 minutes post-injection, averaged, spatially aligned, interpolated to a standard voxel size, intensity normalized, and smoothed to a common resolution of 8-mm full width at half maximum.

We downloaded the baseline CSF A42, t-tau and p-tau data from the ADNI web site (https://www.loni.ucla.edu/ADNI) in December 2009. The CSF collection and transportation protocols are provided in the ADNI procedural manual on https:// www.adni-info.org. Briefly, CSF was collected in the morning after an overnight fast using a 20- or 24-gauge spinal needle, frozen within 1 hour of collection, and transported on dry ice to the ADNI Biomarker Core laboratory at the University of Pennsylvania Medical Center. In this study, CSF A42, CSF t-tau and CSF p-tau are used as the features.

2.2 Image Analysis

Image pre-processing is performed for all MR and PET images. First, we do anterior commissure (AC) posterior commissure (PC) correction on all images, and use the N3 algorithm [27] to correct the intensity inhomogeneity. Next, we do skull-stripping on structural MR images using both brain surface extractor (BSE) [25] and brain extraction tool (BET) [28], followed by manual edition and intensity inhomogeneity correction. After removal of cerebellum, FAST in the FSL package [41] is used to segment structural MR images into three different tissues: grey matter (GM), white matter (WM), and cerebrospinal fluid (CSF). After registration using HAMMER [26], we obtain the subject-labeled image based on a template with 93 manually labeled ROIs. For each of the 93 ROI regions in the labeled MR image, we compute the volume of GM tissue in that ROI region as a feature. For PET image, we first align it to its respective MR image of the same subject using a rigid transformation, and then compute the average intensity of each ROI region in the PET image as a feature. Therefore, for each subject, we totally obtain 93 features from MRI image, other 93 features from PET image, and 3 features from CSF biomarkers.

---

[1] https://www.loni.ucla.edu/ADNI.

3   Multi-task Feature Selection (MTFS)

For imaging modalities such as MRI and PET, even after feature extraction, the number of features (extracted from brain regions) may be still large. Besides, not all features are relevant to the disease under study. So, feature selection is commonly used for dimensionality reduction, as well as for removal of irrelevant features. Different from the conventional single-task feature selection,the multi-task feature selection simultaneously selects a common feature subset relevant to all tasks. This point is especially important for diagnosis of neurological diseases,since multiple regression/classification variables are essentially determined by the same underlying pathology, i.e., the diseased brain regions. Also, simultaneously performing feature selection for multiple regression/classification variables is very helpful to suppress noises in the individual variables.

3.1   Method

Denote $X^{(m)} = [x_1^{(m)}, \ldots, x_i^{(m)}, \ldots, x_N^{(m)}]^T$ as the training data matrix on the m-th modality from N training samples, and $y^{(j)} = [t_1^{(j)}, \ldots, t_i^{(j)}, \ldots, t_N^{(j)}]^T$ as the response vector on the j-th task from the same N training samples. Following the method proposed in [20], linear models are used to model the multi-task feature selection (MTFS) as below:

$$\hat{t}^{(j)}(x^{(m)}, v_j^{(m)}) = (x^{(m)})^T v_j^{(m)}, j = 1, \ldots, T; m = 1, \ldots, M \tag{1}$$

where $v_j^{(m)}$ is the weight vector for the j-th task on the m-th modality, and $x^{(m)}$ is the m-th modal data of a certain subject. The weight vectors for all T tasks form a weight matrix $V^{(m)} = [v_1^{(m)}, \ldots, v_j^{(m)}, \ldots, v_T^{(m)}]$, which can be optimized by the following objective function:

$$
\begin{aligned}
\min_{V^{(m)}} \quad & \frac{1}{2} \sum_{j=1}^{T} \sum_{i=1}^{N} (t_i^{(j)} - \hat{t}^{(j)}(x_i^{(m)}, v_j^{(m)}))^2 + \lambda \sum_{d=1}^{D^{(m)}} V^{(m)} | d_2 \\
= \quad & \frac{1}{2} \sum_{j=1}^{T} (y^{(j)} - X^{(m)} v_j^{(m)})^2 + \lambda \sum_{d=1}^{D^{(m)}} V^{(m)} | d_2
\end{aligned}
\tag{2}
$$

where $V^{(m)}|d$ denotes the d-th row of $V^{(m)}$, $D^{(m)}$ is the dimension of the m-th modal data, and λ is the regularization coefficient controlling the relative contributions of the two terms. Note that λ also controls the sparsity of the linear models, with the high value corresponding to more sparse models (i.e., more values in $V^{(m)}$ are zero). It is easy to show that the above equation reduces to the standard ℓ_1-norm regularized optimization problem in Lasso [30] when there is only one task. In our case, this is a multi-task learning for the given m-th modal data.

The key point of the above objective function of MTFS is the use of ℓ_2-norm for $V^{(m)}|d$, which forces the weights corresponding to the d-th feature (of the m-th modal data) across multiple tasks to be grouped together and tends to select features based on the strength of T tasks jointly. Note that, because of the characteristic of group sparsity, the solution of MTFS results in a weight matrix $V^{(m)}$ whose elements in some rows are all zeros. For feature selection, we just keep those features with non-zero weights. At present, there are many algorithms developed to solve MTFS; in this chapter we adopt the SLEP toolbox [19], which has been shown very effective on many datasets.

3.2 Multimodal Data Fusion and Classification

Now we will present the multiple-kernel SVM which can be used to integrate multiple modalities of biomarkers (i.e., MRI, PET and CSF) for individual classification of AD (or MCI) from normal controls. Suppose that we are given n training samples and each of them is of M modalities. Let $x_i^{(m)}$ denote a feature vector of the m-th modality of the i-th sample, and its corresponding class label be $y_i \in \{1, -1\}$. Multiple-kernel based SVM solves the following primal problem:

$$
\begin{aligned}
&\min_{w^{(m)}, b, \xi} \frac{1}{2} \sum_{m=1}^{M} \beta_m \|w^{(m)}\|^2 + C \sum_{i=1}^{n} \xi_i \\
&\text{s.t.} y_i (\sum_{m=1}^{M} \beta_m ((w^{(m)})^T \phi^{(m)}(x_i^{(m)}) + b)) \geq 1 - \xi_i \\
&\xi_i \geq 0, i = 1, \ldots, n.
\end{aligned}
\tag{3}
$$

where $w^{(m)}$, $\phi^{(m)}$ and $\beta_m \geq 0$ denote the normal vector of hyperplane, the kernel-induced mapping function, and the combining weight on the m-th modality, respectively.

Similarly as in the conventional SVM, the dual form of multiple-kernel SVM can be represented as below:

$$
\begin{aligned}
&\max_{\alpha} \sum_{i=1}^{n} \alpha_i - \frac{1}{2} \sum_{i,j} \alpha_i \alpha_j y_i y_j \sum_{m=1}^{M} \beta_m k^{(m)}(x_i^{(m)}, x_j^{(m)}) \\
&\text{s.t.} \sum_{i=1}^{n} \alpha_i y_i = 0 \\
&0 \leq \alpha_i \leq C, i = 1, \ldots, n.
\end{aligned}
\tag{4}
$$

where $k^{(m)}(x_i^{(m)}, x_j^{(m)}) = \phi^{(m)}(x_i^{(m)})^T \phi^{(m)}(x_j^{(m)})$ is the kernel function for the two training samples on the m-th modality. The symbol n is the number of training samples.

For a new test sample $x = \{x^{(1)}, x^{(2)}, \ldots, x^{(M)}\}$, we first denote $k^{(m)}(x_i^{(m)}, x^{(m)}) = \phi^{(m)}(x_i^{(m)})^T \phi^{(m)}(x^{(m)})$ as the kernel between the new test sample and each training sample on the m-th modality. Then, the decision function for the predicted label can be obtained as below:

$$f(x^{(1)}, x^{(2)}, \ldots, x^{(M)}) = sign(\sum_{i=1}^{n} y_i \alpha_i \sum_{m=1}^{M} \beta_m k^{(m)}(x_i^{(m)}, x^{(m)}) + b). \quad (5)$$

It's easy to show that the multiple-kernel based SVM can be naturally embedded into the conventional single-kernel SVM if we interpret $k(x_i, x_j) = \sum_m \beta_m k^{(m)}(x_i^{(m)}, x_j^{(m)})$ and x_j, and $k(x_i, x) = \sum_m \beta_m k^{(m)}(x_i^{(m)}, x^{(m)})$ as a mixed kernel between the multimodal training sample x_i and the test sample x. In fact, our method can be viewed as a way for a kernel combination which combines multiple kernels into one kernel.

It is worth noting that our formulation of multiple-kernel SVM is similar, but different from the existing multi-kernel learning methods [7, 14, 33]. One key difference is that we do not jointly optimize the weights β_ms together with other SVM parameters (e.g., α) in an iterative way. Instead, we constrain $\sum_m \beta_m = 1$ and use a coarse-grid search through cross-validation on the training samples to find the optimal values. After we obtain the values of β_ms, we use them to combine multiple kernels into a mixed kernel, and then perform the standard SVM using the mixed kernel. The main advantage of our method is that it can be conveniently solved using the conventional SVM solvers, e.g., LIBSVM [5]. As explained above, this kernel combination method can provide a convenient and effective way for fusing various data from different modalities.

3.3 Validation

To evaluate the performance of different methods, we perform two sets of experiments on 186 ADNI baseline MRI, PET, and CSF data, respectively, from 45 AD, 91 MCI (including 43 MCI-C and 48 MCI-NC), and 50 NC. In the first set of experiments, we estimate two clinical variables (including MMSE and ADAS-Cog) and one categorical variable (with class label of AD, MCI or NC) from the baseline brain data of all 186 subjects. It is worth noting that only the baseline data of MRI, PET, and CSF are used in our experiments, but, in order to alleviate the effect of noise in the measured clinical scores, we use the mean clinical score at both baseline and immediate follow-up time points as the ground truth for each subject. The same strategy has also been adopted in [32]. In the second set of experiments, we predict the 2-year changes of MMSE and ADAS-Cog scores and the conversion of MCI to

AD from the baseline brain data of 167 subjects (since 19 subjects do not have the 2-year follow-up MMSE or ADAS-Cogscores and arethus discarded. Also, only the baseline data of MRI, PET, and CSF are used in the experiment, and the corresponding ground truths for the two regression tasks are the MMSE and ADAS-Cog changes from baseline to the 2-year follow-up. For classification task, we will discriminate between MCI-C and MCI-NC subjects, using the baseline MRI, PET, and CSF data.

We use 10-fold cross validation strategy by computing the Pearson's correlation coefficient (for measuring the correlation between the predicted clinical scores and the actual clinical score in the regression tasks) and the classification accuracy (for measuring the proportion of subjects correctly classified in the classification task). Specifically, the whole set of subject samples are equally partitioned into 10 subsets, and each time the subject samples within one subset are selected as the testing samples and all remaining subject samples in the other 9 subsets are used for training the SVM models. This process is repeated for 10 times. It is worth noting that, in Experiment 1, two binary classifiers (i.e., AD vs. NC and MCI vs. NC, respectively) are built. Specifically, for AD versus NC classification, we ignore the MCI subjects at each cross-validation trial and use only the AD and NC subjects. Similarly, for MCI versus NC classification, we ignore the AD subjects at each cross-validation trial and use only the MCI and NC subjects. On the other hand, in Experiment 2, only one binary classifier (i.e., MCI-C vs. MCI-NC) is built involving only the MCI subjects. In both experiments, SVM is implemented using LIBSVM toolbox [5], and linear kernel is used after normalizing each feature vector with unit norm. For all respective methods, the values of the parameters (e.g., λ and β_m) are determined by performing another round of cross-validation on the training data. Also, at preprocessing stage, we perform a common feature normalization step, i.e., subtracting the mean and then dividing the standard deviation (of all training subjects) for each feature value.

3.4 Results

3.4.1 Experiment1: Estimating Clinical Stages (MMSE, ADAS-Cog, and Class Label)

We first estimate the clinical stages, including two regression variables (MMSE and ADAS-Cog) and one classification variable (i.e., class label with a value of AD, MCI or NC), from the baseline MRI, PET, and CSF data. It is worth noting that the original multi-class classification problem is formulated as two binary classification problems, i.e., AD versus NC and MCI versus NC, as mentioned above. Table 2 shows the performances of the proposed method, compared with three methods each using individual modality, as well as the CONCAT method (as detailed below). Specifically, in Table 2, MRI , PET-, and CSF-based methods denote the classification results using only the respective individual modality of data. For MRI-based and PET-based methods, similarly as our MTFS method, they contain two successive steps, i.e., (1) the single-task feature selection method using Lasso (Tibshirani 1996), and (2) the standard SVM for both regression and classification. For CSF-based method, it uses

Table 2 Comparison of performances of five different methods on Experiment1. The reported values are the correlation coefficient (for MMSE and ADAS-Cog regression) and accuracy (for AD vs. NC and MCI vs. NC classification), averaged on 10-fold tests (with standard deviation also reported)

	Correlation coefficient		Classification accuracy	
	MMSE	ADAS-Cog	AD versus NC	MCI versus NC
MRI-based	0.504 ± 0.038	0.609 ± 0.014	0.848 ± 0.026	0.739 ± 0.028
PET-based	0.658 ± 0.027	0.670 ± 0.018	0.845 ± 0.035	0.797 ± 0.023
CSF-based	0.465 ± 0.019	0.474 ± 0.013	0.805 ± 0.022	0.536 ± 0.044
CONCAT	0.658 ± 0.023	0.695 ± 0.011	0.920 ± 0.033	0.800 ± 0.024
Proposed	0.697 ± 0.022	0.739 ± 0.012	0.933 ± 0.022	0.832 ± 0.015

AD = Alzheimer's Disease, NC = Normal Control, MCI = Mild Cognitive Impairment, MMSE = Mini-Mental State Examination, ADAS-Cog = Alzheimer's Disease Assessment Scale-Cognitive Subscale.

the original 3 features without any further feature selection, and performs the standard SVM for both regression and classification. Obviously, MRI-, PET- and CST-based methods all belong to the SMST learning. For comparison, we also implement a simple concatenation method (denoted as CONCAT) for using multi-modal data. In the CONCAT method, we first concatenate 93 features from MRI, 93 features from PET, and 3 features from CSF into a 189 dimensional vector, and then perform the same two steps (i.e., Lasso feature selection and SVM regression/classification) as in MRI-, PET- and CSF-based methods. It is worth noting that the same experimental settings are used in all five methods as compared in Table 2.

As can be seen from Table 2, our proposed MTFS method consistently achieves better performance than other four methods. Specifically, for estimating MMSE and ADAS-Cog scores, our method achieves the correlation coefficients of 0.697 and 0.739, respectively, while the best performance using individual modality is only 0.658 and 0.670 (when using PET), respectively. On the other hand, for AD versus NC and MCI versus NC classification, our method achieves the accuracies of 0.933 and 0.832, respectively, while the best performance using individual modality is only 0.848 (when using MRI) and 0.797 (when using PET), respectively. Table 2 also indicates that our proposed MTFS method consistently outperforms the CONCAT method on each performance measure, although the latter also achieves better performance than three MRI-, PET-, or CSF-based methods in most cases, because of using multi-modal imaging data. However, CSF-based method always achieves the worst performances in all tasks, and is significantly inferior to MRI- and PET-based methods in this experiment. Finally, for each group (i.e., AD, MCI or NC), we compute its average estimated clinical scores using MTFS, with respective values of 24.8 (AD), 25.5 (MCI) and 28.1 (NC) for MMSE, and 14.9 (AD), 13.3 (MCI) and 8.3 (NC) for ADAS-Cog. These results show certain consistency with the actual clinical scores as shown in Table 1.

3.4.2 Experiment 2: Predicting 2-Year MMSE and ADAS-Cog Changes and MCI conversion

In this experiment, we predict the 2-year changes of MMSE and ADAS-Cog scores and the conversion of MCI to AD, from the baseline MRI, PET, and CSF data. Here, we have two regression tasks corresponding to the prediction of the regression variables of MMSE and ADAS-Cog changes from baseline to 2-year follow-up, respectively, and one classification task corresponding to prediction of the classification variable of MCI conversion to AD, i.e., MCI-C versus MCI-NC. It is worth noting that as in Experiment 1, only the baseline MRI, PET, and CSF data are used for all prediction tasks. We use the same subjects as in Experiment 1, except for 19 subjects without 2-year MMSE or ADAS-Cog scores, thus reducing to totally 167 subjects with 40 AD, 80 MCI (38 MCI-C and 42 MCI-NC), and 47 NC that are finally used in Experiment 2. Table 3 shows the performance of the proposed MTFS method compared with three individual-modality based methods and also the CONCAT method, which are the same methods as those used in Experiment 1. Here, for MCI-C versus MCI-NC classification, besides reporting the classification accuracy, we also give other performance measures including sensitivity (i.e., the proportion of MCI-C subjects correctly classified) and the specificity (i.e., the proportion of MCI-NC subjects correctly classified). In addition, we also plot the ROC curves of five different methods for classification between MCI-C and MCI-NC, as shown in Fig. 1. Here, the individual-modality based methods (using MRI, CSF or PET) and the CONCAT method are defined in the same way as in Experiment 1.

Table 3 and Fig. 1 show that, as in Experiment 1, MTFS also consistently outperform the individual-modality based methods and the CONCAT method, on both regression and classification tasks. Specifically, our method achieves the correlation coefficients of 0.511 and 0.531 and the accuracy of 0.739, for predicting the 2-year changes of MMSE and ADAS-Cog scores and the MCI conversion, respectively, while the best performance of individual-modality based methods are 0.434 (when

Table 3 Comparison of performances of five different methods on Experiment 2. The reported values are the correlation coefficient (for regressions of MMSE and ADAS-Cog change) and accuracy, sensitivity and specificity (for MCI-C vs. MCI-NC classification), averaged on 10-fold tests (with standard deviation also reported)

	Correlation coefficient		MCI-C versus MCI-NC
	MMSE change	ADAS-Cog chage	Accuracy
MRI-based	0.419±0.019	0.455±0.037	0.620±0.058
PET-based	0.434±0.027	0.401±0.046	0.639±0.016
CSF-based	0.327±0.018	0.425±0.028	0.518±0.086
CONCAT	0.484±0.009	0.475±0.045	0.654±0.050
Proposed	0.511±0.021	0.531±0.032	0.739±0.038

MCI-C = MCI converter, MCI-NC = MCI non-converter, MMSE = Mini-Mental State Examination, ADAS-Cog = Alzheimer's Disease Assessment Scale-Cognitive Subscale.

Fig. 1 ROC curves of five
different methods:
MRI-based, PET-based,
CSF-based, CONCAT, and
MTFS methods, for
classification between
MCI-C and MCI-NC

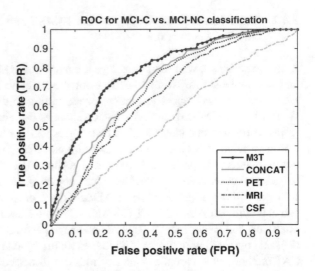

using PET), 0.455 (when using MRI), and 0.639 (when using PET), respectively. In
addition, the area under the ROC curve (AUC) is 0.797 for MCI-C versus MCI-NC
classification with our MTFS method, while the best AUC using the individual-
modality based method is 0.70 (when using PET) and the AUC of the CONCAT
method is 0.729. On the other hand, if comparing Table 3 with Table 2, we can see
that there is a significant decline in the corresponding performances. It implies that
predicting future MMSE and ADAS-Cog changes and the MCI conversion is much
more difficult and challenging than estimating the MMSE and ADAS scores and the
class labels.

4   Manifold Regularized Multi-task Feature Selection (M2TFS)

Multi-task learning aims to improve the performance of learning algorithms by jointly
learning a set of related tasks [2, 21], which is particularly useful when these tasks
have some commonality and are generally slightly under sampled. Based on multi-
task learning framework, Zhang and Shen [39] proposed a feature learning method
to jointly predict the multiple regression and classification variables from multi-
modality data, and achieved state-of-the-art performance in AD classification. Motivated by their work, we proposed a new multi-task feature learning framework to
jointly detect the disease related regions from multi-modality data for classification.
We will introduce manifold regularized multi-task feature learning models, as well
as the corresponding optimization algorithm.

4.1 Manifold Regularized MTFS (M2TFS)

Assume that there are M supervised learning task (i.e., M modalities). Denote $X^m = [x_1^m, x_2^m, \ldots, x_N^m]^T \in R^{N \times d}$ as the training data matrix in the m-th task (i.e., m-th modality) from N training subjects, and $Y = [y_1, y_2, \ldots, y_N]^T \in R^N$ as the response vector from these training subjects, where x_i^m represents the feature vector of the i-th subject in the m-th modality, and $y_i \in \{+1, -1\}$ is the corresponding class label (i.e., patient or NC). It is worth noting that different modalities from the same subject have the same class label. Let $w^m \in R^d$ parameterize a linear discriminant function for task m. Then, the linear multi-task feature selection (MTFS) model [2, 39] is to solve the following objective function:

$$\min_{W} \quad \frac{1}{2} \sum_{m=1}^{M} \|Y - X^m w^m\|_2^2 + \beta \|W\|_{2,1} \tag{6}$$

where $W = [w^1, w^2, \ldots, w^M] \in R^{d \times M}$ is the weight matrix whose row w_j is the vector of coefficients associated with the j-th feature across different tasks. Here, $\|W\|_{2,1} = \sum_{j=1}^{d} \|w_j\|_2$ is the sum of the ℓ_2-norm of the rows of matrix W, as was used in the group-sparsity regularizer [38]. The use of $\ell_{2,1}$-norm encourages the weight matrices with many zero rows. For feature selection, only those features with nonzero coefficients are kept. In other words, this norm combines multiple tasks and ensures that a small number of common features be jointly selected across different tasks. The parameter β is a regularization parameter that balances the relative contributions of the two terms. The larger β value means few features preserved for classification and vice versa. It is easy to show that the problem in Eq. (6) reduces to the ℓ_1-norm regularized optimization problem in the least absolution shrinkage and selection operator (LASSO) [30] when the number of tasks equals to one.

In the MTFS model, a linear mapping function (i.e., $f(x) = w^T x$) was adopted to transform the data from the original high-dimensional space to one-dimensional space. In this model, for each task we only consider the relationship between data and class label, while the mutual dependence among data is ignored, which may result in large deviation seven for very similar data after mapping. To address this issue, we introduced a new regularization item as:

$$\min_{w} \quad \sum_{m=1}^{M} \sum_{i,j}^{N} s_{ij}^m \|f(x_i^m) - f(x_j^m)\|_2^2$$
$$- 2 \sum_{m=1}^{M} (X^m w^m)^T L^m (X^m w^m) \tag{7}$$

where $S^m = [s_{ij}^m]$ denotes a similarity matrix that defines the similarity on task m across different subjects. $L^m = D^m - S^m$ represents combinatorial Laplacian matrix for task m, where D^m is the diagonal matrix defined as $D^m = \sum_{j=1}^{N} S_{ij}^m$. Here, the similarity matrix is defined as:

$$S_{ij}^m = \begin{cases} 1, & \text{if } x_i^m \text{ and } x_j^m \text{ are from the same class} \\ 0, & \text{otherwise} \end{cases} \tag{8}$$

This penalized item can be explained as follows: if x_i^m and x_j^m come from the same class, the distance between $f(x_i^m)$ and $f(x_j^m)$ should be smaller. It is easy to see that Eq. (7) aims to preserve the local neighboring structure of same-class data during the mapping. With the regularizer in Eq. (7), the proposed manifold regularized MTFS model (M2TFS) has the following objective function:

$$\min_{W} \quad \frac{1}{2} \sum_{m=1}^{M} \|Y - X^m w^m\|_2^2 + \beta \|W\|_{2,1} + \gamma \sum_{m=1}^{M} (X^m w^m)^T L^m (X^m W^m) \tag{9}$$

where β and γ are two positive constants. Their values can be determined via inner cross-validation on the training data.

In our proposed M2TFS model, the group sparsity regularizer ensures only a small number of features to be jointly selected from multi-modality data. The Laplacian regularization item preserves the discriminative information of the data from each modality via incorporating the label information of both classes and thus may induce more discriminative features.

4.2 Classification

Following [40], we adopted the multikernel learning (MKL) SVM method for classification. Specifically, for each modality of training subjects, a linear kernel was first calculated based on the features selected by the above proposed method. Then, to combine multiple modality data, we adopted the following MKL technique:

$$k(x, z) = \sum_{m=1}^{M} \mu^m k^m (x^m, z^m) \tag{10}$$

where $k^m(x^m, z^m)$ enotes the kernel function over the m-th modality across subject x and z, and μ^m is a no-negative weight parameter with $\sum_{m=1}^{M} \mu^m = 1$.

In the current studies, the MKL technique used in [40] was applied to combine multiple kernels. The optimal μ^m is determined based on the training subjects through a grid search with the range from 0 to 1 at a step size of 0.1, via another 10-fold cross-validation. Once the optimal μ^m was obtained, the standard SVM can be performed for classification.

4.3 Results

In the current studies, we compared our proposed method with the state-of-the-art multi-modality-based methods, including Multi-modality method proposed in [40] (denoted as MM and MML, corresponding to the method without feature selection and the method using LASSO as feature selection, respectively) and MTFS method [39] (denoted as MTFS). In addition, for more comparisons, we also concatenate all features from MRI and FDG-PET into a long feature vector, and then perform three different feature selection methods, that is, t-test, LASSO and sequential floating forward selection. Finally, the standard SVM with linear kernel was used for classification. The detailed experimental results are summarized in Tables 4, 5, and 6. Figures 2, 3, and 4 plot the ROC curves of four multi-modality-based methods (i.e., MM, MML, MTFS, and the proposed method).

As we can see from Tables 4, 5 and 6 and Figs. 2, 3 and 4, our proposed M2TFS method consistently outperforms the other methods on three classification groups. Specifically, our proposed M2TFS method achieves the classification accuracy of 95.03%, 79.27%, and 68.94% for AD versus NC, MCI versus NC, and MCI-C versus MCI-NC, respectively, while the best classification accuracy of other methods are

Table 4 Classification performance of different methods

	AD versus NC			
	ACC (%)	SEN (%)	SPE (%)	AUC
LASSO	91.02	90.39	91.35	0.95
t-test	90.94	91.57	90.00	0.97
SFFS	86.78	87.06	86.15	0.93
MM	91.65	92.94	90.19	0.96
MML	92.25	92.16	92.12	0.96
MTFS	92.07	91.76	92.12	0.95
M2TFS	95.03	94.90	95.00	0.97

ACC = nACCuracy, SEN = SENsitivity, SPE = SPEcificity

Table 5 Classification performance of different methods

	MCI versus NC			
	ACC (%)	SEN (%)	SPE (%)	AUC
LASSO	73.44	76.46	67.12	0.78
t-test	73.02	78.08	63.08	0.77
SFFS	69.21	82.12	45.38	0.73
MM	74.34	85.35	53.46	0.78
MML	73.84	77.27	66.92	0.77
MTFS	74.17	81.31	60.19	0.77
M2TFS	79.27	85.86	66.54	0.82

ACC = ACCuracy, SEN = SENsitivity, SPE = SPEcificity

Table 6 Classification performance of different methods

	MCI-C versus MCI-NC			
	ACC (%)	SEN (%)	SPE (%)	AUC
LASSO	58.44	52.33	63.04	0.60
t-test	59.11	53.49	63.57	0.64
SFFS	56.28	44.42	64.82	0.55
MM	59.67	46.28	69.64	0.60
MML	61.67	54.19	66.96	0.61
MTFS	61.61	57.21	65.36	0.62
M2TFS	68.94	64.65	71.79	0.70

ACC = ACCuracy, SEN = SENsitivity, SPE = SPEcificity.

Fig. 2 The ROC curves of four multi-modality based methods for the classification of AD versus NC

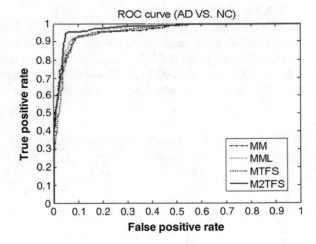

Fig. 3 The ROC curves of four multi-modality based methods for the classification of MCI versus NC

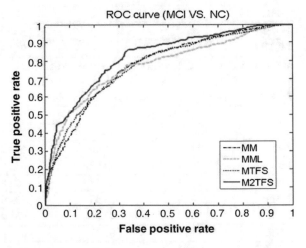

Fig. 4 The ROC curves of
four multi-modality based
methods for the classification
of MCI-C versus MCI-NC

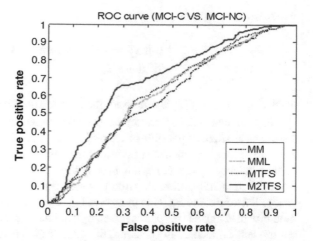

92.25%, 74.34%, and 61.67%, respectively. Also, M2TFS is consistently superior
to other methods in sensitivity measure. High sensitivity is very important for the
purpose of diagnosis, because there are different costs for misclassifying a normal
person to be a patient or misclassifying a patient to be a healthy person. Obviously,
compared with the former, the latter may cause more severe consequences and thus
has higher misclassification cost. Hence, it is advantageous for a classifier to provide
higher sensitivity rate. In addition, the AUC of proposed method, respectively, is
0.97, 0.82, and 0.70 for those classifications, which indicates excellent diagnostic
power. The results show that our proposed M2TFS method can take advantage of
the local neighboring structure information of same-class data to seek out the most
discriminative subset of features.

5   Label-Aligned Multi-task Feature Selection (LAMTFS)

5.1   *Method*

One limitation of the standard multi-task feature selection model is that only the
relationship between modalities of the same subjects is considered, while ignoring
the important relationship among labeled subjects. To address this issue, we introduce
a new term called label-aligned regularization term, which minimizes the distance
between within-class subjects in the feature-reduced space as follows:

$$\Omega = \sum_{i,j}^{N} \sum_{p,q(p \leq q}^{M} \|(w^p)^T x_i^p - (w^q)^T x_j^q\|_2^2 S_{ij} \tag{11}$$

where S_{ij} is defined as:

$$S_{ij} = \begin{cases} 1, \text{ if } x_i^p \text{ and } x_j^q \text{ are from the same class} \\ 0, \text{ otherwise} \end{cases} \tag{12}$$

$\|(w^p)^T x_i^p - (w^q)^T x_j^q\|_2^2 S_{ij}$ measrues the distance between x_i^p and x_j^q in the projected space. It implies that if x_i^p and x_j^q are from the same class, the distance between them should be as small as possible in the projected space. It is worth noting that (1) when $p = q$ the local geometric structure of the same modality data is preserved in the feature-reduced space; (2) when $p < q$ the complementary information provided from different modalities are used to guide the estimation of the feature-reduced space. Therefore, the Eq. (11) preserves the intrinsic label relatedness among multi-modality data and also explores the complementary information conveyed by different modalities. Generally speaking, the goal of (11) is to preserve label relatedness by aligning paired within-class subjects from multiple modalities.

We can obtain the objective function of our label-aligned multi-task feature selection model as below:

$$\min_{W} \quad \frac{1}{2} \sum_{m=1}^{M} \|Y - X^m w^m\|_2^2 + \lambda_1 \|W\|_{2,1} + \lambda_2 \sum_{i,j}^{N} \sum_{p,q(p \leq q)}^{M} \|(w^p)^T x_i^p - (w^q)^T x_j^q\|_2^2 S_{ij} \tag{13}$$

where λ_1 and λ_2 are the two positive constants that control the sparseness and the degree of preserving the distance between subjects, respectively. From (13), we can not only jointly select a subset of common features from multi-modality data, but also preserve label relatedness by aligning paired within-class subjects. our proposed method can preserve not only the multi-modality relationship from the same subject, but also the correlation across modalities between different subjects.

5.2 Experiments and Results

The classification results of AD versus NC and MCI versus NC produced by different methods are listed in Tables 7 and 8. As can be seen, our proposed method consistently achieves better performance than other methods for the classification between AD/MCI patients and normal controls. Specifically, for classifying AD from NC, our proposed method achieves a classification accuracy of 95.95%, while the best accuracy of other methods is only 92.25% (obtained via single modality feature selection by lasso, denoted as SMFS). In addition, for classifying MCI from NC, our proposed method achieves a classification accuracy of 80.26%, while the best accuracy of other methods is only 74.34% (obtained by Baseline). Furthermore, we perform the significance test using paired t-test on the classification accuracies between our proposed method and other compared methods, with the corresponding

Table 7 Classification performance of different methods

	AD versus NC			
	ACC (%)	SEN (%)	SPE (%)	AUC
LASSO	91.02	90.39	91.35	0.95
t-test	90.94	91.57	90.00	0.97
Baseline	91.65	92.94	90.19	0.96
SMFS	92.25	92.16	92.12	0.96
MMFS	92.07	91.76	92.12	0.95
LAMTFS	95.95	95.10	96.54	0.97

ACC = ACCuracy, SEN = SENsitivity, SPE = SPEcificity.

Table 8 Classification performance of different methods

	MCI versus NC			
	ACC (%)	SEN (%)	SPE (%)	AUC
LASSO	73.44	76.46	67.12	0.78
t-test	73.02	78.08	63.08	0.77
Baseline	74.34	85.35	53.46	0.78
SMFS	73.84	77.27	66.92	0.77
MMFS	74.17	81.31	60.19	0.77
LAMTFS	80.26	84.95	70.77	0.81

ACC = ACCuracy, SEN = SENsitivity, SPE = SPEcificity.

results given in Tables 7 and 8. We can see that our proposed method is significantly better than the compared methods (i.e., the corresponding p values are very small).

For further validation, in Figs. 5 and 6 we plot the ROC curves of four multi-modality based classification methods for AD/MCI versus NC classification. Figures 5 and 6 show that our proposed method consistently achieves better classification performances than other multi-modality based methods for both AD versus NC and MCI versus NC classifications. Specifically, our method achieves the area under the ROC curve (AUC) of 0.97 and 0.81 for AD versus NC and MCI versus NC classifications, respectively, showing better classification ability compared with other methods.

The classification results for MCI-C versus MCI-NC are shown in Table 9. As can be seen from Table 9, our proposed method consistently outperforms other methods in MCI-converter classification. Specifically, our proposed method achieves a classification accuracy of 69.78%, while the best one of other methods is only 61.67%, which is obtained by SMFS. The classification accuracy of our proposed method is significantly ($p < 0.001$) higher than any compared methods.

Figure 7 plots the corresponding ROC curves of four multi-modality based methods for MCI-C versus MCI-NC classification. We can see from Fig. 7 that the superior classification performance is obtained by our proposed method. Table 9 lists the area under the ROC curve (AUC) of different classification methods. AUC achieved by

Fig. 5 The ROC curves of four multi-modality based methods for the classification of AD versus NC

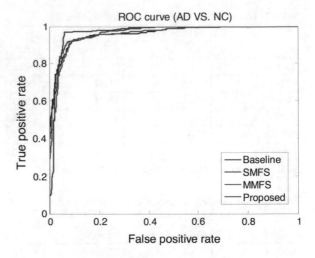

Fig. 6 The ROC curves of four multi-modality based-methods for the classification of MCI versus NC

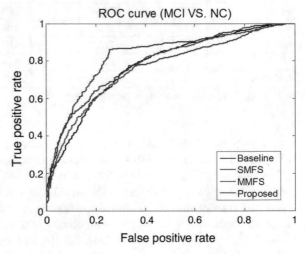

Table 9 Classification performance of different methods

| | MCI-C versus MCI-NC | | | |
	ACC (%)	SEN (%)	SPE (%)	AUC
LASSO	58.44	52.33	63.04	0.60
t-test	59.11	53.49	63.57	0.64
Baseline	59.67	46.28	69.64	0.60
SMFS	61.67	54.19	66.96	0.61
MMFS	61.61	57.21	65.36	0.62
LAMTFS	69.78	66.74	71.43	0.69

ACC = ACCuracy, SEN = SENsitivity, SPE = SPEcificity

Fig. 7 The ROC curves of
four multi-modality based
methods for the classification
of MCI-C versus MCI-NC

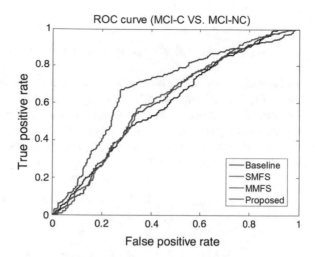

our proposed method is 0.69 for MCI-C versus MCI-NC classification, while the
best one of other methods is only 0.64, obtained by t-test, indicating the outstanding
classification performance of our proposed method.

6   Discriminative Multi-task Feature Selection (DMTFS)

In MTFS model, a linear function (i.e., $f(x) = w^T x$) was used to map the data from
the original high-dimensional feature space to one-dimensional space. This model
only focuses on the relationship between label and subject, and thus ignores the
distribution information of subjects from each modality, such as the compactness of
intra-class subjects and the separability of inter-class subjects. This kind of information may help induce the more discriminative features and thus further improve the
classification performance.

6.1   Method

To address this problem, inspired by some recent works [4, 35], we propose a new discriminative regularization term to preserve the distribution information of subjects.
To be specific, in each modality, for each subject x_i^m, we first seek its k nearest neighbors, i.e., $n(x_i^m) = \{x_i^{m,1}, x_i^{m,2}, \ldots, x_i^{m,k}\}$, and define two disjoint subject subsets as
follows:

$$n_w(x_i^m) = \{x_i^{m,l} | \text{if } x_i^{m,l} \text{ and } x_i^m \text{ belong to same class}, 1 \leq l \leq k\} \qquad (14)$$

$$n_b(x_i^m) = \{x_i^{m,l} | \text{if } x_i^{m,l} \text{ and } x_i^m \text{ belong to different class, } 1 \leq l \leq k\} \tag{15}$$

where $n_w(x_i^m)$ includes the neighbors that have the same label with the subject x_i^m, and $n_b(x_i^m)$ contains the neighbors having different labels with the subject x_i^m. Then, to discover discriminative structure and geometrical information of the data, we construct two graphs, i.e., intra-class graph G_w^m and inter-class graph G_b^m, with each subject as a node for both graphs. Let Z_w^m and Z_b^m denote the weight matrices of G_w^m and G_b^m, respectively. We define:

$$Z_{w,ij}^m = \begin{cases} 1, & |\text{if } x_j^m \in n_w(x_i^m) \text{ or } x_i^m \in n_w(x_j^m) \\ 0, & |\text{otherwise} \end{cases} \tag{16}$$

$$Z_{b,ij}^m = \begin{cases} 1, & |\text{if } x_j^m \in n_b(x_i^m) \text{ or } x_i^m \in n_b(x_j^m) \\ 0, & |\text{otherwise} \end{cases} \tag{17}$$

Then, to preserve the discriminative and structural information of two graphs during linear mapping, we introduce a new discriminative regularization term as:

$$Q(W) = \sigma S_w - (1 - \sigma) S_b \tag{18}$$

where

$$\begin{aligned} S_w &= \sum_{m=1}^{M} \sum_{i,j}^{N} \| f(x_i^m) - f(x_j^m) \|^2 Z_{w,ij}^m \\ &= 2 \sum_{m=1}^{M} (w^m)^T (X^m)^T L_w^m X^m w^m \end{aligned} \tag{19}$$

and

$$\begin{aligned} S_b &= \sum_{m=1}^{M} \sum_{i,j}^{N} \| f(x_i^m) - f(x_j^m) \|^2 Z_{b,ij}^m \\ &= 2 \sum_{m=1}^{M} (w^m)^T (X^m)^T L_b^m X^m w^m \end{aligned} \tag{20}$$

here, $L_w^m = D_w^m - Z_w^m$ and $L_b^m = D_b^m - Z_b^m$ represent intra-class and inter-class Laplacian matrices for the m-th modality, respectively. $D_{w,ii}^m = \sum_{j=1}^{N} Z_{w,ij}^m$ and $D_{b,ii}^m = \sum_{j=1}^{N} Z_{b,ij}^m$ are the corresponding diagonal matrices. σ is a positive constant which controls the relative importance of both terms.

With the regularizer, our proposed discriminative multi-task feature selection model (DMTFS) has the following objective function:

$$\min_{w} \quad \frac{1}{2}\|Y - X^m w^m\|_2^2 + \lambda\|W\|_{2,1} + \sum_{m=1}^{M}(w^m)^T(X^m)^T[\sigma L_w^m - (1-\sigma)L_b^m]X^m w^m$$

$$(21)$$

6.2   Experimental Results

We compare our proposed DMTFS method with several other methods, including multi-task feature selection method (denoted as MTFS) [39], and multi-modal classification method proposed in [40] using the least absolution shrinkage and selection operator (Lasso) as feature selection (denoted as MML). For further comparison, we also concatenate the MRI and PET features into a long feature vector, followed by the sequential forward floating selection (SFFS) [24] for feature selection, and then using the standard SVM for classification. Tables 10 and 11 list the comparison of different methods for AD/MCI classifications. Figures 8 and 9 plots the ROC curves of different methods.

We can see that our proposed method outperforms the other methods in all performance measures for both AD and MCI classifications. Specifically, our method achieves the classification accuracies of 95.92% and 82.13% for AD versus NC and MCI versus NC, respectively, while the best accuracies of other methods are only

Table 10   Classification performance of different methods

	AD versus NC			
	ACC (%)	SEN (%)	SPE (%)	AUC
SFFS	86.78	87.06	86.15	0.93
MML	92.25	92.16	92.12	0.96
MTFS	92.07	91.76	92.12	0.95
DMTFS	95.92	94.71	97.12	0.97

ACC = ACCuracy, SEN = SENsitivity, SPE = SPEcificity.

Table 11   Classification performance of different methods

	MCI versus NC			
	ACC (%)	SEN (%)	SPE (%)	AUC
SFFS	69.21	82.12	45.38	0.73
MML	73.84	77.27	66.92	0.77
MTFS	74.17	81.31	60.19	0.77
DMTFS	82.13	87.68	71.54	0.82

ACC = ACCuracy, SEN = SENsitivity, SPE = SPEcificity.

Fig. 8 The ROC curves of
four multi-modality based
methods for the classification
of AD versus NC

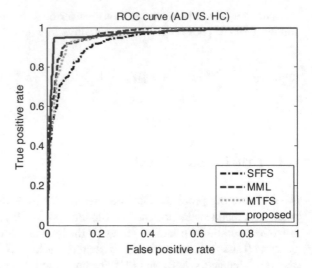

Fig. 9 The ROC curves of
four multi-modality based
methods for the classification
of MCI versus NC

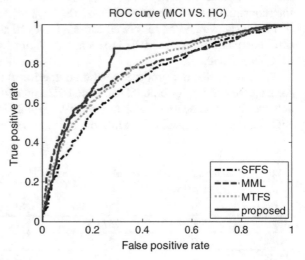

92.07% and 74.17%, respectively. In addition, our method achieves high AUC values
of 0.97 and 0.82 for AD versus NC and MCI versus NC, respectively, showing better
diagnostic power than the other methods for AD/MCI classifications.

On the other hand, we also perform experiments on classifying MCI converters (MCI-C) from MCI non-converters (MCI-NC), with the corresponding results
shown in Table 12 and Fig. 10. As can be seen from Table 12 and Fig. 10, our proposed method achieves better classification performances than other methods for
MCI-C versus MCI-NC classification. Specifically, our proposed method achieves a
classification accuracy of 71.12% for MCI-C versus MCI-NC classification, which
is nearly 10% higher than the best result by other methods.

Table 12 Classification performance of different methods

| | MCI-C versus MCI-NC | | | |
	ACC (%)	SEN (%)	SPE (%)	AUC
SFFS	56.28	44.42	64.82	0.55
MML	61.67	54.19	66.96	0.61
MTFS	61.61	57.21	65.36	0.62
DMTFS	71.12	67.21	73.93	0.68

ACC = ACCuracy, SEN = SENsitivity, SPE = SPEcificity.

Fig. 10 The ROC curves of four multi-modality based methods for the classification of MCI-C versus MCI-NC

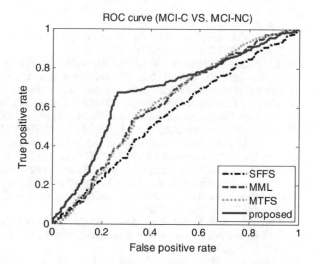

7 Conclusion

We have reviewed four latest multi-task feature learning methods for classification of Alzheimer's Disease. Specifically, the MTFS approach can effectively estimate the MMSE and ADAS-Cog scores and the classification label in both AD versus NC and MCI versus NC classifications, and can also predict the 2-year MMSE and ADAS-Cog changes and the classification label in MCI-C versus MCI-NC classification. The manifold regularized MTFS method can exploit the distribution information of data to build the multi-task feature learning method for jointly selecting features from multimodalities of data. With the help of manifold regularization term, the M2TFS method can seek out the most informative feature subset. By introducing the label-aligned regularization term into the multi-task learning framework, the LAMTFS algorithm can utilize the relationships across both modalities and subjects to seek out the most discriminative features subset. The discriminative multi-task feature selection method is different from the existing multi-modality based feature selection methods which can explores both the distribution information of intra-class subjects and inter-class subjects.

References

1. Apostolova, L.G., Hwang, K.S., Andrawis, J.P., Green, A.E., Babakchanian, S., Morra, J.H., Cummings, J.L., Toga, A.W., Trojanowski, J.Q., Shaw, L.M., et al.: 3d pib and csf biomarker associations with hippocampal atrophy in adni subjects. Neurobiol. Aging **31**(8), 1284–1303 (2010)
2. Argyriou, A., Evgeniou, T., Pontil, M.: Convex multi-task feature learning. Mach. Learn. **73**(3), 243–272 (2008)
3. Brookmeyer, R., Johnson, E., Ziegler-Graham, K., Arrighi, H.M.: Forecasting the global burden of alzheimers disease. Alzheimer's dementia **3**(3), 186–191 (2007)
4. Cai, D., He, X., Zhou, K., Han, J., Bao, H.: Locality sensitive discriminant analysis. In: IJCAI, pp. 708–713 (2007)
5. Chang, C.C., Lin, C.J.: Libsvm: a library for support vector machines. ACM Trans. Intell. Syst. Technol. (TIST) **2**(3), 27 (2011)
6. Chincarini, A., Bosco, P., Calvini, P., Gemme, G., Esposito, M., Olivieri, C., Rei, L., Squarcia, S., Rodriguez, G., Bellotti, R., et al.: Local mri analysis approach in the diagnosis of early and prodromal alzheimer's disease. NeuroImage **58**(2), 469–480 (2011)
7. Ckriet, G., Deng, M., Cristianini, N., NOBLE, W.: Rernel-based data fusion and its application to protein function prediction in yeast. Biocomputing 300 (2004)
8. Dai, Z., Yan, C., Wang, Z., Wang, J., Xia, M., Li, K., He, Y.: Discriminative analysis of early alzheimer's disease using multi-modal imaging and multi-level characterization with multi-classifier (m3). Neuroimage **59**(3), 2187–2195 (2012)
9. Drzezga, A., Lautenschlager, N., Siebner, H., Riemenschneider, M., Willoch, F., Minoshima, S., Schwaiger, M., Kurz, A.: Cerebral metabolic changes accompanying conversion of mild cognitive impairment into alzheimer's disease: a pet follow-up study. Eur. J. Nucl. Med. Mol. Imaging **30**(8), 1104–1113 (2003)
10. Fan, Y., Resnick, S.M., Wu, X., Davatzikos, C.: Structural and functional biomarkers of prodromal alzheimer's disease: a high-dimensional pattern classification study. Neuroimage **41**(2), 277–285 (2008)
11. Foster, N.L., Heidebrink, J.L., Clark, C.M., Jagust, W.J., Arnold, S.E., Barbas, N.R., DeCarli, C.S., Turner, R.S., Koeppe, R.A., Higdon, R., et al.: Fdg-pet improves accuracy in distinguishing frontotemporal dementia and alzheimer's disease. Brain **130**(10), 2616–2635 (2007)
12. Higdon, R., Foster, N.L., Koeppe, R.A., DeCarli, C.S., Jagust, W.J., Clark, C.M., Barbas, N.R., Arnold, S.E., Turner, R.S., Heidebrink, J.L., et al.: A comparison of classification methods for differentiating fronto-temporal dementia from alzheimer's disease using fdg-pet imaging. Stat. Med. **23**(2), 315–326 (2004)
13. Hinrichs, C., Singh, V., Mukherjee, L., Xu, G., Chung, M.K., Johnson, S.C., Initiative, A.D.N., et al.: Spatially augmented lpboosting for ad classification with evaluations on the adni dataset. Neuroimage **48**(1), 138–149 (2009)
14. Hinrichs, C., Singh, V., Xu, G., Johnson, S.: Mkl for robust multi-modality ad classification. In: Medical Image Computing and Computer-Assisted Intervention–MICCAI 2009, pp. 786–794. Springer (2009)
15. Huang, S., Li, J., Ye, J., Wu, T., Chen, K., Fleisher, A., Reiman, E.: Identifying alzheimer's disease-related brain regions from multi-modality neuroimaging data using sparse composite linear discrimination analysis. In: Advances in Neural Information Processing Systems, pp. 1431–1439 (2011)
16. Jie, B., Zhang, D., Cheng, B., Shen, D.: Manifold regularized multitask feature learning for multimodality disease classification. Hum. Brain Mapp. **36**(2), 489–507 (2015)
17. Landau, S., Harvey, D., Madison, C., Reiman, E., Foster, N., Aisen, P., Petersen, R., Shaw, L., Trojanowski, J., Jack, C., et al.: Comparing predictors of conversion and decline in mild cognitive impairment. Neurology **75**(3), 230–238 (2010)

18. Liu, F., Wee, C.Y., Chen, H., Shen, D.: Inter-modality relationship constrained multi-modality multi-task feature selection for alzheimer's disease and mild cognitive impairment identification. NeuroImage **84**, 466–475 (2014)
19. Liu, J., Ji, S., Ye, J., et al.: Slep: Sparse Learning with Efficient Projections, vol. 6, no. 491. Arizona State University (2009)
20. Obozinski, G., Taskar, B., Jordan, M.: Multi-task feature selection. Technical Report, Statistics Department, UC Berkeley (2006)
21. Obozinski, G., Taskar, B., Jordan, M.I.: Joint covariate selection and joint subspace selection for multiple classification problems. Stat. Comput. **20**(2), 231–252 (2010)
22. Oliveira Jr, P.P.d.M., Nitrini, R., Busatto, G., Buchpiguel, C., Sato, J.R., Amaro Jr, E.: Use of SVM methods with surface-based cortical and volumetric subcortical measurements to detect alzheimer's disease. J. Alzheimer's Dis. **19**(4), 1263–1272 (2010)
23. Orrù, G., Pettersson-Yeo, W., Marquand, A.F., Sartori, G., Mechelli, A.: Using support vector machine to identify imaging biomarkers of neurological and psychiatric disease: a critical review. Neurosci. Biobehav. Rev. **36**(4), 1140–1152 (2012)
24. Pudil, P., Novovičová, J., Kittler, J.: Floating search methods in feature selection. Pattern Recogn. Lett. **15**(11), 1119–1125 (1994)
25. Shattuck, D.W., Sandor-Leahy, S.R., Schaper, K.A., Rottenberg, D.A., Leahy, R.M.: Magnetic resonance image tissue classification using a partial volume model. NeuroImage **13**(5), 856–876 (2001)
26. Shen, D., Davatzikos, C.: Hammer: hierarchical attribute matching mechanism for elastic registration. IEEE Trans. Med. Imaging **21**(11), 1421–1439 (2002)
27. Sled, J.G., Zijdenbos, A.P., Evans, A.C.: A nonparametric method for automatic correction of intensity nonuniformity in mri data. IEEE Trans. Med. Imaging **17**(1), 87–97 (1998)
28. Smith, S.M.: Fast robust automated brain extraction. Hum. Brain Mapp. **17**(3), 143–155 (2002)
29. Sui, J., Adali, T., Yu, Q., Chen, J., Calhoun, V.D.: A review of multivariate methods for multimodal fusion of brain imaging data. J. Neurosci. Methods **204**(1), 68–81 (2012)
30. Tibshirani, R.: Regression shrinkage and selection via the lasso. J. R. Stat. Soc. Ser B (Methodological) 267–288 (1996)
31. Walhovd, K., Fjell, A., Dale, A., McEvoy, L., Brewer, J., Karow, D., Salmon, D., Fennema-Notestine, C., Initiative, A.D.N., et al.: Multi-modal imaging predicts memory performance in normal aging and cognitive decline. Neurobiol. Aging **31**(7), 1107–1121 (2010)
32. Wang, Y., Fan, Y., Bhatt, P., Davatzikos, C.: High-dimensional pattern regression using machine learning: from medical images to continuous clinical variables. Neuroimage **50**(4), 1519–1535 (2010)
33. Wang, Z., Chen, S., Sun, T.: Multik-mhks: a novel multiple kernel learning algorithm. IEEE Trans. Pattern Anal. Mach. Intell. **30**(2), 348–353 (2008)
34. Westman, E., Simmons, A., Zhang, Y., Muehlboeck, J.S., Tunnard, C., Liu, Y., Collins, L., Evans, A., Mecocci, P., Vellas, B., et al.: Multivariate analysis of mri data for alzheimer's disease, mild cognitive impairment and healthy controls. Neuroimage **54**(2), 1178–1187 (2011)
35. Xue, H., Chen, S., Yang, Q.: Discriminatively regularized least-squares classification. Pattern Recogn. **42**(1), 93–104 (2009)
36. Ye, J., Wu, T., Li, J., Chen, K.: Machine learning approaches for the neuroimaging study of alzheimer's disease. Computer **44**(4), 99–101 (2011)
37. Ye, T., Zu, C., Jie, B., Shen, D., Zhang, D., Initiative, A.D.N., et al.: Discriminative multi-task feature selection for multi-modality classification of alzheimers disease. Brain Imaging Behav. 1–11 (2015)
38. Yuan, M., Lin, Y.: Model selection and estimation in regression with grouped variables. J. R. Stat. Soc. Ser. B (Statistical Methodology) **68**(1), 49–67 (2006)
39. Zhang, D., Shen, D., Initiative, A.D.N., et al.: Multi-modal multi-task learning for joint prediction of multiple regression and classification variables in alzheimer's disease. NeuroImage **59**(2), 895–907 (2012)

40. Zhang, D., Wang, Y., Zhou, L., Yuan, H., Shen, D., Initiative, A.D.N., et al.: Multimodal classification of alzheimer's disease and mild cognitive impairment. Neuroimage **55**(3), 856–867 (2011)
41. Zhang, Y., Brady, M., Smith, S.: Segmentation of brain mr images through a hidden markov random field model and the expectation-maximization algorithm. IEEE Trans. Med. Imaging **20**(1), 45–57 (2001)
42. Zu, C., Jie, B., Liu, M., Chen, S., Shen, D., Zhang, D., Initiative, A.D.N., et al.: Label-aligned multi-task feature learning for multimodal classification of alzheimers disease and mild cognitive impairment. Brain Imaging Behav. 1–12 (2015)

A Comparative Study of Modern Machine Learning Approaches for Focal Lesion Detection and Classification in Medical Images: BoVW, CNN and MTANN

Nima Tajbakhsh and Kenji Suzuki

Abstract Two dominant classes of modern approaches for the detection and classification of focal lesions are a bag of visual words and end-to-end learning machines. In this study, we reviewed and compared these approaches for lung nodule detection, colorectal polyp detection, and lung nodule classification in CT images. Specifically, we considered massive-training artificial neural networks (MTANNs) and convolutional neural networks (CNNs) as representatives of end-to-end learning machines, and Fisher vectors as a representative of the bag of visual words. We first compared CNNs with Fisher vectors in nodule detection, nodule classification, and polyp detection, concluding that the best performing CNN model achieved comparable performance to that of Fisher vectors. We also analyzed the performance of CNNs with varying depths for the 3 studied applications. Our experiments showed that the CNN architectures with 3 or 4 convolutional layers were more effective than shallower architectures, but we did not observe a further performance gain by using deeper architectures. We then compared CNNs with MTANNs, concluding that MTANNs outperformed CNNs for nodule detection and classification particularly given limited training data. Specifically, for nodule detection, the MTANNs generated 0.08 false positives per section at 100% sensitivity, which was significantly ($p < 0.05$) lower than the best performing CNN model with 0.67 false positives per section at the same level of sensitivity. We showed that the best performing CNN model achieved comparable performance to that of Fisher vectors in the 3 studied applications, and that MTANNs outperformed CNNs in nodule detection and classification, especially given limited training data.

N. Tajbakhsh (✉) · K. Suzuki
Medical Imaging Research Center & Department of Electrical and Computer Engineering,
Illinois Institute of Technology,
3440 S. Dearborn St., Chicago, IL 60616, USA
e-mail: ntajbakh@iit.edu

K. Suzuki
e-mail: ksuzuki@iit.edu

© Springer International Publishing AG 2018
K. Suzuki and Y. Chen (eds.), *Artificial Intelligence in Decision Support Systems for Diagnosis in Medical Imaging*, Intelligent Systems Reference Library 140,
https://doi.org/10.1007/978-3-319-68843-5_2

1 Introduction

Computer-aided focal lesion detection and classification are well-studied topics in the field of medical imaging. The former consists of detecting a small abnormality given a medical image whereas the latter consists of determining the type or severity of lesions given a lesion example. Development of computer-aided detection and classification systems has been a very active area of research over the past few decades, resulting in a large body of published research and a number of successful commercial systems. Nowadays, these systems provide decision support in clinical settings and have proved highly effective in reducing the misdiagnoses of various diseases.

With recent advancements in the fields of computer vision and machine learning, the literature has witnessed a new generation of lesion detectors that can be tailored with less efforts for a given application or modality without having to change the core technology or principles. Two dominant categories of such approaches for focal lesion detection and classification are (1) end-to-end learning machines wherein the input images are mapped directly to the desired labels; and (2) a bag of visual words with modern encoding schemes wherein the mapping from images to the target labels is established through the use of an intermediate feature space. The first approach has shown promising performance for a variety of medical vision tasks but is often criticized as a black-box model whose training requires a large number of labeled examples. The second approach is relatively more transparent but has a large number of influencing hyper-parameters.

In this study, we reviewed and compared three modern approaches for focal lesion detection and classification, of which massive-training artificial neural networks (MTANNs) [1] and convolutional neural networks (CNNs) [2] represent the category of end-to-end learning methods, and Fisher vectors [3] represent the category of a bag of visual words. Due to recent popularity of CNNs in medical image analysis, we first analyzed the performance of CNNs of varying depths in comparison with Fisher vectors for lung nodule detection, lung nodule classification, and colorectal polyp detection in CT. We then compared the performance of CNNs with MTANNs for nodule detection and classification in CT.

The rest of the chapter is organized as follows: In Sect. 2, we briefly explain the theory and principles behind MTANNs, CNNs, and Fisher vectors. We describe the databases used in our experiments in Sect. 3. The base candidate generation systems for the applications under this study are briefly explained in Sect. 4. We present the experimental results in Sect. 5, discussions in Sect. 6, and conclude the chapter in Sect. 7.

2 Methods

2.1 Massive-Training Artificial Neural Networks (MTANNs)

As the extension of neural filters [4, 5], MTANNs can accommodate various pattern recognition tasks [1, 6, 7] such as detection of focal lesions and classification of lesion types. MTANNs come at 2 major models: (1) 2D MTANNs, which are designed for processing 2D images, and (2) 3D MTANNs, which are the generalized form of 2D MTANNs and are designed for processing volumetric data. The first appearance of 2D MTANNs dates back in 2002 when they were developed for the reduction of false positives in computerized detection of lung nodules in low-dose computed tomography (CT) in a slice-by-slice fashion. The use of 2D MTANNs was further extended to a number of applications including the separation of bones from soft tissue in chest x-ray (CXR) [1] and the distinction between benign and malignant lung nodules on 2D CT slices [6]. The 3D MTANNs were first developed in 2006 for removing a particular source of false positives (i.e., rectal tubes) in computer-aided detection of polyps in CT colonography [7]. The success of 3D MTANNs in removing rectal tubes set the foundation for the subsequent 3D MTANN-based systems [8–11] for computer-aided detection of polyps.

An MTANN employs an ANN regression model that is capable of operating on pixel data directly. In the applications to focal lesion detection and classification, an MTANN adopted a shallow network [7–10] because low-level and mid-level representations of patterns were sufficient for those tasks, though it is capable of having a deeper network. A mixture of expert MTANNs utilizes an ensemble of multiple MTANNs with a combiner. This is because one single ANN regression model has a limited learning capacity and thus may not learn all the essential features needed to distinguish a lesion with a large appearance variability from non-lesion structures. Hence, the first step in the design of multiple MTANNs is to divide the non-lesion class into a number of sub-classes and then train each of the MTANNs to distinguish between the lesion class and each of the non-lesion sub-classes. During the test stage, each case receives a score from each of the MTANNs in the ensemble. To produce the final score, the outputs of individual MTANNs for each case are combined by the combiner such as averaging, a logical AND operator, or an additional ANN called an integration ANN. The architecture of each ANN in the MTANNs consists of hidden layers (typically one layer for focal lesion applications) with sigmoid activation functions and 1 output layer with a linear activation function. In the following, we explain how an ANN regression model is trained in the 2D MTANN framework.

Figure 1 illustrates the training process. The inputs to the MTANN in the training process are a set of regions of interest (ROIs) and the corresponding "teaching" (desired) images that have the same size as the ROIs (precisely, the teaching image size is smaller than the ROI size by a half of the image patch size). Each pixel in the teaching image indicates the likelihood of the corresponding pixel in the input ROI to be the pattern of interest (e.g., a lesion). A negative ROI is extracted away from a lesion, and thus the corresponding teaching image is black. A positive ROI is

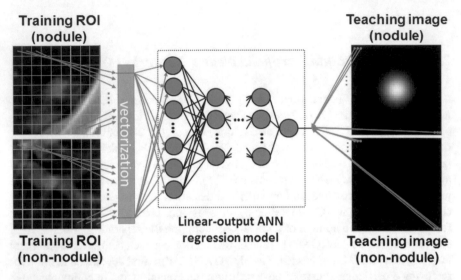

Fig. 1 Schematic overview of MTANN training. To avoid clutter in the figure, non-overlapping patches are depicted in the region of interest (ROI). In practice, the image patches are densely extracted from each ROI, resulting in a massive set of training patches

centered at a lesion's location; and thus, the corresponding teaching image contains a certain distribution such as a 2D Gaussian function in its center. Mathematically, a teaching image is defined as follows:

$$T(v) = \begin{cases} exp\{(v - \mu)^T \Sigma^{-1}(v - \mu)\}, & \text{for a lesion} \\ 0, & \text{otherwise,} \end{cases}$$

where $v = (x, y)$ indicates the location of a pixel with respect to the origin, μ denotes the center of the ROI, and Σ denotes the covariance matrix. Because lesions can generally appear in arbitrary shapes in medical images, it is common to use a diagonal covariance matrix with equal variance in each direction $\Sigma = diag(\sigma)$, where σ determines the pace of decay in the lesion likelihood as we deviate from the center of the ROI.

Once the training ROIs and the corresponding teaching images are constructed, the actual pairs of training samples and outputs are extracted. Training samples are overlapping or non-overlapping subregions (patches) that are extracted from the input ROI. If subregions are extracted at all locations in the input ROI, the centers of consecutive (overlapping) subregions differ by just one pixel. All pixel values in each of the subregions are entered as input to the ANN, whereas one pixel from the teacher image is entered into the output unit in the ANN as the teaching value. This single pixel is chosen at the location in the teacher image that corresponds to the center of the input subregion. Therefore, the training set from the ith input ROI, R_i, is represented by:

$$\mathscr{I}_{R_i} = \{I_s(x,y)|x,y \in R_i\} = \{I_1, I_2, \dots, I_k\}$$

$$\mathscr{T}_{R_i} = \{T_s(x,y)|x,y \in R_i\} = \{T_1, T_2, \dots, T_k\}$$

where $\mathscr{I}_R$ and $\mathscr{T}_R$ denote the set of training image patches and the corresponding teaching outputs, respectively. Also, I_1 denotes the first image patch extracted from the top left corner of the ROI that has been reshaped in the form of a vector, and T_1 denotes the corresponding teaching value for I_1. An ROI of size $N \times N$ allows for extraction of $k = (N - n + 1)^2$ subimages where n is the size of each subimage along x and y directions. The final massive training set is formed as the union of the training samples and the corresponding teaching values collected from each training ROI. Mathematically,

$$\mathscr{I} = \bigcup_i \mathscr{I}_{R_i}, \quad \mathscr{T} = \bigcup_i \mathscr{T}_{R_i}$$

During the test stage, each MTANN in the ensemble is applied to a test ROI in a convolutional fashion, producing a confidence map with the same size as the input ROI, if appropriate image boarder padding is applied. To convert the confidence map into a single score for each ROI, the confidence map is multiplied with the same 2D Gaussian function used during the training stage, and then the resulting confidence values are summed. The choice of a 2D Gaussian function is motivated by the fact that a lesion is a focal object; and thus, pixels that are located farther away from the center pixel should contribute less to the lesion likelihood than do the nearer pixels. Next, the scores generated by different MTANNs for an ROI is combined by using averaging, the logical AND, or the integration ANN in order to produce the final score for the given ROI.

2.2 Convolutional Neural Networks (CNNs)

A CNN can be viewed as a simplified version of the Neocognitron model [12–14], which was proposed to simulate the human visual system in 1980 [12]. CNNs initially appeared in the early 1990s [15, 16], but they did not enjoy much popularity at the time due to limited computational resources. However, with the advent of powerful graphics processing unit (GPU) computing and abundance of labeled training data, CNNs have once again emerged as a powerful feature extraction and classification tool, yielding record-breaking results in major computer vision challenges. The success of CNNs in computer vision has widely inspired investigators in the medical imaging community, resulting in a number of publications in a short period of time [17–24], which collectively demonstrates the effectiveness of CNNs for a variety of medical imaging tasks.

CNNs are so-named due to the convolutional layers in their architectures. Convolutional layers are responsible for detecting certain local features in all locations of their input images. To detect local structures, each node in a convolutional layer is connected to only a small subset of spatially connected neurons in the input image channels. To enable the search for the same local feature all over the input channels, the connection weights are shared between the nodes in the convolutional layers. Each set of shared weights is called a *kernel*, or a *convolution kernel*. Thus, a convolutional layer with n kernels, learns to detect n local features whose strength across the input images is visible in the resulting n feature maps. To reduce computational complexity and achieve a hierarchical set of image features, each sequence of convolution layers is followed by a *pooling layer*. The max pooling layer reduces the size of feature maps by selecting the maximum feature response in overlapping or non-overlapping local neighborhoods, discarding the exact location of such maximum responses. As a result, max pooling can further improve translation invariance. CNNs typically consist of several pairs of convolutional and pooling layers, followed by a number of consecutive 1×1 convolutional layers (a.k.a., fully connected), and finally a *softmax layer*, or a *regression layer*, to generate the desired outputs. In more modern CNN architectures, to achieve more computational efficiency, the pooling layer replaced with a convolution layer with a stride larger than 1. A CNN typically has a large number of convolutional and fully connected layers; therefore, it is not uncommon for a CNN to contain millions or billions of weights in its architecture.

A CNN is commonly trained by minimizing the logistic cost function $\mathcal{L} = -\sum_n log(P_n(W)) + \lambda W^2$ where W denotes the network weights, P_n is the probability that nth training sample belongs to the true class, and λ is the regularization parameter that helps prevent over-fitting when the number of weights are larger than the number of training samples. We use stochastic gradient descent to minimize the above cost function. Due to the limited memory on the GPUs, the cost function is computed for mini batches of data rather than the entire training set at once. Prior to training, the weights in the network must be initialized. In this study, we used the method suggested in [25], which is commonly known as Xavier. In this initialization scheme, the weights connected to neuron l are uniformly drawn from the interval $[-u, u]$ where $u = \sqrt{\frac{3}{n_l}}$ and n_l is the number of the incoming weights. This scheme ensures that the network gradient will not vanish nor explode as it back-propagates through the network.

2.3 Bag of Visual Words with Fisher Encoding

The BoVW paradigm [26] consists of representing images using a dictionary of visual words and an encoding scheme. The original encoding scheme suggested for BoVW was histogram encoding. However, Fisher encoding [3] has recently emerged as a more powerful alternative, yielding superior results for various computer vision tasks. Due to its tremendous success, BoVW with Fisher encoding is now commonly used as a baseline performance for competitive performance evaluation. Very recently, BoVW with Fisher encoding was also adopted by the medical imaging community, demonstrating promising performance for various medical image analysis tasks [27–30].

The training phase of BoVW begins with extracting a large number of local descriptors from allover training images. A common choice of the local descriptor is SIFT features [31]. After the descriptors are extracted, it is advantageous to reduce their dimension by means of the principle component analysis (PCA). We denote D as the dimension of descriptors after applying the PCA. The Gaussian mixture model (GMM) powered by the expectation maximization algorithm is then used to find K clusters in D dimensional feature space. Each cluster or visual word C_i is represented by a Gaussian function with average $\mu_i \in \mathbb{R}^D$, covariance matrix $\Sigma_i \in \mathbb{R}^{D \times D}$, and a prior $w_i \in \mathbb{R}$. The resulting K clusters $\{(\mu_i, \Sigma_i, w_i)|i = 1, 2, \ldots, K\}$ constitute the dictionary of visual words.

After the dictionary is constructed, a Fisher vector is computed for each training image. Let $X = \{x_i \in \mathbb{R}^D | i = 1, 2, \ldots, N\}$ denote a set of N local descriptors extracted from a training image. To obtain the corresponding Fisher vector, all descriptors are compared against each word in the dictionary; and then, the average and standard deviation of the resulting distances are computed using the following formula

$$m_c = \frac{1}{|X|\sqrt{w_c}} \sum_{x_i \in X} u_{ic} \left[\frac{x_i - \mu_c}{\sigma_c} \right] \tag{1}$$

$$s_c = \frac{1}{|X|\sqrt{2w_c}} \sum_{x_i \in X} u_{ic} \left[\frac{(x_i - \mu_c)^2}{\sigma_c^2} - 1 \right] \tag{2}$$

where $\sigma_c = diag(\Sigma_c) \in \mathbb{R}^D$ is a vector containing the diagonal elements of the covariance matrix, and u_{ic} is the soft assignment of x_i to the cth visual word in the dictionary that is compute as follows

$$u_{ic} = \frac{p(x_i|\mu_c, \Sigma_c)w_c}{\sum_{j=1}^{K} p(x_i|\mu_j, \Sigma_j)w_j} \quad \forall, c = 1, 2, 3 \ldots, K$$

The Fisher vector for a given image is then formed by concatenating the average and standard deviations vectors computed for each visual word, $f = \{m_1^T, s_1^T, \ldots, m_K^T, s_K^T\} \in \mathbb{R}^{2KD}$ with K being the number of visual words and D being the number of elements in the dimension-reduced descriptors. This is in contrast to histogram encoding whereby a K dimensional feature vector is generated for each image.

The Fisher vector described above is effective for texture analysis purpose; however, it can be further tailored for object detection tasks by including spatial information. Note that the original Fisher encoding does not consider spatial information, ignoring the locations from which the descriptors are extracted. To increase the discrimination power of Fisher vectors, it is customary to split an image into a number of sub-regions, compute a Fisher vector for each sub-region, and then concatenate these Fisher vectors to form the final Fisher vector. This spatial pooling scheme results in a higher dimensional feature space, but also adds to the discrimination power of the Fisher vectors. The resulting vectors can be then used to train a pattern classifier such as random forest.

In the test phase, a dense set of descriptors is extracted from a test image. The descriptors undergo the dimension reduction transformation and are then grouped according to the region division scheme used in the training stage. The Fisher vectors computed for each group of local descriptors are concatenated; and the resulting vector is then fed to the classifier to predict the label for the test image.

3 Datasets

3.1 Database for Lung Nodule Detection

We used a database of low-dose thoracic helical CT (LDCT) [32, 33] acquired from 31 patients, who participated voluntarily in a lung cancer screening program between 1996 and 1999 in Nagano, Japan. This database consists of 38 scans with a total of 1057 sections (slices) of the size 512×512 pixels. The scans were acquired under a low-dose protocol of 120 kVp with 25 or 50 mA. Each section has 10 mm thickness and the pixel sizes within the sections vary between 0.586 and 0.684 mm. An experienced chest radiologist annotated 50 lung nodules in the scans, of which 38 nodules were confirmed lung cancers that had been "missed" during the initial clinical interpretation. The remaining 12 nodules in the scans were classified as "confirmed benign" (n = 8), "suspected benign" (n = 3), or "suspected malignant" (n = 1). The above nodule classification was made through biopsy or by follow-up over a period of up to 2 years. We used this database in this study, because the lesions in the database have histopathological confirmations, and because it has very challenging nodules that had been missed by expert radiologists. Figure 2a shows examples of nodules from this database.

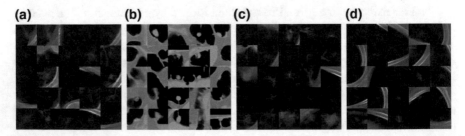

Fig. 2 Examples from **a** our nodule detection database, **b** polyp detection database, and **c, d** nodule classification database. Panel (**a**) shows non-solid (ground-glass) nodules and part-solid nodules that are major sources of false negatives. Panel (**b**) shows examples of flat, sessile, and pedunculated polyps. Panel (**c**) shows examples of malignant nodules and panel (**d**) shows examples of benign nodules

3.2 Database for Colorectal Polyp Detection

We used a database of 146 CT colonography (CTC) scans collected at the University of Chicago Medical Center. The scans were acquired from 73 patients in both supine and prone positions. Each CTC dataset consists of sections of the size 512×512 pixels, with an in-plane pixel size of 0.5–0.7 mm. The section thickness varies from one dataset to another, covering a range from 2.5 to 5.0 mm. This database contains 28 unique polyps, 15 of which are 5–9 mm and 13 are 10–25 mm in size. The locations of the polyps in the datasets were established by use of the optical colonoscopy reports that were performed on the same day as CT colonography. Figure 2b shows examples of polyps from this database.

3.3 Database for Lung Nodule Classification

We used a nodule database [32] consisting of 76 histopathologically confirmed lung cancers in 73 patients and 413 benign nodules in 342 patients, who participated voluntarily in a lung cancer screening program between 1996 and 1999 in Nagano, Japan. The nodule size ranged from 3 to 29 mm. Of the 76 primary lung cancers, 22 (28.9%) nodules were identifiable in a single section, 37 (48.7%) nodules in two sections, and 17 (22.3%) nodules in three sections. The 413 benign nodules consisted of 265 (64.2%) nodules in a single section, 133 (32.2%) in two sections, and 15 (3.6%) nodules in three sections. We used this database in this study, because all lesions in the database have histopathological confirmations, and because classification of nodules in LDCT is a very challenging task even for expert radiologists. Figure 2c, d shows examples of malignant and benign nodules from this database.

4 Candidate Generation and Data Augmentation

For nodule detection, we first applied a base computer-aided detection (CADe) scheme [1], consisting of gray-level-based lung segmentation, feature extraction and analysis, and linear-discriminant-analysis-based classification, to the entire database. The CADe scheme generated 1128 candidates with 50 true positives and 1078 false positives. These candidates were used for training and testing the MTANNs, CNNs, and Fisher vectors. For MTANNs, we extracted an ROI around each candidate, but for CNNs and Fisher vectors we extracted multiple ROIs around each candidate by performing data augmentation. Specifically, we extracted square patches at 6 scales, 40 translations from the candidate locations, and 8 orientations from each candidate, resulting in a total of 1920 image patches for each candidate. Note that, due to relatively large thickness of sections (slices), we chose to use gray-scale 2D patches for our experiments.

For polyp detection, we applied a base CADe scheme [34, 35], consisting of a Bayesian neural network with geometric and texture features. When applied to the 146 CTC datasets, the candidate generation method achieved 96.4% by-polyp sensitivity with 3.1 FPs per patient. These candidates were used for training and testing the MTANNs, CNNs, and Fisher vectors. For MTANNs, we extracted an ROI around each candidate, but for CNNs and Fisher vectors we extracted multiple ROIs around each candidate by performing data augmentation. Given a candidate in slice z, we first selected the following set of channels from the original dataset: (1) slices $z - 2, z, z + 2$; (2) slices $z - 4, z, z + 4$, and (3) slices $z - 6, z, z + 6$. By doing so, the CT dataset around each polyp candidate reduced to 3 datasets each with only 3 slices. From each reduced volume, we then extracted square patches at 4 scales, with 5 translations, in 20 random orientations uniformly selected from 0° to 360°, resulting in a total of 1200 variations for each polyp candidate.

For nodule classification, an experienced chest radiologist determined the center of each nodule in the section wherein the nodule appeared the largest (if the nodule appeared in more than 1 section). The selected sections along with the nodule centers were used for extracting ROIs for training and testing the MTANNs, CNNs, and Fisher vectors. For MTANNs, we used the original ROIs, but for CNNs and Fisher vectors we generated multiple ROIs by performing data augmentation. We extracted ROIs at 3 scales, 40 translations from the center of the ROI, in 8 orientations, resulting in a total of 960 variations for each ROI.

5 Experiments

We employed a free-response receiver-operating-characteristic (FROC) analysis [36] for nodule and polyp detection and a receiver-operating-characteristic (ROC) analysis for nodule classification with the malignant nodules being the target (positive) class. We used JAFROC analysis [37] to compare the FROC curves and bootstrapping to compare the area under the ROC curves. The statistical analyses were performed in R version 3.2.1 using RJafroc [38] and pAUC [39] packages. For training CNNs, we used the Caffe library [40], which is arguably one of the most reliable and popular open source implementations of CNNs. We also used the open source implementation of Fisher vectors [41] and our private implementation of MTANNs.

5.1 CNNs Versus Fisher Vectors

We used 5-fold cross validation for all experiments presented in this section. Specifically, we divided the candidates and ROIs generated in Sect. 4 into 5 disjoint subsets at lesion-level and then used 4 subsets for training and the remaining subset for testing. This process was repeated 5 times and the resulting classification scores were concatenated to plot the performance curves.

We used the CNN architecture shown in Fig. 3, which is further detailed in Table 1. We first studied performance improvement or degradation due to the network depth. For this purpose, we incrementally removed the convolutional layers from the above architecture starting from the end. Namely, we first removed layer 9, then layers 7 and 8, and then layers 5 and 6, and so on. The resulting architectures after incremental layer removal are shown in Tables 1b–e. Note that each time a convolutional layer was removed, the size of the receptive field of the last convolutional layer (fully connected layer) increased by a factor of 2. We refer to the architecture that has all the layers as $d = 5$, and refer to the architecture with 1 less convolutional layer as $d = 4$, and so on.

We experimentally found out that careful selection of the learning rate is the key to successful training of CNNs with varying depths. Specifically, relatively large learning rates not only enabled the fast convergence of deep CNNs but also resulted in higher classification performance than what could be achieved by lower learning rates. On the other hand, we realized that the same large learning rates could cause severe convergence issues for shallower CNNs. In our experiments, we used a learning rate of 10^{-3} for the networks in Table 1a, b, a learning rate of 10^{-5} for the networks in Tables 1c, d, and a learning rate of 10^{-6} for the network in Table 1e. We also used a regularization parameter (weight decay) of $\lambda = 0.0005$ and a momentum of 0.9 in all the experiments.

Figure 4 shows the performance curves for each of the studied applications when the network depth changes from 1 to 5. For nodule detection, the analysis of variance (ANOVA) based on the JAFROC analysis showed that there was a statistically significant difference between the CNNs with varying depths. Specifically, we observed that the CNN with 3, 4, and 5 convolutional layers significantly outperformed the CNN with 1 convolutional layer ($p < 0.05$). The other differences between CNNs were not statistically significant though. For polyp detection and nodule classification, we obtained no statistically significant differences among CNNs with varying depths. These results may suggest that high level semantic features embedded in the late layers of a deep CNN may not be essential for focal lesion detection or classification.

We further compared the performance of the CNN-based systems with that of Fisher vectors. The parameters of the handcrafted approach were determined through

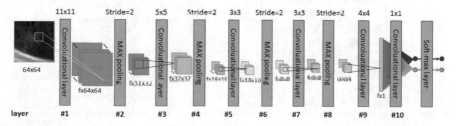

Fig. 3 Schematic overview of the CNN architecture that is incrementally pruned in our experiments

Table 1 The CNN architectures used in our experiments. The last fully connected layer (fc) can also be viewed as a convolutional layer, but we choose to consider it as the classification layer rather than a convolutional feature extraction layer; hence, the complete architecture is assumed to have 5 convolutional layers ($d = 5$)

(a)	5 convolutional layers ($d = 5$)					
Layer	Type	Input	Kernel	Stride	Pad	Output
0	Input	$64 \times 64 \times 3$	N/A	N/A	N/A	$64 \times 64 \times 3$
1	Convolution	$64 \times 64 \times 3$	11×11	1	5	$32 \times 64 \times 64$
2	Max pooling	$32 \times 64 \times 64$	2×2	2	0	$32 \times 32 \times 32$
3	Convolution	$32 \times 32 \times 32$	5×5	1	2	$32 \times 32 \times 32$
4	Max pooling	$32 \times 32 \times 32$	2×2	2	0	$32 \times 16 \times 16$
5	Convolution	$32 \times 16 \times 16$	3×3	1	2	$32 \times 16 \times 16$
6	Max pooling	$32 \times 16 \times 16$	2×2	2	0	$32 \times 8 \times 8$
7	Convolution	$32 \times 8 \times 8$	3×3	1	2	$32 \times 8 \times 8$
8	Max pooling	$32 \times 8 \times 8$	2×2	2	0	$32 \times 4 \times 4$
9	Convolution	$32 \times 4 \times 4$	4×4	1	0	32×1
10	fc	32×1	1×1	1	0	2×1
(b) 4 convolutional layers ($d = 4$)						
0	Input	$64 \times 64 \times 3$	N/A	N/A	N/A	$64 \times 64 \times 3$
1	Convolution	$64 \times 64 \times 3$	11×11	1	5	$f \times 64 \times 64$
2	Max pooling	$32 \times 64 \times 64$	2×2	2	0	$32 \times 32 \times 32$
3	Convolution	$32 \times 32 \times 32$	5×5	1	2	$32 \times 32 \times 32$
4	Max pooling	$32 \times 32 \times 32$	2×2	2	0	$32 \times 16 \times 16$
5	Convolution	$32 \times 16 \times 16$	3×3	1	2	$32 \times 16 \times 16$
6	Max pooling	$32 \times 16 \times 16$	2×2	2	0	$32 \times 8 \times 8$
7	Convolution	$32 \times 8 \times 8$	3×3	1	2	$32 \times 8 \times 8$
8	Max pooling	$32 \times 8 \times 8$	2×2	2	0	$32 \times 4 \times 4$
9	fc	32×1	4×4	1	0	2×1

(continued)

Table 1 (continued)

Layer	Type	Input	Kernel	Stride	Pad	Output
(c) 3 Convolutional layers ($d = 3$)						
0	Input	$64 \times 64 \times 3$	N/A	N/A	N/A	$64 \times 64 \times 3$
1	convolution	$64 \times 64 \times 3$	11×11	1	5	$32 \times 64 \times 64$
2	Max pooling	$32 \times 64 \times 64$	2×2	2	0	$32 \times 32 \times 32$
3	Convolution	$32 \times 32 \times 32$	5×5	1	2	$32 \times 32 \times 32$
4	Max pooling	$32 \times 32 \times 32$	2×2	2	0	$32 \times 16 \times 16$
5	Convolution	$32 \times 16 \times 16$	3×3	1	2	$32 \times 16 \times 16$
6	Max pooling	$32 \times 16 \times 16$	2×2	2	0	$32 \times 8 \times 8$
7	fc	32×1	8×8	1	0	2×1
(d) 2 convolutional layers ($d = 2$)						
0	Input	$64 \times 64 \times 3$	N/A	N/A	N/A	$64 \times 64 \times 3$
1	Convolution	$64 \times 64 \times 3$	11×11	1	5	$32 \times 64 \times 64$
2	Max pooling	$32 \times 64 \times 64$	2×2	2	0	$32 \times 32 \times 32$
3	Convolution	$32 \times 32 \times 32$	5×5	1	2	$32 \times 32 \times 32$
4	Max pooling	$32 \times 32 \times 32$	2×2	2	0	$32 \times 16 \times 16$
5	fc	32×1	16×16	1	0	2×1
(e) 1 convolutional layer ($d = 1$)						
0	Input	$64 \times 64 \times 3$	N/A	N/A	N/A	$64 \times 64 \times 34$
1	Convolution	$64 \times 64 \times 3$	11×11	1	5	$32 \times 64 \times 64$
2	Max pooling	$32 \times 64 \times 64$	2×2	2	0	$32 \times 32 \times 32$
3	fc	32×1	32×32	1	0	2×1

the use of an inner validation set. Specifically, we split each of the 5 training sets into a smaller training set containing 80% of the training data and a validation set containing 20% of the training data, and then tuned the parameters to maximize the performance on the validation set. The tuned models were then evaluated on the corresponding test folds.

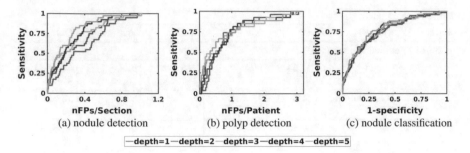

Fig. 4 Impact of the network depth on the performance of **a** lung nodule detection, **b** polyp detection, and **c** nodule classification

Table 2 Comparison between the AUCs of the CNN models with varying depths and the model based on the Fisher vectors for nodule classification

Model	AUC
Fisher vectors [3]	AUC = 0.798 (95% CI: 0.767 to 0.868)
d = 1	AUC = 0.766 (95% CI: 0.706 to 0.826)
d = 2	AUC = 0.760 (95% CI: 0.699 to 0.821)
d = 3	AUC = 0.771 (95% CI: 0.711 to 0.831)
d = 4	AUC = 0.776 (95% CI: 0.719 to 0.834)
d = 5	AUC = 0.791 (95% CI: 0.735 to 0.847)

For lung nodule detection, we obtained the best performance by building a dictionary with $K = 180$ visual words after reducing the dimension of the SIFT descriptor to $D = 10$ using the PCA. We also used spatial pyramid pooling to include spatial information in the resulting Fisher vectors. Specifically, we split each image into 4 non-overlapping quadrants, computed a Fisher vector for each quadrant as well as one for the entire image, and then concatenated the resulting 5 Fisher vectors to obtain the final descriptor, $f \in \mathbb{R}^{10KD}$. For lung nodule classification and polyp detection, we used a dictionary of $K = 60$ visual words after reducing the dimension of the SIFT descriptor to $D = 30$. To include spatial information, we employed the same spatial pooling scheme that we used for lung nodule detection. For classification, we used a random forest classifier with 100 fully grown trees for all 3 applications.

The JAFROC analysis for lung nodule detection showed that the handcrafted approach outperformed the CNN with 1 convolutional layer. We also observed that the handcrafted approach did not outperform CNNs with at least 2 convolutional layers. For polyp detection, we observed that the JAFROC figure of merit for the CNNs and handcrafted approach were never statistically different. ROC analysis for nodule classification showed that the handcrafted approach achieved an AUC comparable to that of the CNNs with varying depths. Table 2 compares the AUCs with 95% confidence interval. Therefore, the CNNs with at least 2 convolutional layers performed on a par with the Fisher vectors for the three studied applications.

5.2 CNNs Versus MTANNs

To rigorously evaluate MTANNs and CNNs for nodule detection and classification, we conducted our experiments in 2 scenarios. We refer to the first scenario as "division" wherein the object proposal or lesion candidates were split into disjoint training and test sets. In the division scenario, candidates were split according to the schemes suggested in [1, 6], which reserved the majority of samples for testing. This evaluation scenario allows for a stringent evaluation of machine-learning models that are trained based on limited training data. We refer to the second scenario as "5-fold" wherein the test set of the division scenario was first divide into 5 disjoint subsets in the lesion-level; and then, the resulting subsets were added to the training set of the division scenario in a 5-fold cross validation manner. That is, 4 subsets were added to the training set; and the remaining subset was used for testing. This process was repeated 5 times, resulting in 5 classification models, each of which generates predictions for the corresponding test subset. By collecting the predictions generated for each of the 5 test subsets, a performance curve was generated for the whole test set. Through this evaluation scenario, we can study how the increase in the size of training set impacts the performance of the classification models (both scenarios have the same test set). Figure 5 illustrates how the image data were divided into training and tests sets for the division and 5-fold scenarios.

We used 3 distinct CNN architectures in our experiments: a shallow CNN (2-conv-layer CNN), a relatively deep CNN (6-conv-layer CNN) whose deviations are commonly used in medical imaging applications, and a deep CNN (9-conv-layer CNN) called AlexNet that is popular in the computer vision community. These 3 architectures are shown in Fig. 6 and are further detailed in Table 1. For the AlexNet, in addition to training from scratch, we considered fine-tuning of the pre-trained AlexNet model that was available in Caffe. This pre-trained model had been trained using 1.2 million images labeled with 1000 semantic classes.

The architectures of MTANNs were chosen according to the corresponding publications [1, 6]. For lung nodule detection, we used the architecture suggested in [1], which consisted of 9 MTANNs: 5 MTANNs were trained to distinguish nodules from various-sized vessels; and 4 MTANNs were applied to eliminate some other opacities. Each MTANN in the ensemble consisted of 1 hidden layer with 25 neurons, and it was trained with subimages of size 9×9 extracted from 10 nodule ROIs and 10 non-nodule ROIs. In the test stage, the output of each MTANN was binarized by a pre-specified threshold; and then, the resulting binary outputs were combined using a logical AND operator. For lung nodule classification, we used the architecture suggested in [6], which consisted of 6 MTANNs with 20 neurons in their single hidden layers. Each MTANN was trained with subimages of size 9×9 extracted from 10 malignant nodule ROIs and 10 benign ROIs. In the test stage, the output of each MTANN was fed to an integration ANN to produce the final confidence score. The integration ANN had 1 hidden layer with 4 neurons in it. One of the authors (K. S.), who was also the first author of those publications, helped reproduce the exact results reported in [1, 6].

Fig. 5 Training and
evaluation protocols used in
our experiments. **a** The
division protocol where the
database is split into disjoint
training and testing sets. **b**
The 5-fold protocol wherein
the training set is the union
of the training set of the
division protocol and 4/5 of
the test set of the division
protocol. The test set consists
of the remaining 1/5 of the
test set of the division
protocol

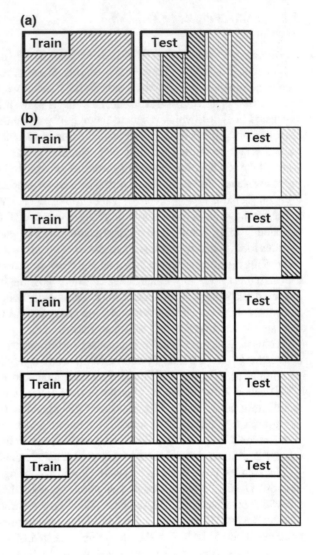

Figure 7 shows FROC curves for nodule detection. The confidence intervals for
the FROC plots were computed according to the method suggested in [42]. Figure
7a compares the performance of the MTANNs and CNNs in the division scenario.
As can be seen, the performance of the MTANNs are higher than that of CNNs in
most of the operating points with a significant margin ($p < 0.05$). As indicated by
the overlapping error bars, the difference between the three CNN architectures was
not significant at any of the operating points, which suggests that deep architectures
become ineffective given limited training data. However, as shown in Fig. 7b, the
performance gap between MTANNs and CNNs becomes less evident when CNNs
were trained and evaluated in the 5-fold cross validation scenario. The improved per-

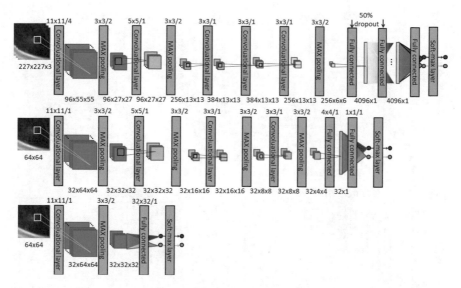

Fig. 6 Schematic overview of the CNN architectures used for comparison against MTANNs. **a** A deep CNN (AlexNet) with 9 convolutional layers. **b** A relatively deep CNN with 6 convolutional layers. **c** A shallow CNN with 2 convolutional layers

formance is attributed to the use of larger training sets available in the 5-fold cross validation scenario. Noteworthy, at 100% sensitivity, MTANNs generate 0.08 false positives per section, which is significantly higher than the best performing CNN with 0.67 false positives per section (p < 0.05). Figure 7c compares the performance of each CNN architecture in the division and 5-fold scenarios. Clearly, the performance improvement is more substantial for deeper architectures, which suggests that deeper architectures can more effectively leverage the additional training instances than the shallower architectures.

Figure 8 compares the top 30 "difficult" false positives generated by the MTANNs and the best performing CNN (9-conv-layer FT CNN) for lung nodule detection. The ROIs are shown in an increasing level of difficulty, namely, from the top left to bottom right ROI, the level of difficulty changes from easier to the most difficult to distinguish from nodules. The false positives of the MTANNs were collected at an operating point where 100% sensitivity was achieved. At this operating point, the MTANNs generated 85 false positives or equivalently 0.08 false positives per section. Similarly, the operating point of the CNN was chosen as the point at which the CNN achieved 100% sensitivity with 713 false positives (0.67 false positives per section). As seen from Fig. 8, the majority of the top false positives generated by the MTANNs and CNN include the chest wall, indicating that false positive sources tend to be near the chest wall. Some of the false positives look like lung nodules to our eyes, although they were not confirmed as lung nodules by radiologists in their reviews.

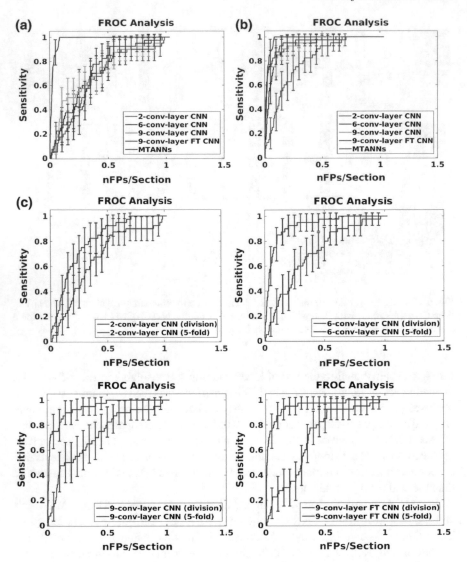

Fig. 7 Evaluation of lung nodule detection. Comparison between MTANNs and 3 CNN architectures in **a** the division protocol and **b** 5-fold protocol. **c** Performance comparison for each CNN architecture using the division and 5-fold protocols

Figure 9 shows ROC curves for nodule classification. The confidence intervals for the ROC plots were computed according to the method suggested in [42]. Figure 9a shows the ROC curves for the MTANNs and each of the CNN architectures when applied to the test ROIs in the division scenario. As can be seen, CNNs with varying depths performed comparably, yielding no significant performance improvement compared to each other. However, the MTANNs achieved a substantial improvement over the CNN-based systems, particularly at the optimal operating points located

(a)   **(b)**

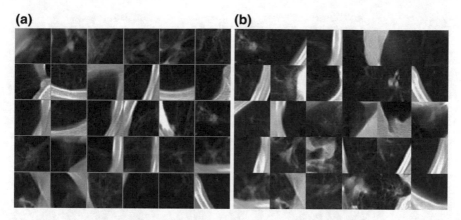

Fig. 8 Top 30 "difficult" false positives generated by the **a** MTANNs and **b** fine-tuned AlexNet (9-conv-layer FT CNN) for nodule detection in the 5-fold cross validation scenario

Table 3 AUCs with 95% confidence intervals for the MTANNs and CNNs trained for nodule classification using the 5-fold cross validation

Learning machine	AUC
MTANNs	0.8806 (95% CI: 0.8389 to 0.9223)
2-conv-layer CNN	0.7709 (95% CI: 0.7079 to 0.8272)
6-conv-layer CNN	0.7813 (95% CI: 0.7189 to 0.8306)
9-conv-layer CNN	0.7685 (95% CI: 0.7025 to 0.8311)
9-conv-layer FT CNN	0.7755 (95% CI: 0.7120 to 0.8270)

around the elbow of the ROC plot. Figure 9b shows the ROC curves for the 5-fold scenario. As with the division scenario, CNN-based systems perform closely yet inferior to that of the MTANNs. For a quantitative comparison, we tabulate the area under the curve (AUC) with 95% confidence intervals for each model in Table 3. As can be seen, the MTANNs yields a significantly higher AUC than the listed CNN-based models ($p < 0.5$), but as indicated by overlapping intervals, different variants of CNNs perform comparably. Figure 9c compares the performance of each CNN architecture in the division and 5-fold scenarios. The increased number of training samples in the 5-fold scenario did not improve nodule classification performance significantly.

Figure 10 shows the top 20 "easy-to-classify" and "hard-to-classify" malignant and benign nodules according to the malignancy scores produced by the MTANNs and the fine-tuned AlexNet (9-conv-layer FT CNN) in the 5-fold cross validation scenario. Figure 10a and b show easy-to-classify malignant nodules. As shown, both models, and to a larger degree the MTANNs, tend to assign a larger malignancy score to a larger malignant nodule. Figure 10c and d show easy-to-classify benign nodules. In this case, both models assign lower malignancy scores to smaller nodules. These observations suggest that the size of nodules has been considered by both models as

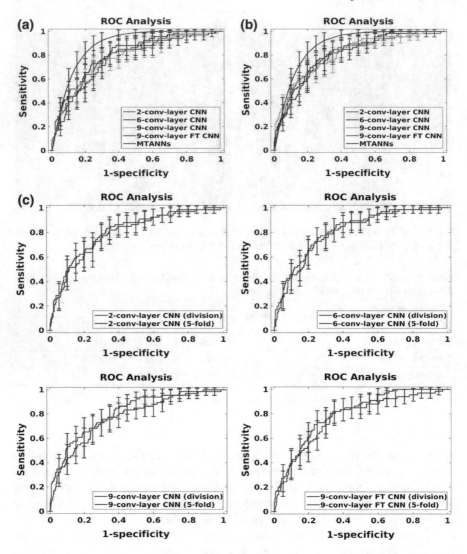

Fig. 9 Evaluation of lung nodule classification. Comparison between the MTANNs and 3 CNN architectures in **a** the division protocol and **b** 5-fold protocol. **c** Performance comparison for each CNN architecture using the division and 5-fold protocols

a distinguishing feature for distinction between malignant and benign nodules. That makes sense, because malignant nodules tend to be larger than benign nodules in nature. However, as shown in Fig. 10e and f, heavy reliance on the size of nodules has led to the misclassification of small malignant nodules as benign. Similarly, as shown in Fig. 10e and f, large benign nodules were misclassified as malignant by both machine-learning models.

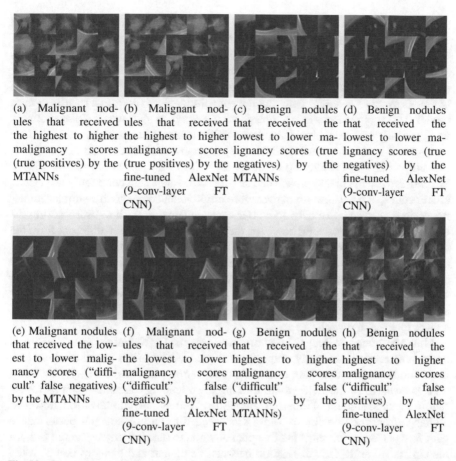

(a) Malignant nod-
ules that received
the highest to higher
malignancy scores
(true positives) by the
MTANNs

(b) Malignant nod-
ules that received
the highest to higher
malignancy scores
(true positives) by the
fine-tuned AlexNet
(9-conv-layer FT
CNN)

(c) Benign nodules
that received the
lowest to lower ma-
lignancy scores (true
negatives) by the
MTANNs

(d) Benign nodules
that received the
lowest to lower ma-
lignancy scores (true
negatives) by the
fine-tuned AlexNet
(9-conv-layer FT
CNN)

(e) Malignant nodules
that received the low-
est to lower malig-
nancy scores ("diffi-
cult" false negatives)
by the MTANNs

(f) Malignant nod-
ules that received
the lowest to lower
malignancy scores
("difficult" false
negatives) by the
fine-tuned AlexNet
(9-conv-layer FT
CNN)

(g) Benign nodules
that received the
highest to higher
malignancy scores
("difficult" false
positives) by the
MTANNs)

(h) Benign nodules
that received the
highest to higher
malignancy scores
("difficult" false
positives) by the
fine-tuned AlexNet
(9-conv-layer FT
CNN)

Fig. 10 Compassion between easy- and hard-to-classify malignant and benign nodules. According to panels (**a**)–(**d**), both machine-learning models use the size of nodules as a characteristic feature to distinguish between malignant and benign nodules. However, heavy reliance on the size of nodules has led to misclassification of small malignant nodules as benign (see panels (**e**) and (**f**)) and misclassification of large benign nodules as malignant (see panels (**g**) and (**h**))

6 Discussion

In Sect. 5.1, we showed that the performance of best performing CNN was comparable to that of the handcrafted approach based on Fisher vectors. This, however, is not an unprecedented finding. For instance, Ginneken et al. in [43] showed that the performance of a CNN model was only comparable to a handcrafted approach even though the combination of both approaches yielded higher performance than that of each individual approach. The similar performance between the deep models and Fisher vectors is further justified by the recent studies [44–46] in the computer vision literature where Fisher vectors and CNNs are shown to be similar in spirit. Nevertheless, we could have probably achieved higher performance than the handcrafted approach by means of more customized CNNs architectures; however, an exhaustive model search was not feasible given the time-consuming training process of CNNs and the extent of the presented experiments.

In Sect. 5.1, we also studied the impact of network depth on the performance of CNNs by incrementally removing the convolutional layers from a relatively deep model. This approach was also adopted by Zeiler et al. in [47], where a deep network was gradually pruned to obtain shallower architectures. Alternatively, we could take an approach based on recursive CNNs [48]. A recursive CNN consists of a convolution and pooling layer followed by multiple copies of the same convolutional layer. We chose to use the first approach because it is consistent with commonly used CNN architectures, and because we expect more intuitive outcomes with a simpler implementation. The recursive networks offer a systematic approach to investigating the impact of the network depth; however, their layouts are relatively different from the commonly used CNN architectures in the literature. Therefore, findings derived from the recursive networks may not be intuitive to a wide range of CNN users. The benefit of the layer removal approach is that it is intuitive and consistent with how a designer would shrink a network. Nevertheless, it would still be interesting to study how an approach based on recursive networks would corroborate our findings obtained using a layer removal approach.

Our experiments in Sect. 5.2 demonstrated that the CNNs trained using the 5-fold cross validation substantially outperformed the CNNs trained in the division scenario for the nodule detection task. This observation was consistent with the common knowledge in the field where training deep leaning machines such as CNNs requires a large amount of labeled training data. For nodule classification, however, a change from the division to 5-fold scenario led to an insignificant performance gain for the CNNs. We attribute this phenomenon to the challenging nature of nodule classification. In fact, distinction between malignant and benign nodules using visual characteristics is a difficult task even for human experts. This is confirmed by an observer performance study [49] based on the same nodule database, which reported a low AUC of 0.56 for the average performance of five radiologists and an AUC of 0.63 when the radiologists were shown relevant (similar) examples of benign and malignant nodules provided by a content-based image retrieval system. Referring to Table 3, we find it interesting that both the CNNs and MTANNs achieved significantly higher performance than that of the average human observers.

In Sect. 5.2, we based the comparison between CNNs and MTANNs on the applications for which MTANNs had previously shown promising performance. This is because our study was to investigate whether the state-of-the-art deep learning machines such as the CNNs, which are well-established in the computer-vision field, could outperform the MTANNs as a well-established machine-learning model for medical vision tasks. This is an interesting research question because the CNNs are currently considered as a panacea that can outperform the previously suggested solutions for a variety of medical imaging applications. However, in this study, we demonstrated that the use of the CNNs was not as effective as the MTANNs for lung nodule detection and classification. Given the relatively similar characteristics of focal lesions, our conclusion may also generalize to similar tasks such as polyp detection, breast mass detection, and liver tumor detection, where the low-level and mid-level features captured by MTANNs are adequate for accurate detection. However, we would also like to emphasize that the conclusions reached in this study may not generalize to more complex medical vision tasks such as image plane recognition [50] or pathology identification [51], where high-level semantic features extracted by deep CNNs are indispensable.

To provide a deeper comparison between CNNs and MTANNs, we would like to further discuss these two learning machines in terms of learned feature hierarchies, handling of sample uncertainty, and reliance on the size of the training set.

- *Learned feature hierarchies*: Consider an MTANN that has a hidden layer with k nodes and an output layer with 1 output node. Further assume that the above MTANN is trained using $d \times d$ image patches. During the training phase, $k \times d \times d$ weights will be learned between the input and the hidden layer, which can be viewed as learning k filters of size $d \times d$; k weights will be learned between the hidden layer and the output layer, which can be viewed as learning a fusion rule for combining the k filter responses in order to produce the desired output. Therefore, each MTANN in an ensemble learns k low-level features and the corresponding combination rule. During the test phase, the likelihood of being a lesion is computed for small $d \times d$ regions in an ROI; and then, the resulting likelihood values for lesion parts are aggregated using a Gaussian function. Therefore, the MTANNs never attempt to detect the entire lesion at once, rather, they learn to detect lesion parts using low-level features; and then, aggregate the predictions in a weighted manner to compute an overall lesion score for the whole ROI. CNNs, on the other hand, not only learn the low-level features but also extract the mid-level and high-level features in order to produce a likelihood value for a given ROI.
  The distinction between the above-explained feature hierarchies can contribute to the higher performance of the MTANNs for focal lesion detection. In Fig. 8, we showed that the majority of the top false positives generated by the MTANNs and CNN appeared around the chest wall. However, examining the remaining top false positives generated by the two models reveals that the CNN-based model shows a higher degree of reliance on the presence of chest walls than does the classification model based on the MTANNs. This is because a CNN tends to extract semantic features from ROIs. This together with the presence of the chest wall in the training ROIs has led to the inclusion of chest walls as a characteristic feature of the lung nodules. On the other hand, the MTANNs tend to extract the low-level features and use a Gaussian function centered in the middle of each ROI for weighted averaging of the scores, which makes the MTANNs more agnostic to image information located in the border areas (chest wall).
- *Handling of sample uncertainty*: In Sects. 2.1 and 2.2, we explained that CNNs take the original ROIs with the corresponding binary labels for training, but MTANNs receive small image patches from the ROIs and the corresponding continuous outputs ranged between 0 and 1. Therefore, the CNNs learn a classification model, but MTANNs learn a regression model. This seemingly subtle difference

can contribute to the superior performance of the MTANNs. This is because a CNN treats all the training samples equally regardless of their levels of uncertainty; as a result, the decision boundary can be readily affected by the presence of hard-to-classify training samples [52]. One way to overcome this limitation is to score the ROIs according to their level of difficulty. However, a manual approach is both subjective and expensive, and an automatic approach is still an immature area of research [53]. In the MTANNs, however, the uncertainty associated with difficult training samples is embedded in the continuous teaching values. Basically, the positive patches that are selected farther from the lesion location are considered hard-to-classify samples; and thus, they receive smaller likelihoods of being a lesion. Therefore, the proper handling of uncertainty in the MTANNs could contribute to its higher performance.

- *Reliance on the size of the training set*: MTANNs differ from CNNs in that they require only a small number of training ROIs. This is indeed a major advantage of the MTANNs over CNNs, which makes them particularly suitable for medical imaging applications where it is difficult and expensive to obtain a large number of labeled training data. This advantage stems from the fact that the MTANNs do not learn directly from the ROIs, rather, from small image patches, which can be effortlessly collected from a few training ROIs [54]. Furthermore, modeling appearance variability in small image patches is relatively less challenging than that of large ROIs, further decreasing the number of samples required for training the MTANNs. In contrast, the CNNs directly learn from the training ROIs; and thus, one must obtain a large number of training ROIs through either acquiring new cases or performing data augmentation. The former is difficult and expensive because lesions are not found frequently in medical images, and because they require expert annotations. The latter is computationally cheap, but the resulting training samples are highly correlated. Therefore, it can only partially compensate for insufficient training ROIs. This can be seen in Fig. 7b where the inclusion of additional unique training ROIs in the 5-fold cross validation scenario substantially improved the performance of the CNNs trained in the division scenario, even though sufficient data augmentation had been performed in the division scenario.

7 Conclusion

In this study, we compared two dominant classes of modern machine learning approaches in the detection and classification of focal lesions, namely, a bag of visual words and end-to-end learning machines. We based our comparisons on three well-studied applications in medical imaging: lung nodule detection, colorectal polyp detection, and lung nodule classification, all in CT images. We considered MTANNs and CNNs as representatives of end-to-end learning machines, and Fisher vectors as a representative of a bag of visual words. We first compared CNNs with Fisher vectors, concluding that the best performing CNN model achieved comparable performance to that of Fisher vectors. We also analyzed the performance of CNNs with varying depths. Our experiments showed that the CNN architectures with 3 or 4 convolutional layers were more effective than shallower architectures, but we did not observe a further performance gain by using deeper architectures. We then compared CNNs with MTANNs, concluding that MTANNs outperformed CNNs in nodule detection and classification particularly given limited training data. Specifically, for nodule detection, the MTANNs generated 0.08 false positives per section at 100% sensitivity, which was significantly ($p < 0.05$) lower than the best performing CNN model with 0.67 false positives per section at the same level of sensitivity. For nodule classification, the MTANNs yielded an AUC of 0.8806 (95% CI: 0.8389 to 0.9223), which was significantly ($p < 0.05$) higher than the best performing CNN model with an AUC of 0.7755 (95% CI: 0.7120 to 0.8270). We further theoretically compared the MTANNs and CNNs and discussed the possible reasons for the superiority of the MTANNs.

References

1. Suzuki, K., Armato III, S.G., Li, F., Sone, S., Doi, K.: Massive training artificial neural network (mtann) for reduction of false positives in computerized detection of lung nodules in low-dose computed tomography. Med. Phys. **30**(7), 1602–1617 (2003)
2. Krizhevsky, A., Sutskever, I., Hinton, G.E.: Imagenet classification with deep convolutional neural networks. In: Advances in Neural Information Processing Systems, pp. 1097–1105 (2012)
3. Perronnin, F., Sánchez, J., Mensink, T.: Improving the fisher kernel for large-scale image classification. In: Computer Vision–ECCV 2010, pp. 143–156. Springer (2010)
4. Suzuki, K., Horiba, I., Sugie, N.: Efficient approximation of neural filters for removing quantum noise from images. IEEE Trans. Signal Process. **50**(7), 1787–1799 (2002)
5. Suzuki, K., Horiba, I., Sugie, N., Nanki, M.: Neural filter with selection of input features and its application to image quality improvement of medical image sequences. IEICE Trans. Inf. Syst. **85**(10), 1710–1718 (2002)
6. Suzuki, K., Li, F., Sone, S., et al.: Computer-aided diagnostic scheme for distinction between benign and malignant nodules in thoracic low-dose ct by use of massive training artificial neural network. IEEE Trans. Med. Imag. **24**(9), 1138–1150 (2005)
7. Suzuki, K., Yoshida, H., Näppi, J., Dachman, A.H.: Massive-training artificial neural network (mtann) for reduction of false positives in computer-aided detection of polyps: suppression of rectal tubes. Med. Phys. **33**(10), 3814–3824 (2006)
8. Suzuki, K., Yoshida, H., Näppi, J., Armato III, S.G., Dachman, A.H.: Mixture of expert 3d massive-training anns for reduction of multiple types of false positives in cad for detection of polyps in ct colonography. Med. Phys. **35**(2), 694–703 (2008)
9. Suzuki, K., Rockey, D.C., Dachman, A.H.: Ct colonography: advanced computer-aided detection scheme utilizing mtanns for detection of missed polyps in a multicenter clinical trial. Med. Phys. **37**(1), 12–21 (2010)
10. Suzuki, K., Zhang, J., Xu, J.: Massive-training artificial neural network coupled with laplacian-eigenfunction-based dimensionality reduction for computer-aided detection of polyps in ct colonography. IEEE Trans. Med. Imag. **29**(11), 1907–1917 (2010)
11. Xu, J.-W., Suzuki, K.: Massive-training support vector regression and gaussian process for false-positive reduction in computer-aided detection of polyps in ct colonography. Med. Phys. **38**(4), 1888–1902 (2011)
12. Fukushima, K.: Neocognitron: a self-organizing neural network model for a mechanism of pattern recognition unaffected by shift in position. Biol. Cybern. **36**(4), 193–202 (1980)

13. Fukushima, K.: Neocognitron capable of incremental learning. Neural Netw. **17**(1), 37–46 (2004)
14. Deutsch, S.: A simplified version of kunihiko fukushima's neocognitron. Biol. Cybern. **42**(1), 17–21 (1981)
15. LeCun, Y., Boser, B., Denker, J.S., Henderson, D., Howard, R.E., Hubbard, W., Jackel, L.D.: Backpropagation applied to handwritten zip code recognition. Neural Comput. **1**(4), 541–551 (1989)
16. Le Cun, B.B., Denker, J.S., Henderson, D., Howard, R.E., Hubbard, W., Jackel, L.D.: Handwritten digit recognition with a back-propagation network. In: Advances in Neural Information Processing Systems. Citeseer (1990)
17. Tajbakhsh, N., Gotway, M.B., Liang, J.: Computer-aided pulmonary embolism detection using a novel vessel-aligned multi-planar image representation and convolutional neural networks. In: Medical Image Computing and Computer-Assisted Intervention MICCAI 2015 (2015)
18. Shen, W., Zhou, M., Yang, F., Yang, C., Tian, J.: Multi-scale convolutional neural networks for lung nodule classification. In: Ourselin, S., Alexander, D.C., Westin, C.-F., Cardoso, M.J. (eds.), Information Processing in Medical Imaging. Lecture Notes in Computer Science, vol. 9123, pp. 588–599. Springer International Publishing (2015)
19. Roth, H., Lu, L., Seff, A., Cherry, K., Hoffman, J., Wang, S., Liu, J., Turkbey, E., Summers, R.: A new 2.5d representation for lymph node detection using random sets of deep convolutional neural network observations. In: Golland, P., Hata, N., Barillot, C., Hornegger, J., Howe, R. (eds.), Medical Image Computing and Computer-Assisted Intervention MICCAI 2014. Lecture Notes in Computer Science, vol. 8673, pp. 520–527. Springer International Publishing (2014)
20. Tajbakhsh, N., Gurudu, S.R., Liang, J.: A comprehensive computer-aided polyp detection system for colonoscopy videos. In: Information Processing in Medical Imaging, pp. 327–338. Springer (2015)
21. Zhang, W., Li, R., Deng, H., Wang, L., Lin, W., Ji, S., Shen, D.: Deep convolutional neural networks for multi-modality isointense infant brain image segmentation. NeuroImage **108**, 214–224 (2015)
22. Havaei, M., Davy, A., Warde-Farley, D., Biard, A., Courville, A., Bengio, Y., Pal, C., Jodoin, P.-M., Larochelle, H.: Brain tumor segmentation with deep neural networks (2015). arXiv:1505.03540
23. Tajbakhsh, N., Shin, J.Y., Gurudu, S.R., Hurst, R.T., Kendall, C.B., Gotway, M.B., Liang, J.: Convolutional neural networks for medical image analysis: Fine tuning or full training? IEEE Trans. Med. Imag. **35**, 1299–1312 (2016)
24. Tajbakhsh, N., Gurudu, S.R., Liang, J.: Automatic polyp detection in colonoscopy videos using an ensemble of convolutional neural networks. In: 2015 IEEE 12th International Symposium on Biomedical Imaging (ISBI), pp. 79–83. IEEE (2015)
25. Glorot, X., Bengio, Y.: Understanding the difficulty of training deep feedforward neural networks. In: International Conference on Artificial Intelligence and Statistics, pp. 249–256 (2010)
26. Fei-Fei, L., Perona, P.: A bayesian hierarchical model for learning natural scene categories. In: IEEE Computer Society Conference on Computer Vision and Pattern Recognition, 2005. CVPR 2005, vol. 2, pp. 524–531. IEEE (2005)
27. Song, Y., Cai, W., Zhang, F., Huang, H., Zhou, Y., Feng, D.D.: Bone texture characterization with fisher encoding of local descriptors. In: 2015 IEEE 12th International Symposium on Biomedical Imaging (ISBI), pp. 5–8. IEEE (2015)
28. Kwitt, R., Hegenbart, S., Rasiwasia, N., Vécsei, A., Uhl, A.: Do we need annotation experts? a case study in celiac disease classification. In: Medical Image Computing and Computer-Assisted Intervention–MICCAI 2014, pp. 454–461. Springer (2014)
29. Twinanda, A.P., De Mathelin, M., Padoy, N.: Fisher kernel based task boundary retrieval in laparoscopic database with single video query. In: Medical Image Computing and Computer-Assisted Intervention–MICCAI 2014, pp. 409–416. Springer (2014)
30. Manivannan, S., Wang, R., Trucco, E.: Inter-cluster features for medical image classification. In: Medical Image Computing and Computer-Assisted Intervention–MICCAI 2014, pp. 345–352. Springer (2014)

31. Lowe, D.G.: Object recognition from local scale-invariant features. In: The Proceedings of the Seventh IEEE International Conference on Computer vision, 1999, vol. 2, pp. 1150–1157. IEEE (1999)
32. Sone, S., Takashima, S., Li, F., Yang, Z., Honda, T., Maruyama, Y., Hasegawa, M., Yamanda, T., Kubo, K., Hanamura, K., et al.: Mass screening for lung cancer with mobile spiral computed tomography scanner. The Lancet **351**(9111), 1242–1245 (1998)
33. Li, F., Sone, S., Abe, H., MacMahon, H., Armato, S.G., Doi, K.: Lung cancers missed at low-dose helical ct screening in a general population: comparison of clinical, histopathologic, and imaging findings 1. Radiology **225**(3), 673–683 (2002)
34. Näppi, J., Yoshida, H.: Feature-guided analysis for reduction of false positives in cad of polyps for computed tomographic colonography. Med. Phys. **30**(7), 1592–1601 (2003)
35. Yoshida, H., Näppi, J.: Three-dimensional computer-aided diagnosis scheme for detection of colonic polyps. IEEE Trans. Med. Imag. **20**(12), 1261–1274 (2001)
36. Egan, J.P., Greenberg, G.Z., Schulman, A.I.: Operating characteristics, signal detectability, and the method of free response. J. Acoust. Soc. Am. **33**(8), 993–1007 (1961)
37. Chakraborty, D.P., Berbaum, K.S.: Observer studies involving detection and localization: modeling, analysis, and validation. Med. Phys. **31**(8), 2313–2330 (2004)
38. Zhai, X., Chakraborty, D.: RJafroc: Analysis of Data Acquired Using the Receiver Operating Characteristic Paradigm and Its Extensions (2015). R package version 0.1.1
39. Robin, X., Turck, N., Hainard, A., Tiberti, N., Lisacek, F., Sanchez, J.-C., Mller, M.: Proc: an open-source package for r and s+ to analyze and compare roc curves. BMC Bioinform. **12**(77) (2011)
40. Jia, Y., Shelhamer, E., Donahue, J., Karayev, S., Long, J., Girshick, R., Guadarrama, S., Darrell, T.: Caffe: convolutional architecture for fast feature embedding (2014). arXiv:1408.5093
41. Vedaldi, A., Fulkerson, B.: VLFeat: an open and portable library of computer vision algorithms (2008). http://www.vlfeat.org/
42. Edwards, D.C., Kupinski, M.A., Metz, C.E., Nishikawa, R.M.: Maximum likelihood fitting of froc curves under an initial-detection-and-candidate-analysis model. Med. Phys. **29**(12), 2861–2870 (2002)
43. van Ginneken, B., Setio, A.A., Jacobs, C., Ciompi, F.: Off-the-shelf convolutional neural network features for pulmonary nodule detection in computed tomography scans. In: 2015 IEEE 12th International Symposium on Biomedical Imaging (ISBI), pp. 286–289, April 2015
44. Simonyan, K., Vedaldi, A., Zisserman, A.: Deep fisher networks for large-scale image classification. In: Advances in Neural Information Processing Systems, pp. 163–171 (2013)
45. Sydorov, V., Sakurada, M., Lampert, C.: Deep fisher kernels-end to end learning of the fisher kernel gmm parameters. In: Proceedings of the IEEE Conference on Computer Vision and Pattern Recognition, pp. 1402–1409 (2014)
46. Perronnin, F., Larlus, D.: Fisher vectors meet neural networks: A hybrid classification architecture. In: Proceedings of the IEEE Conference on Computer Vision and Pattern Recognition, pp. 3743–3752 (2015)
47. Zeiler, M.D., Fergus, R.: Visualizing and understanding convolutional networks. In: Computer Vision–ECCV 2014, pp. 818–833. Springer (2014)
48. Eigen, D., Rolfe, J., Fergus, R., LeCun, Y.: Understanding deep architectures using a recursive convolutional network (213). arXiv:1312.1847
49. Li, Q., Li, F., Shiraishi, J., Katsuragawa, S., Sone, S., Doi, K.: Investigation of new psychophysical measures for evaluation of similar images on thoracic computed tomography for distinction between benign and malignant nodules. Med. Phys. **30**(10), 2584–2593 (2003)
50. Margeta, J., Criminisi, A., Cabrera Lozoya, R., Lee, D.C., Ayache, N.: Fine-tuned convolutional neural nets for cardiac mri acquisition plane recognition. Comput. Methods Biomech. Biomed. Eng. Imag. Vis., 1–11 (2015)
51. Bar, Y., Diamant, I., Wolf, L., Greenspan, H.: Deep learning with non-medical training used for chest pathology identification, vol. 9414, pp. 94140V–94140V–7 (2015)

52. Kobetski, M., Sullivan, J.: Improved boosting performance by explicit handling of ambiguous positive examples. In: Pattern Recognition Applications and Methods. Advances in Intelligent Systems and Computing, vol. 318, pp. 17–37 (2015)
53. Ba, J., Caruana, R.: Do deep nets really need to be deep? In: Advances in Neural Information Processing Systems, pp. 2654–2662 (2014)
54. Suzuki, K., Doi, K.: How can a massive training artificial neural network (mtann) be trained with a small number of cases in the distinction between nodules and vessels in thoracic ct? 1. Acad. Radiol. **12**(10), 1333–1341 (2005)

Introduction to Binary Coordinate Ascent: New Insights into Efficient Feature Subset Selection for Machine Learning

Amin Zarshenas and Kenji Suzuki

Abstract Feature selection has been an active area of research in machine learning area, and a number of techniques have been developed for selecting an optimal or sub-optimal subset of features, because it is a major factor to determine the performance of a machine-learning technique. In this study, we propose and develop a novel optimization technique, namely, a binary coordinate ascent (BCA) algorithm inspired by the coordinate descent algorithm. The BCA algorithm is an iterative deterministic local optimization approach that can be coupled with wrapper, filter, or hybrid feature selection (FS) techniques. The algorithm searches throughout the space of binary coded input variables by iteratively optimizing the objective function in each dimension at a time. We investigated our BCA approach in a wrapper-based FS framework for the task of classification. In this framework, area under the receiver-operating-characteristic (ROC) curve (AUC) is used as the criterion to find the best subset of features. We evaluated our BCA-based FS in optimization of features for support vector machine, multilayer perceptron, and Naïve Bayes classifiers with five publicly available datasets. Our experimental datasets are distinct in terms of the number of attributes (ranging from 18 to 60), and the number of classes (binary or multi-class classification). The efficiency in terms of the number of subset evaluations was improved substantially (by factors of 5–40) compared with two popular FS meta-heuristics, i.e., sequential forward selection (SFS) and sequential floating forward selection (SFFS), while the classification performance for unseen data was maintained.

Keywords Machine learning · Classification · Feature subset selection
Attribute selection · Wrapper · Optimization · Supervised learning
Heuristic · Pattern recognition

A. Zarshenas (✉) · K. Suzuki
Medical Imaging Research Center & Department of Electrical
and Computer Engineering, Illinois Institute of Technology,
3440 S. Dearborn St., Chicago, IL 60616, USA
e-mail: mzarshen@hawk.iit.edu

K. Suzuki
e-mail: ksuzuki@iit.edu

© Springer International Publishing AG 2018
K. Suzuki and Y. Chen (eds.), *Artificial Intelligence in Decision Support Systems for Diagnosis in Medical Imaging*, Intelligent Systems Reference Library 140,
https://doi.org/10.1007/978-3-319-68843-5_3

1 Introduction

Feature selection (FS) in classification and regression has been an active area of research in machine learning. FS plays an important role in machine learning and data mining, because it is a major factor to determine the performance of a machine-learning technique [22]. Because of its importance, a number of investigators have studied and developed various techniques. The goal of an FS technique is to select an optimal or sub-optimal subset of features that makes a machine-learning technique the highest performance for a specific task (e.g., classification) [11]. A number of surveys have been published in literature to review the efficacy and efficiency of FS techniques in different machine-learning tasks [5, 15, 22, 33, 34]. FS for classification, which is the main focus of this study, was surveyed in detail in [15, 34]. In the context of medical image analysis and specifically the computer-aided detection (CADe) field [46–48], FS has long been an active area of research [4, 21, 27, 31, 40]. A large number of investigators have applied FS methods in classification tasks in their applications to improve the performance of their systems [13, 48, 49].

FS techniques can be generally categorized into filter, wrapper, hybrid, and embedded methods [45, 51]. Filter methods use a measurement to assign meaningful scores to different combinations of features, i.e., subsets of features, without using the knowledge on the employed classifier. Correlation criteria [30] and mutual information (MI) [3] are two of the most popular measurements used in this type of technique, in order to determine the usefulness of feature subsets. On the other hand, wrapper methods utilize an algorithmic-dependent measurement to examine the usefulness of feature subsets in an iterative manner [29]. Hybrid methods exploit both filter and wrapper methods in a single context in a way to boost up the FS algorithm. A hybrid feature selection technique was used for detection of prostate cancer in a trance-rectal ultrasound (TRUS) image-based CAD system [36]. Unlike the mentioned categories, embedded techniques such as decision trees [42] and L1-support-vector-machine (SVM) [57] accomplish their goal by directly including FS as a part of the optimization objective of the learning algorithm.

The wrappers have been used widely for classification because they often obtained superior performance as they find feature subsets better suited with a pre-determined classifier [34]. In general, there are three main factors that describe a wrapper procedure: a type of the classifier, a feature subset evaluation criterion, and an optimization technique to find the best combination of features. Several evaluation criteria such as accuracy [26, 32], a false-positive (FP) elimination rate [7, 8], and area under the receiver-operating-characteristic (ROC) curve (AUC) [9, 37, 44, 53, 54] have been used widely. Meta-heuristics including sequential and randomized techniques have been studied extensively and utilized in order to find the optimum or a sub-optimum subset of features. Genetic algorithms (GA) [7, 52], particle swarm optimization (PSO) [28, 39], and simulated annealing (SA) [16, 32, 38] are few examples of randomized search strategies used widely in FS. A wrapper feature selection technique based on the PSO was proposed for prostate cancer analysis in TRUS images [39]. Despite progress made through a randomized graph-based optimization approach, they are not fully satisfactory as they either yield a solution away from the optimum or they are computationally impractical [41]. There exist popular and commonly used deterministic search strategies, designed specifically for the task of FS, as alternatives that try to overcome the above mentioned problems, such as sequential forward selection (SFS) [11, 15, 18] and sequential forward floating selection (SFFS) [26, 41]. To discriminate breast tumors in ultrasonic images, an AdaBoost-algorithm-based ensemble classifier was coupled with an SFS technique [50]. An SFFS technique was combined with multiple classifiers to improve the correct classification rate (CCR) in grading for prostatic carcinoma in pathological images [26].

This study is based on [55], where we propose and develop a novel optimization technique, namely, a binary coordinate ascent (BCA) algorithm, inspired by the popular coordinate descent algorithm [25, 35], for efficiently solving combinatorial optimization problems. Our BCA optimization algorithm, as a deterministic local optimization approach, starts its search from an initial point in the space with binary representation of input variables and continuous output values. It iteratively updates the solution by optimizing the given cost function at each individual coordinate, one at a time. In this study, we investigated our BCA approach in a wrapper-based FS framework for the task of classification in order to reduce a huge number of subset evaluations needed in earlier existing FS techniques. We use a binary representation of feature subsets to set up the requirements for our BCA algorithm in FS for classification. In order to find the best (i.e., optimum or sub-optimum) subset of features, AUC of a classifier which quantifies the generalization performance of a classification system, obtained in a 10-fold cross validation (CV) manner, is set as the evaluation criterion to determine the usefulness of different subsets. To examine the consistency of our wrapper-based BCA approach, we investigated the efficiency and performance of our proposed method coupled with SVMs [14], multilayer perceptron (MLP) [24], and naïve Bayes (NB) [56] classifiers. In order to reduce the risk of overfitting while performing assessment of FS methods [43], an independent test set was used for comparisons of our proposed algorithm with two of the most popular FS techniques, i.e., the SFS and SFFS. To our knowledge, no investigator has proposed the BCA algorithm or developed an FS algorithm based on the BCA algorithm before.

2 Methods

2.1 Coordinate Descent Algorithm

Coordinate descent (CD) algorithm [35] is one of the most popular non-derivative optimization techniques that have been used widely to solve a variety of optimization problems including quadratic programming. It has been employed in machine-learning community for different tasks such as for training SVMs [25]. Convergence of the CD algorithm to the global optimum is guaranteed under specific assumptions such as convexity of the objective function and its smoothness, but such assumptions cannot always be made in real applications. Without following all of those assumptions, CD is capable of finding a local optimum. The CD algorithm can be formulated as follows:

$$X_i^{k+1} = \text{argmin}_{a \in R} J\left(X_1^{k+1}, \ldots, X_{i-1}^{k+1}, a, X_{i+1}^k, \ldots, X_N^k\right) \tag{1}$$

where N is the number of dimensions of the input variables, $J(.): R^N \to R$ is the objective function, and X_i^k is the ith variable of the solution at the kth iteration. Without loss of generality, we can formulate the coordinate ascent (CA) algorithm by considering the maximization of the negative of the objective function J in Eq. (1). CD is motivated by the hypothesis that one can find the local optimum of an objective function by minimizing it along each coordinate, one at a time. If optimality assumptions are not followed, CD results are subject to the choice of initialization as well as other local search methods.

2.2 Binary Coordinate Ascent Algorithm

In a variety of programming problems, a binary representation of input variables is possible, and it can be used to encode the input space [10]. FS is one of the problems that can be represented in a binary variable framework, which was the main motivation for the proposed method. The general form of an unconstrained programming problem of maximizing a continuous objective function in a binary variable framework is given by:

$$X^* = \text{argmax}_{X \in B^N} J(X), \ B = \{0, 1\}. \tag{2}$$

The problem in Eq. (2) is a special case of integer programming; therefore, an exhaustive search can possibly be performed if the number of variables is not too large, but the problem is considered as one of the NP-hard problems in computational complexity theory [22]. As a result, a variety of suboptimal solution techniques such as evolutionary-algorithm-based optimizations [2] and swarm-based algorithms [6] have been used widely to deal with these problems. However, most of these either stochastic or deterministic heuristics are computationally expensive; thus, they require minor or major modifications for the task of FS. Motivated by the given facts, we propose a new version of the CA algorithm, suitable for solving these types of problems in terms of efficiency and efficacy, namely, a binary coordinate ascent (BCA) algorithm. Unlike the CA algorithm that requires defining a search line optimization approach through single coordinates, the BCA employs a zero-one switch strategy to find the local optimum along each coordinate, one at a time. The detailed pseudocode of our BCA optimization algorithm is given in Table 1.

In the given algorithm in Table 1, the BCA starts its search from an initial point, i.e., the binary vector of all zeroes at the origin. We discuss the choice of the initial point that depends on the application requirements in a later section. The BCA then

Table 1 Pseudocode of our BCA optimization algorithm for combinatorial optimization in a binary representation framework

BCA optimization algorithm

Initialization:

Set $X^* = (0, 0, ..., 0)^T$, where $X^* \in \{0, 1\}^N$ // *vector of all zeroes as the initial solution*

Set $Y^* = J(X^*)$ // *initial value of the objective function to be maximized*

Set Δ // Δ *and Stop variables are defined for convergence criterion*

Stop = 0

while (*Stop* = 0)

        for ($i = 1 : N$)

                $X = X^*$

                $X_i = not(X_i^*)$ // *not(0) = 1 and not(1) = 0*

                if ($J(X) > J(X^*)$)

                        $X^* = X$

                end

        end

        $Y = J(X^*)$ // *objective function value for the current solution*

        if ($|Y^* - Y| < \Delta$) // *stopping criterion, i.e., convergence of the objective function value*

                Stop = 1

        end

        $Y^* = Y$

end

Output:

Final solution (X^*, Y^*)

updates the solution to the optimization problem through maximizing the objective function at each coordinate individually. A zero-one switching strategy is used to find the maximum along a single coordinate. Once the BCA completes the search through all coordinates, the solution (i.e., maximum) Y^* is updated. The algorithm stops when there is no more significant change in the optimum objective function value. Other stopping criteria such as the number of iterations could be employed, as the BCA performs in an any-time programming algorithm manner. Eventually, the algorithm returns a pair of Y^* and X^* as the final maximum and argument of the maximum, respectively. Although the BCA is designed explicitly for the task of FS, the algorithm can be performed in any programming problem with a binary representation of input variables and continuous objective function values, given the fact that there is no initial assumption about the objective function $J(.)$ in the methodology.

2.3   BCA-Based Wrapper FS

Based on our BCA optimization approach, we propose a fast wrapper FS algorithm with two variants of initialization strategies: one starting with an empty set of features, namely, BCA-Zero; and the other with a filter-based initialization scheme, namely, BCA-Filter. In order to set up the FS problem to be solved with the BCA optimization algorithm, we first represent feature subsets in a binary fashion. In this framework, each feature subset is represented as a binary vector of length N, where N is the total number of initial input features (i.e., the number of attributes), and each element corresponds to one of the input features. An element of this vector is one only if the corresponding feature to that element is included in the feature subset corresponding to that binary vector.

In this scenario, we can represent the FSS problem using Eq. (2) having X and $J(.)$ be the binary-encoded feature subsets and the performance of a pre-determined classifier, respectively. An example of the state diagram to visualize FS in a binary fashion for the case of N = 4 is given in Fig. 1. In the figure, nodes represent feature subsets (the total of 2^N solutions exist), while edges connect feature subsets with a Hamming distance of one, i.e., a shift between these subsets can be made by adding or removing only one feature. The directed edges shown on the graph correspond to the scanning directions through which the BCA algorithm examines candidates and selects feature subsets, for an example shown in the small table included in Fig. 1. Note that the objective function values in the table are hand-picked and are used for the purpose of illustration only.

The block diagram of our proposed wrapper FS algorithm is shown in Fig. 2. In BCA-Zero approach, our FS algorithm starts its search from an empty set of features, i.e., a vector of all zeroes in a binary representation fashion. The BCA algorithm iteratively adds and removes features to and from the selected subset of

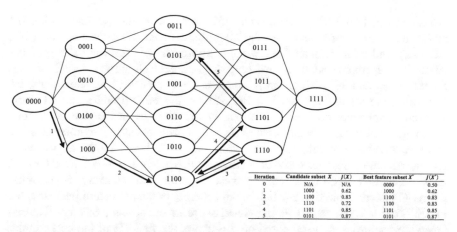

Iteration	Candidate subset X	J(X)	Best feature subset X*	J(X*)
0	N/A	N/A	0000	0.50
1	1000	0.62	1000	0.62
2	1100	0.83	1100	0.83
3	1110	0.72	1100	0.83
4	1101	0.85	1101	0.85
5	0101	0.87	0101	0.87

Fig. 1 State diagram for visualizing feature subset selection in a binary representation framework. In this example, the diagram shows all combinations of feature subsets in a four-dimensional binary space, i.e., the total number of features is four. The directed edges shown on the graph correspond to the scanning directions through which the BCA algorithm examines candidates and selects feature subsets based on the example shown in the table

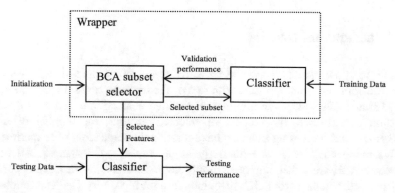

Fig. 2 Block diagram of our proposed wrapper FS algorithm employing the BCA optimization algorithm

features based on the objective function values. In fact, at each iteration, the BCA ensures whether existence of a feature, in a given subset of features, improves or drops the classification performance. In our implementation, AUC, which approximates the generalization performance of a learning algorithm properly by estimating the probability that a classifier ranks a randomly chosen positive instance higher than a randomly chosen negative instance [19], is used as the objective function $J(.)$. Indeed, the objective function is the validation performance of a pre-determined classifier obtained by 10-fold CV on a validation set. Once the algorithm converges to the final solution, i.e., the best subset of features, a classifier is trained and tested on the entire validation set and an independent testing set, respectively, in order to evaluate the algorithm. To examine the consistency in efficiency and performance of our wrapper approach with the choice of the classifier, in our implementations, we employed three well-known classifiers, i.e., SVM, MLP, and NB, which are distinct in their strategies to learn a model. Regarding the second scheme, i.e., BCA-Filter, the FS procedure and all corresponding implementation details are exactly the same as that of the BCA-Zero, except that in this case, a filter-based strategy is utilized to select the initial subset of features, instead of starting from the empty set of features. To do so, we use a ranking scheme of features based on a classifier-dependent score calculated for each feature individually. In other words, for each feature independently, we calculate the AUC (i.e., the objective function in our scheme) of the pre-determined classifier in a 10-fold CV fashion, as its individual score in the absence of other features. Once the features are ranked based on this score, the first T% of the best features (i.e., the highest AUCs) are selected in the initial subset of features. T is a variable set by a user and needs a prior knowledge of the dataset such as the total number of features. In our experiments, T is set to 20%, based on the number of attributes of the datasets that we experiment on.

3 Experimental Results

In order to show the efficiency and performance of our proposed BCA FS algorithm, we compared our algorithm with two of the most popular FS techniques, i.e., SFS [18] and SFFS [41]. We did the comparative evaluation in terms of the classification performance, the number of selected features, the number of subset evaluations, and processing time. To have a rational comparison, we experimented on five independent datasets with fairly large numbers of instances. All of the datasets, which are either binary or multi-class classification tasks, are publicly available and obtained from UCI machine-learning repository [1]. The number of dataset attributes ranges from 18 to 60 excluding the class attribute. The full description of the datasets is summarized in Table 2.

In order to examine the consistency of the performance of the proposed algorithm with the choice of the pre-determined classifier in a wrapper FS framework, we coupled both the proposed algorithms and the reference techniques with three different classifiers, namely, the SVM, MLP, and NB. These classifiers were selected because they are distinct in terms of their nature of learning of a model. LIBSVM [12] and WEKA [23] packages were utilized for implementation of these learning algorithms in our experiments. All classifier parameters in our implementations were set to default values of these libraries. In order to reduce the risk of overfitting while performing FS [43], we employed independent test sets for evaluation of each approach. We extracted approximately 70% of samples from

Table 2 Description of the datasets used in our comparative evaluation experiments

Data set	#instances	Number of attributes	Attribute types	#Classes	Application
Sonar	208	60	Numerical	2	Discriminate between metal and rock objects
Parkinson	195	22	Numerical	2	Discriminate healthy people from those with Parkinson
Breast cancer	569	30	Numerical	2	Breast cancer diagnostic
Segmentation	2310	19	Numerical	7	Image segmentation by classification
Climate	540	18	Numerical	2	Predict climate model simulation outcome (fail or succeed)

each dataset as a training set, randomly and in a stratified manner, while we kept the rest for testing purpose. In other words, each FS method was executed on the training data using a 10-fold CV strategy. Once the best subset of features (i.e., the best validation performance) was obtained, a model was then trained on the entire training set, using only selected features, and tested on the independent test set.

The performance results represented by AUC values as well as the number of selected features obtained for the proposed algorithms and the two reference methods, using three classifiers on five datasets, are shown in Table 3. We performed statistical analysis on the results obtained for each classifier separately. In this study, we followed the statistical analysis methodology recommended in [17, 20]. Namely, Friedman test was utilized to statistically compare the results obtained for all four approaches for each classifier, separately. If a significant difference with a confidence level of 0.05 was detected, we proceeded to the pair-wise comparison of approaches using the non-parametric Wilcoxon signed rank test. We use the notations N_B and S_B under the results of method A, when there was no significant or a significant difference between method A and B, respectively. Our experiments showed that none of the three statistical tests obtained significance; thus, we did not proceed to pairwise comparisons. Therefore, the performance, in terms of AUC values, of the proposed methods is considered comparable to that of the SFS and SFFS techniques. The average rank of each approach obtained by the Friedman ranking method is also depicted in Table 3 for a better understanding of the comparisons. Note that the best AUC and the best number of selected features should result in ranks of 4 and 1, respectively. Moreover, one can see that there is no substantial difference between the two variants of the proposed algorithm in terms of the classification performance. To have a better insight into the performance evaluation results, we illustrate the bar chart of the AUC values obtained in our experiments in Fig. 3. The visual results of Fig. 3 are consistent with our previous analysis. The same comparison and statistical analysis methodology was also applied for the number of selected features obtained for each method. Results showed that there was

Table 3 Comparisons of the classification performance (in terms of AUC) as well as the number of selected features (#Feats) of our BCA algorithms with zero and filter-based initialization schemes with that of the SFS and SFFS FS techniques for five datasets using SVM, MLP, and NB classifiers. AUC results on independent (unseen) test data as well as the number of selected features (#Feats) are reported

Dataset	BCA-Zero		BCA-Filter		SFS		SFFS	
	AUC	#Feats	AUC	#Feats	AUC	#Feats	AUC	#Feats
SVM								
Sonar	0.779	17	0.743	17	0.756	9	0.744	10
Parkinson	0.855	6	0.855	6	0.855	6	0.855	6
Breast cancer	0.997	15	0.998	10	0.997	12	0.997	12
Segmentation	0.988	8	0.990	8	0.989	6	0.989	6
Climate	0.974	10	0.978	9	0.973	12	0.974	10
Mean ± SD	0.918 ± 0.10	11.2 ± 4.7	0.913 ± 0.11	10 ± 4.2	0.914 ± 0.10	9 ± 3.0	0.912 ± 0.11	8.8 ± 2.7
Average rank	2.4	3.2	3.1	2.3	2.2	2.3	2.3	2.2
	N_B, N_C, N_D	N_B, N_C, N_D	N_A, N_C, N_D	N_A, N_C, N_D	N_A, N_B, N_D	N_A, N_B, N_D	N_A, N_B, N_C	N_A, N_B, N_C
MLP								
Sonar	0.880	18	0.897	16	0.797	8	0.839	17
Parkinson	0.767	4	0.705	8	0.796	12	0.776	12
Breast cancer	0.999	12	0.998	9	0.997	5	0.998	18
Segmentation	0.992	15	0.982	11	0.989	14	0.994	18
Climate	0.973	11	0.962	5	0.959	14	0.953	10
Mean ± SD	0.92 ± 0.10	12 ± 5.2	0.909 ± 0.12	9.8 ± 4.1	0.908 ± 0.10	10.6 ± 4.0	0.912 ± 0.10	15 ± 3.7
Average rank	3.2	2.8	2.3	1.6	2	2.3	2.5	3.3
	N_B, N_C, N_D	N_B, N_C, N_D	N_A, N_C, N_D	N_A, N_C, N_D	N_A, N_B, N_D	N_A, N_B, N_D	N_A, N_B, N_C	N_A, N_B, N_C
NB								
Sonar	0.802	16	0.734	11	0.664	14	0.783	8
Parkinson	0.680	6	0.672	6	0.680	6	0.680	6
Breast cancer	0.998	10	0.999	9	0.998	12	0.998	9

(continued)

Table 3 (continued)

Dataset	BCA-Zero		BCA-Filter		SFS		SFFS	
	AUC	#Feats	AUC	#Feats	AUC	#Feats	AUC	#Feats
Segmentation	0.982	8	0.979	8	0.982	8	0.982	8
Climate	0.978	10	0.978	10	0.977	10	0.977	10
Mean ± SD	0.888 ± 0.14	10 ± 3.7	0.872 ± 0.16	8.8 ± 1.9	0.860 ± 0.17	10 ± 3.2	0.884 ± 0.14	8.2 ± 1.5
Average rank	3.1	2.9	2.3	2.2	2.1	2.9	2.5	2
	N_B, N_C, N_D	N_B, N_C, N_D	N_A, N_C, N_D	N_A, N_C, N_D	N_A, N_B, N_D	N_A, N_B, N_D	N_A, N_B, N_C	N_A, N_B, N_C

Note when considering the results for pair-wise statistical analysis, the BCA-Zero, BCA-Filter, SFS and SFFS are assigned letters of A, B, C, and D, respectively. N_B or S_B under the results of method A indicate that there is no significant or a significant difference between method A and B, respectively

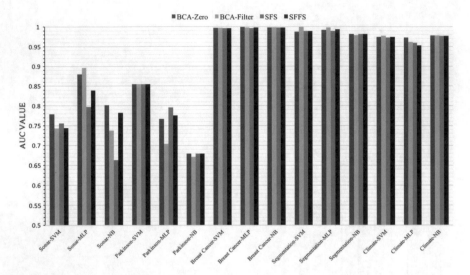

Fig. 3 Bar chart for visual comparison of the testing classification performance (in terms of AUC values) of our BCA algorithm with zero and filter-based initializations with that of the SFS and SFFS FS techniques

no statistically significant difference between experimental methods in terms of the number of selected features. Nonetheless, one might notice that the BCA-Filter found a smaller subset of features on average, compared with that of the BCA-Zero. This result makes sense because the BCA-Filter employs the more sophisticated initialization strategy.

Table 4 shows the number of feature subset evaluations (i.e., the number of trials before selecting the best feature subset) and the algorithm running time, for both our proposed algorithms and the reference FS techniques. All timing results were obtained on a workstation running the Ubuntu.

Linux 14.04 operating system with Intel Core i7-4790 K @ 4.0 GHz CPU and 16 GB RAM. Results show that the number of subset evaluations was reduced substantially by factors of approximately 7 and 40 on average, when comparing our BCA-Filter to the SFS and SFFS techniques, respectively. Comparing our BCA-Zero with the SFS and SFFS techniques, the number of subset evaluations was reduced approximately by factors of 5 and 26 on average, respectively. Looking at Table 4, one can see that the processing speed was also improved substantially by the proposed algorithms, which is consistent with our analysis of the number of subset evaluations. Similar statistical analysis methodology discussed earlier was used to examine the significance for the timing and the number of subset evaluation results. In this case, all p-values obtained by the Friedman tests were less than 0.05, yielding to reject the null hypothesis in favor of the alternative hypothesis, i.e., there exist some significant differences in the obtained results.

Table 4 Comparisons of the computational complexity (in terms of the number of subset evaluations) as well as the timing results (in minutes) of our BCA algorithms with zero and filter-based initialization schemes with that of the SFS and SFFS FS techniques for five datasets using SVM, MLP, and NB classifiers

Dataset	BCA-Zero		BCA-Filter		SFS		SFFS	
	Time	#subset	Time	#subset	Time	#subset	Time	#subset
SVM								
Sonar	5.08	540	2.03	180	17.29	1830	110.53	9567
Parkinson	0.69	88	0.64	66	1.93	253	6.43	792
Breast cancer	1.58	90	1.17	60	7.59	465	32.15	1676
Segmentation	7.15	57	8.90	57	21.90	190	113.30	886
Climate	1.12	90	0.62	36	1.94	171	7.70	597
Mean ± SD	3.12 ± 2.8	173 ± 205	2.67 ± 3.5	79.8 ± 57	10.13 ± 9.1	581.8 ± 707	54.02 ± 53.8	2703.6 ± 3858
Average rank	1.8	1.9	1.2	1.1	3	3	4	4
	N_B, S_C, S_D	N_B, S_C, S_D	N_A, S_C, S_D	N_A, S_C, S_D	S_A, S_B, S_D	S_A, S_B, S_D	S_A, S_B, S_C	S_A, S_B, S_C
MLP								
Sonar	9.33	300	4.01	120	87.70	1830	1531.6	16094
Parkinson	0.84	66	0.83	44	4.18	253	30.24	408
Breast cancer	7.36	150	4.20	90	24.48	465	427.83	5364
Segmentation	28.81	57	28.90	76	59.32	190	416.13	1005
Climate	2.07	54	1.82	54	5.62	171	46.30	1042
Mean ± SD	9.68 ± 11.3	125.4 ± 105	7.95 ± 11.8	76.8 ± 30	36.26 ± 36.3	581.8 ± 707	490.42 ± 613	4782.6 ± 6627
Average rank	1.8	1.7	1.2	1.3	3	3	4	4
	N_B, S_C, S_D	N_B, S_C, S_D	N_A, S_C, S_D	N_A, S_C, S_D	S_A, S_B, S_D	S_A, S_B, S_D	S_A, S_B, S_C	S_A, S_B, S_C
NB								
Sonar	1.37	240	1.56	240	10.90	1830	64.00	9343
Parkinson	0.44	88	0.31	44	1.22	253	6.48	1158
Breast cancer	0.91	120	0.84	90	3.58	465	16.34	1796
Segmentation	0.89	57	1.12	57	2.86	190	7.71	453
Climate	0.26	36	0.37	36	1.18	171	3.29	430
Mean ± SD	0.77 ± 0.4	108.2 ± 80	0.84 ± 0.5	93.4 ± 85	4.15 ± 4.0	581.8 ± 707	19.56 ± 25	2636 ± 3792
Average rank	1.4	1.7	1.6	1.3	3	3	4	4
	N_B, S_C, S_D	N_B, S_C, S_D	N_A, S_C, S_D	N_A, S_C, S_D	S_A, S_B, S_D	S_A, S_B, S_D	S_A, S_B, S_C	S_A, S_B, S_C

Note when considering the results for pair-wise statistical analysis, the BCA-Zero, BCA-Filter, SFS and SFFS are assigned letters of A, B, C, and D, respectively. N_B or S_B under the results of method A indicate that there is no significant or a significant difference between method A and B, respectively

Therefore, we proceeded to the non-parametric Wilcoxon signed rank test. The pair-wise statistical analysis confirmed that differences between the timing and the number of subset evaluation results of either of our BCA-Zero or BCA-Filter algorithms were significant, with a significance level of 0.1, with respect to those of obtained by either of the SFS or SFFS techniques. We also compared the SFS and SFFS techniques and found that the difference between these two techniques in terms of the running time and the number of subset evaluations was statistically significant. Moreover, we compared the two variants of our proposed approach, i.e., the BCA-Zero and BCA-Filter. They were comparable in terms of timing results, whereas there was a slight improvement in terms of the number of subset evaluations for the case of the BCA-Filter. This was achieved by sacrificing some processing time for the algorithm initialization through the filter FS process. Statistical analysis confirmed the fact that there was no significant difference between the BCA-Zero and BCA-Filter. Note that, although we performed statistical analysis to confirm our comparisons, one might easily see from Table 4 that the SFS and SFFS techniques were assigned the third and the fourth ranks, respectively, by the Friedman ranking method in all experiments. Moreover, to have a better insight into the improvement of the number of subset evaluations achieved by the two variants of the proposed method, we illustrate the bar chart of the number of subset evaluations in Fig. 4.

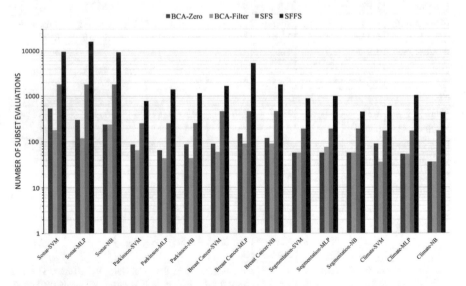

Fig. 4 Bar chart for visual comparison of the number of wrapper subset evaluations in our BCA algorithm with zero and filter-based initializations with that in the SFS and SFFS FS techniques. Note the log scale in the vertical axis

4 Discussion

In general, there is not a strong reason to believe that better approaches might overlap in selecting the best subset of features, without having the knowledge of the ground truth features. However, we believe it useful to analyze the selected features for the methods to gain insight into the characteristics of the methods. Table 5 shows the results of the pair-wise analysis of overlapping features for the four approaches, i.e., the BCA-Zero, BCA-Filter, SFS, and SFFS. The number of overlapping features alone may not necessarily provide an accurate similarity measure for this particular purpose, as it does not consider the length of each subset; therefore, we used the Jaccard similarity (JS) metric for feature analysis, i.e., the ratio of the size of the intersection of two sets divided by the size of their union. Looking at the average JS metrics depicted in Table 5, one might see that there is a

Table 5 Analysis of overlapping features between each pair of algorithms (BCA-Zero, BCA-Filter, SFS, and SFFS). Similarities of the selected feature subsets are compared in terms of the Jaccard similarity (JS)

Dataset	BCA-Zero/ BCA-Filter	BCA-Zero/ SFS	BCA-Zero/ SFFS	BCA-Filter/ SFS	BCA-Filter/ SFFS	SFS/ SFFS
SVM						
Sonar	0.478	0.444	0.588	0.368	0.500	0.357
Parkinson	1.000	1.000	1.000	1.000	1.000	1.000
Breast cancer	0.563	0.500	0.500	0.467	0.467	1.000
Segmentation	1.000	0.556	0.556	0.556	0.556	1.000
Climate	0.583	0.833	1.000	0.750	0.583	0.833
Mean ± SD	0.725 ± 0.25	0.667 ± 0.24	0.729 ± 0.25	0.628 ± 0.25	0.621 ± 0.22	0.838 ± 0.28
MLP						
Sonar	0.214	0.130	0.207	0.263	0.320	0.250
Parkinson	0.333	0.231	0.333	0.427	0.333	0.714
Breast Cancer	0.167	0.133	0.364	0.167	0.421	0.150
Segmentation	0.368	0.526	0.737	0.667	0.611	0.789
Climate	0.455	0.563	0.500	0.357	0.500	0.600
Mean ± SD	0.307 ± 0.12	0.317 ± 0.21	0.428 ± 0.20	0.376 ± 0.19	0.437 ± 0.12	0.501 ± 0.28
NB						
Sonar	0.421	0.429	0.500	0.563	0.583	0.467
Parkinson	0.714	0.714	0.714	0.714	0.714	1.000
Breast cancer	0.727	0.692	0.583	0.500	0.636	0.500
Segmentation	0.778	1.000	1.000	0.778	0.778	1.000
Climate	1.000	0.818	0.818	0.818	0.818	1.000
Mean ± SD	0.728 ± 0.21	0.730 ± 0.21	0.723 ± 0.20	0.675 ± 0.14	0.706 ± 0.10	0.793 ± 0.28

better match between the SFS and SFFS techniques than between these two and the proposed algorithms, i.e., the SFS obtained similar features to those obtained by the SFFS. However, all JS values in pair-wise comparisons were comparable, indicating the pair-wise overlap of the selected features was comparable. This does not necessary show the effectiveness of any of these approaches. However, an interesting result can be depicted by considering the JS similarities obtained for the case of the MLP classifier and comparing them to those obtained for the SVM and NB classifiers. Most of the JS results obtained for the MLP were smaller than those of the SVM and NB classifiers. This difference can be understood by considering MLP classifiers as one of the learning algorithms with a built-in FS capability through optimization of the weights of the neural network. To gain more insight into the feature analysis results, we illustrate the selected features obtained by the four experimental methods (i.e., the BCA-Zero, BCA-Filter, SFS, and SFFS) for the case of Climate dataset in Fig. 5. The results for this single dataset was picked for the ease of illustration, while the results for all other datasets followed a same fashion. The results shown in Fig. 5 are consistent with our previous discussion that the selected feature subsets obtained by different methods are more distinct for the case of MLP. To continue with this discussion, we first introduce following notations for the case of Climate dataset with the total number of 18 attributes.

- Ω: the set of all features where $\Omega := \{f_1, f_2, \ldots, f_{17}, f_{18}\}$,
- **B**: best subset of features (ground truth) where $\mathbf{B} \subseteq \Omega$
- $\Theta(c, m)$: selected subset by classifier c and method m, where $c \in \{SVM, MLP, NB\}$, $m \in \{BCA\text{-}Zero, BCA\text{-}Filter, SFS, SFFS\}$, and $\Theta \subseteq \Omega$
- $D(c, m)$: difference subset for classifier c and method m where $D(c, m) = \Theta(c, m) - \mathbf{B}$

In addition, to simplify the problem, we make two hypotheses: first, the subset **B** is given and equals to $\{f_1, f_2, f_{13}, f_{14}\}$ (the squares with darkest gray tone in Fig. 5); second, the best subset **B** is a subset of $\Theta(c, m)$ ($\mathbf{B} \subseteq \Theta(c, m)$) for all combinations of c and m, i.e., in all experiments (out of 12) the resulting subset of features contains the ground truth best features with potentially additional redundant or non-relevant features. Based on the results shown in Fig. 5 and Table 5, one can see that the set intersections between the four difference subsets $D(MLP, m)$ were smaller than those for the SVM and NB cases. As a result, we may conclude that the MLP performance (i.e., classification performance) was robust with respect to the difference subset. We believe that if the variation in difference subset D for the SVM and NB was high, the variation in the obtained performance for the experimental methods would be high as well; therefore, we may conclude that with comparable performance, there is a higher chance of obtaining overlapping features for the case of the SVM and NB than that of the MLP, when applying different FS techniques.

We saw earlier that the BCA-Zero and BCA-Filter algorithms outperformed the SFS and SFFS techniques in terms of the number of subset evaluations. We investigated the complexity of these approaches with theoretical and experimental

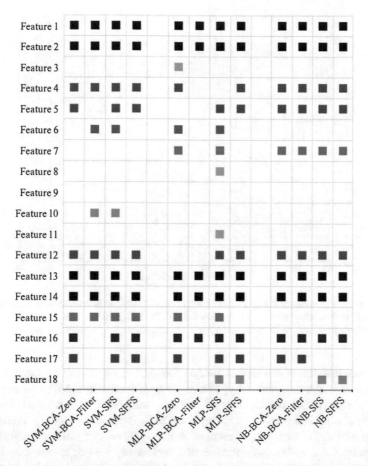

Fig. 5 Selected features obtained by the four experimental algorithms (BCA-Zero, BCA-Filter, SFS, and SFFS) for the case of Climate dataset. The gray level of the square for a selected feature corresponds to the number of times that the feature was selected through 12 (three classifiers and four algorithms) independent experiments, where the darker gray tone corresponds to more experiments

formula of the number of subset evaluations $f(N)$ as a function of the number of input attributes N. The formula for the case of the SFS technique is deterministic and can be derived analytically. For the case of the proposed algorithms and SFFS technique, we utilized regression to find experimental formulas. We fit two linear models and a quadratic polynomial to the data obtained by the proposed algorithms and the SFFS technique, correspondingly. The three experimental expressions as well as the analytical function (for the SFS) are shown in Fig. 6. The error bars in Fig. 6 show the exact data obtained through our experiments. For example, the error bar on the SFFS curve at $N = 60$ is obtained on the Sonar dataset with 60 attributes using the SVM, MLP, and NB classifiers (total of 3 points). Taking the

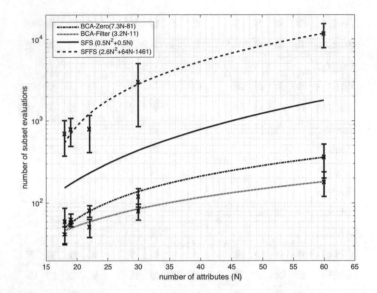

Fig. 6 Number of wrapper subset evaluations as a function of the number of input attributes (N). Linear and non-linear fitted function curves for the BCA algorithms with zero and filter-based initializations, SFS, and SFFS techniques are illustrated. Note the log scale in the vertical axis

hypothesis that the actual points indeed follow the approximated curves, which might be in fact a reasonable hypothesis by a subjective evaluation of Fig. 6, we might conclude that the number of subset evaluations for the BCA-Zero and BCA-Filter algorithms follow a linear complexity, with some scaling factor (3–8), with respect to the number of input attributes N. Having a similar judgment and considering the exact formula for the SFS technique, we might conclude that the SFS and SFFS techniques both follow a quadratic complexity formula with respect to N, and there is a scaling factor (approximately 2) for the case of the SFFS technique.

To have more insights into the reason why BCA-based FS algorithms are linear, whereas the SFS and SFFS techniques are quadratic, we consider the graph-based representation of feature subsets (an example for $N = 4$ was shown in Fig. 1). Using the binary representation of feature subsets, we can represent feature subsets for any dataset with N number of attributes, as a graph with $N + 1$ layers, where Lth layer contains $\binom{N}{L}$ subsets. The SFS method starts searching from the subset of all 0 s ($L = 0$) and scans the graph in a greedy-algorithm-based manner through the last layer ($L = N$). In other words, once the SFS technique finds the best subset of Lth layer, it searches throughout the N-L candidates in the $L + 1$th layer; thus, the total number of subset evaluations is quadratic with respect to N. The SFFS technique follows the same greedy approach, except that it allows the backward search through the previous layers while performing the graph search. Note that regardless of what layer the best subset of features is located in, the SFS and SFFS techniques scan all layers for at least once, where for each layer L, an order of N evaluations is required for a forward or backward search. BCA-based FS algorithms overcome the problem of computational complexity by reducing the number of evaluations needed to pass over a layer in the graph search, i.e., when in layer L, only one subset of either L + 1th layer (adding a feature) or L − 1th layer (removing a feature) will be examined. In fact, BCA-based FS follows a line search strategy through the graph. Moreover, one might notice that the BCA algorithm does not necessary scan all the layers. To make it clearer, consider the example of Sonar dataset with 60 features. One can see from Table 3 that the number of selected features obtained by four methods and three classifiers were all less than 30% of N; therefore, about 70% of layers were redundantly scanned by the SFS and SFFS techniques. On the other hand, BCA-based FS never goes far away from the optimal or sub-optimal subsets in its search space; thus, substantially more efficient.

From the comparisons of computational complexity represented in Table 4, one might notice that the speed ratio (the ratio between the running times) is not exactly the same as the ratio of the number of subset evaluations. The reason is twofold: the first is that the time complexity of learning algorithms is not a constant, and it is a function of number of input features; the second is that the length of the feature subsets evaluated through the FS methods in this study, is not necessary a constant.

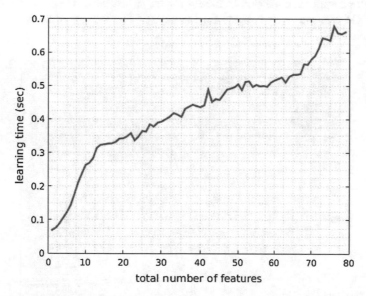

Fig. 7 Time complexity of the SVM classifier with respect to the number of input features to the learning algorithm. The average time required by the SVM classifier to evaluate a feature subset, with a specific length of features, through the 10-fold CV process is shown. The average time for a feature subset of F features was calculated by averaging over all subsets of length F that have been met through the FS process by the SFS technique. A private dataset with 79 attributes was used for this experiment

As an example, we show the time complexity curve for the SVM classifier in Fig. 7. Note that the curve shows the average time required by the SVM classifier to evaluate a feature subset, with a specific length of features, through the 10-fold CV process. Following these observations, one might notice that among two FS methods, the one with a larger number of subset evaluations can be potentially faster, given that the time complexity of the learning algorithm for the subsets that it evaluated were small enough, correspondingly. Based on this reasoning, we may conclude that it is always a wiser choice to initiate the BCA algorithm by an empty set of features (BCA-Zero) or through a filter-based approach (BCA-filter), rather than a full set of features, when enough knowledge about the dataset is not provided. Note that although the BCA-Filter approach requires an additional of N (number of attributes) subset evaluations for initialization, the total time needed for initialization is small, as all of these subsets contain only one feature. Moreover, the initialization of the BCA-Filter might improve the convergence rate of the BCA algorithm by starting the search from a subset which is potentially closer to the local optima than the empty set of features is most of sequential search techniques have to be executed completely in order to obtain a sub-optimum point as the best subset of features. As mentioned earlier, our BCA optimization algorithm is an anytime iterative algorithm, i.e., it can be stopped earlier by considering early stopping criteria. Figure 8 illustrates the trend of the objective function (AUC) maximization through the iterations (i.e., the subset candidates) for BCA-Zero and BCA-Filter algorithms for an example case of the FS for the Sonar dataset and SVM classifier. This single case was only selected for the ease of illustration, while curves for all

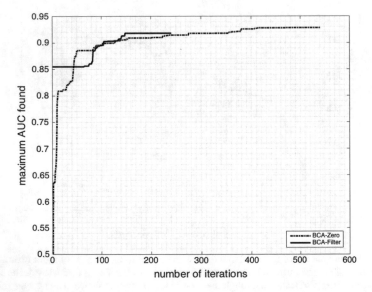

Fig. 8 Optimization trend of the objective AUC function over the number of iterations in our BCA optimization algorithm—The figure shows the trend for the case of the Sonar dataset and the SVM classifier

other BCA-based FS experiments followed the same trend. In this example, for BCA-Zero with a total of 540 iterations, there was almost no significant improvement of the objective function after the 400th iteration; therefore, one might stop the algorithm at this point based on the application needs. The similar case exists for the BCA-Filter as well. Note that the first N (here N is 60) iterations of the BCA-Filter is reserved for initialization, thus, no any-time property at this region. We might also consider this property as one of the limitations of our BCA optimization algorithm. In other words, our BCA algorithm might end up in a local

Table 6 Validation performance comparison of our BCA algorithms with zero and filter-based initializations with the SFS and SFFS FS techniques for five datasets using the SVM, MLP, and NB classifiers

Dataset	BCA-Zero	BCA-Filter	SFS	SFFS
SVM				
Sonar	0.93	0.91	0.93	0.93
Parkinson	0.95	0.95	0.95	0.95
Breast cancer	0.99	0.99	0.99	0.99
Segmentation	0.99	0.99	0.99	0.99
Climate	0.96	0.95	0.95	0.96
Mean $\pm$ SD	0.96 $\pm$ 0.03	0.96 $\pm$ 0.03	0.96 $\pm$ 0.03	0.96 $\pm$ 0.03
Average rank	2.8	2	2.4	2.8
	N_B, N_C, N_D	N_A, N_C, N_D	N_A, N_B, N_D	N_A, N_B, N_C
MLP				
Sonar	0.96	0.96	0.96	0.99
Parkinson	0.99	0.99	0.99	0.99
Breast cancer	0.99	0.99	0.99	0.99
Segmentation	0.99	0.99	0.99	0.99
Climate	0.95	0.97	0.95	0.98
Mean $\pm$ SD	0.98 $\pm$ 0.02	0.98 $\pm$ 0.01	0.98 $\pm$ 0.02	0.99 $\pm$ 0.01
Average rank	2.2	2.5	2.2	3.1
	N_B, N_C, N_D	N_A, N_C, N_D	N_A, N_B, N_D	N_A, N_B, N_C
NB				
Sonar	0.93	0.93	0.92	0.94
Parkinson	0.95	0.95	0.95	0.95
Breast cancer	0.99	0.99	0.99	0.99
Segmentation	0.99	0.99	0.99	0.99
Climate	0.95	0.95	0.95	0.95
Mean $\pm$ SD	0.96 + 0.03	0.96 $\pm$ 0.03	0.96 $\pm$ 0.03	0.96 $\pm$ 0.02
Average rank	2.5	2.5	2.2	2.8
	N_B, N_C, N_D	N_A, N_C, N_D	N_A, N_B, N_D	N_A, N_B, N_C

Note when considering the results for pair-wise statistical analysis, the BCA-Zero, BCA-Filter, SFS and SFFS are assigned letters of A, B, C, and D, respectively. N_B or S_B under the results of method A, indicate that there is no significant or a significant difference between method A and B, respectively

optimum such that there is no way of improving the objective functions even by increasing the number of iterations. In fact, this is a common limitation of most local search methods. This can be studied further for the case of our BCA optimization algorithm by considering techniques that make trade-off between the number of iterations and the objective function results. For the classification application, we showed that even though this limitation exists, the performance results were convincing while significant reductions in the computational complexity were obtained.

In Sect. 3, we investigated the performance of each algorithm based on its AUC obtained on an independent test set, but we did not discuss the results obtained in the 10-fold CV scheme on the validation set through the FS process. Table 6 shows the performance comparison on the validation test. Our exploration indicated that the validation results were also comparable. To confirm that, we performed statistical analysis with the methodology we used earlier. There was no statistically significant difference among our comparisons of the validation AUC results. In fact, we might conclude that our BCA optimization algorithm successfully obtained a local optimum in the space of feature subsets with the objective function value (i.e., the validation AUC) comparable to that of the SFS and SFFS techniques, while reducing the number of iterations substantially. Investigating those validation results, one might notice that although some approaches reached a better AUC on the validation set, the corresponding performance on the independent test set was lower. This is consistent with the study on the performance evaluation of the FS techniques, conducted in [43].

5 Conclusion

We proposed and developed an efficient iterative deterministic local optimization algorithm, namely, binary coordinate ascent (BCA). Our BCA algorithm can be utilized in the optimization frameworks with a binary representation of the input variables and continuous objective function values. To study the efficiency and the performance of our BCA optimization algorithm, we investigated this algorithm for the task of FS in classification applications. To this end, we first represented the space of feature subsets using binary vectors of 0s and 1s. Based on that, we proposed two efficient wrapper-based FS techniques, namely, BCA-Zero and BCA-Filter. The task of our wrapper-based FS approaches was to find the best subset of features in terms of the AUC. We experimented on five publicly available datasets using three classifiers, i.e., the SVM, MLP, and NB, and compared the performance and efficiency results of our proposed algorithms with those of two of the most popular FS techniques, i.e., the SFS and SFFS. The performance analysis demonstrated that the AUC results and the number of selected features for our proposed algorithms were comparable to those of the SFS and SFFS techniques. Investigating the efficiency of the approaches, we demonstrated that with our BCA optimization algorithm, the number of subset evaluations and the processing time of the FS algorithm were reduced substantially, compared with those of the SFS and SFFS techniques. We also performed statistical analysis for all of the experiments and comparisons. Statistical results confirmed that our proposed BCA-based FS algorithms reduced the computational complexity significantly while preserving the performance. In fact, we found that our BCA-based algorithms follow a linear complexity (the number of subset evaluations) with respect to the number of input attributes, whereas the SFS and SFFS techniques follow a quadratic form. Correspondingly, one can use the BCA optimization algorithm as an efficient alternative approach in applications in which efficiency is a requirement, specifically in FS for classification of datasets with a high number of input attributes.

Acknowledgements The authors are grateful to Nima Tajbakhsh, Yisong Chen, Nazanin Makkinejad, Junchi Liu, and other members in the Suzuki Lab for their valuable suggestions and discussions.

References

1. Bache, K., Lichman, M.: UCI Machine Learning Repository. University of California, School of Information and Computer Science, Irvine, CA (2013)
2. Banzhaf, W., Nordin, P., Keller, R., Francone, F.: Genetic Programming: An Introduction. Morgan Kaufmann Publishers, San Francisco (1998)
3. Battiti, R.: Using mutual information for selecting features in supervised neural net learning. IEEE Trans. Neural Netw. **5**, 537–550 (1994). https://doi.org/10.1109/72.298224
4. Bogoni, L., Cathier, P.: Computer-aided detection (CAD) for CT colonography: a tool to address a growing need (2014)
5. Bolón-Canedo, V., Sánchez-Maroño, N., Alonso-Betanzos, A.: A review of feature selection methods on synthetic data. Knowl. Inf. Syst. **34**, 483–519 (2013). https://doi.org/10.1007/s10115-012-0487-8
6. Bonabeau, E., Dorigo, M., Theraulaz, G.: Swarm Intelligence: From Natural to Artificial Systems. Oxford University Press (1999)
7. Böröczky, L., Zhao, L., Lee, K.P.: Feature subset selection for improving the performance of false positive reduction in lung nodule CAD. IEEE Trans. Inf. Technol. Biomed. **10**, 504–511 (2006). https://doi.org/10.1109/TITB.2006.872063
8. Campadelli, P., Casiraghi, E., Artioli, D.: A fully automated method for lung nodule detection from postero-anterior chest radiographs. IEEE Trans. Med. Imaging **25**, 1588–1603 (2006). https://doi.org/10.1109/TMI.2006.884198
9. Canul-Reich, J., Hall, L.O., Goldgof, D., Eschrich, S.A.: Feature selection for microarray data by AUC analysis. In: IEEE International Conference on Systems, Man, and Cybernetics 2008 (SMC 2008), pp. 768–773. https://doi.org/10.1109/ICSMC.2008.4811371
10. Cavazzuti, M.: Optimization Methods: From Theory to Scientific Design and Technological Aspects in Mechanics. Springer Science & Business Media (2012)
11. Chandrashekar, G., Sahin, F.: A survey on feature selection methods. Comput. Electr. Eng. **40**, 16–28 (2014). https://doi.org/10.1016/j.compeleceng.2013.11.024
12. Chang, C., Lin, C.: LIBSVM: a library for support vector machines. ACM Trans. Intell. Syst. Technol. **2**, 27 (2011)
13. Chen, S., Suzuki, K., MacMahon, H.: Development and evaluation of a computer-aided diagnostic scheme for lung nodule detection in chest radiographs by means of two-stage nodule enhancement with support vector classification. Med. Phys. **38**, 1844–1858 (2011). https://doi.org/10.1118/1.3561504

14. Cortes, C., Vapnik, V.: Support-vector networks. Chem. Biol. Drug Des. **297**, 273–297 (2009). https://doi.org/10.1111/j.1747-0285.2009.00840.x
15. Dash, M., Liu, H.: Feature selection for classification. Sience **1**, 131–156 (1997)
16. Debuse, J.C.W., Smith, V.J.R.: Feature subset selection within a simulated annealing data mining algorithm. J. Intell. Inf. Syst. **9**, 57–81 (1997)
17. Demšar, J.: Statistical comparisons of classifiers over multiple data sets. J. Mach. Learn. Res. **7**, 1–30 (2006). https://doi.org/10.1016/j.jecp.2010.03.005
18. Devijver, P., Kittler, J.: Pattern Recognition: A Statistical Approach. Prentice Hall (1982)
19. Fawcett, T.: An introduction to ROC analysis. Pattern Recognit. Lett. **27**, 861–874 (2006)
20. Garcia, S., Herrera, F.: An extension on "statistical comparisons of classifiers over multiple data sets" for all pairwise comparisons. J. Mach. Learn. Res. **9**, 2677–2694 (2008)
21. Graña, M., Termenon, M., Savio, A.: Computer aided diagnosis system for Alzheimer disease using brain diffusion tensor imaging features selected by Pearson's correlation. Neurosci. Lett. **502**, 225–229 (2011)
22. Guyon, I., Elisseeff, A.: An introduction to variable and feature selection. J. Mach. Learn. Res. **3**, 1157–1182 (2003). https://doi.org/10.1023/A:1012487302797
23. Hall, M., Frank, E., Holmes, G.: The WEKA data mining software: an update. ACM SIGKDD Explor. Newsl. **11**, 10–18 (2009)
24. Haykin, S.: Neural Networks: A Comprehensive Foundation, 2nd edn. Prentice Hall (1998)
25. Hsieh, C.-J., Chang, K.-W., Lin, C.-J., et al.: A dual coordinate descent method for large-scale linear SVM. In: Proceedings of the 25th International Conference on Machine Learning—ICML'08, pp. 408–415. https://doi.org/10.1145/1390156.1390208
26. Huang, P.-W., Lee, C.-H.: Automatic classification for pathological prostate images based on fractal analysis. IEEE Trans. Med. Imaging **28**, 1037–1050 (2009). https://doi.org/10.1109/TMI.2009.2012704
27. Hupse, R., Karssemeijer, N.: The effect of feature selection methods on computer-aided detection of masses in mammograms. Phys. Med. Biol. **55**, 2893 (2010)
28. Kennedy, J., Eberhart, R.: Particle swarm optimization. In: Proceedings of IEEE International Conference on Neural networks, vol. 4, pp. 1942–1948 (1995). https://doi.org/10.1109/ICNN.1995.488968
29. Kohavi, R., Kohavi, R.: Wrappers for feature subset selection. Artif. Intell. **97**, 273–324 (1997). https://doi.org/10.1016/S0004-3702(97)00043-X
30. Lazar, C., Taminau, J., Meganck, S., et al.: A survey on filter techniques for feature selection in gene expression microarray analysis. IEEE/ACM Trans. Comput. Biol. Bioinform. **9**, 1106–1119 (2012). https://doi.org/10.1109/TCBB.2012.33
31. Lee, M., Boroczky, L., Sungur-Stasik, K.: Computer-aided diagnosis of pulmonary nodules using a two-step approach for feature selection and classifier ensemble construction. Artif. Intell. Med. **50**, 43–53 (2010)
32. Lin, S.-W., Lee, Z.-J., Chen, S.-C., Tseng, T.-Y.: Parameter determination of support vector machine and feature selection using simulated annealing approach. Appl. Soft Comput. **8**, 1505–1512 (2008). https://doi.org/10.1016/j.asoc.2007.10.012
33. Liu, H., Motoda, H.: Feature Selection for Knowledge Discovery and Data Mining. Springer Science & Business Media (2012)
34. Liu, H., Yu, L., Member, S.S., et al.: Toward integrating feature selection algorithms for classification and clustering. Knowl. Data Eng. IEEE Trans. **17**, 491–502 (2005). https://doi.org/10.1109/TKDE.2005.66
35. Luo, Z.Q., Tseng, P.: On the convergence of the coordinate descent method for convex differentiable minimization. J. Optim. Theor. Appl. **72**, 7–35 (1992). https://doi.org/10.1007/BF00939948
36. Maggio, S., Palladini, A., De Marchi, M., et al.: Predictive deconvolution and hybrid feature selection for computer-aided detection of prostate cancer. IEEE Trans. Med. Imaging **29**, 455–464 (2010). https://doi.org/10.1109/TMI.2009.2034517

37. Marrocco, C., Duin, R.P.W., Tortorella, F.: Maximizing the area under the ROC curve by pairwise feature combination. Pattern Recognit. **41**, 1961–1974 (2008). https://doi.org/10.1016/j.patcog.2007.11.017
38. Meiri, R., Zahavi, J.: Using simulated annealing to optimize the feature selection problem in marketing applications. Eur. J. Oper. Res. **171**, 842–858 (2006). https://doi.org/10.1016/j.ejor.2004.09.010
39. Mohamed, S.S., Salama, M.M.A.: Prostate cancer spectral multifeature analysis using TRUS images. IEEE Trans. Med. Imaging **27**, 548–556 (2008). https://doi.org/10.1109/TMI.2007.911547
40. Newell, D., Nie, K., Chen, J., Hsu, C.: Selection of diagnostic features on breast MRI to differentiate between malignant and benign lesions using computer-aided diagnosis: differences in lesions. Eur. Radiol. **20**, 771–781 (2010)
41. Pudil, P., Novovičová, J., Kittler, J.: Floating search methods in feature selection. Pattern Recognit. Lett. **15**, 1119–1125 (1994). https://doi.org/10.1016/0167-8655(94)90127-9
42. Quinlan, J.R.: Induction of decision trees. Mach. Learn. **1**, 81–106 (1986). https://doi.org/10.1007/BF00116251
43. Reunanen, J.: Overfitting in making comparisons between variable selection methods. J. Mach. Learn. Res. **3**, 1371–1382 (2003). https://doi.org/10.1162/153244303322753715
44. Sahiner, B., Petrick, N., Chan, H.P., et al.: Computer-aided characterization of mammographic masses: accuracy of mass segmentation and its effects on characterization. IEEE Trans. Med. Imaging **20**, 1275–1284 (2001). https://doi.org/10.1109/42.974922
45. Somol, P., Novovicová, J., Pudil, P.: Efficient feature subset selection and subset size optimization. Pattern Recognit. Recent Adv. 1–24 (2010). https://doi.org/10.5772/9356
46. Suzuki, K.: Machine Learning in Computer-Aided Diagnosis: Medical Imaging Intelligence and Analysis. IGI Global, Hershey, PA (2012)
47. Suzuki, K.: A review of computer-aided diagnosis in thoracic and colonic imaging. Quant. Imaging Med. Surg. **2**, 163–176 (2012)
48. Suzuki, K.: Machine learning in computer-aided diagnosis of the thorax and colon in CT: a survey. IEICE Trans. Inf. Syst. **96**, 772–783 (2013)
49. Suzuki, K., Zarshenas, M., Liu, J., et al.: Development of computer-aided diagnostic (CADx) system for distinguishing neoplastic from nonneoplastic lesions in CT Colonography (CTC): toward CTC beyond detection. In: 2015 IEEE International Conference on Systems, Man, and Cybernetics, pp. 2262–2266. IEEE (2015)
50. Takemura, A., Shimizu, A., Hamamoto, K.: Discrimination of breast tumors in ultrasonic images using an ensemble classifier based on the Adaboost algorithm with feature selection. IEEE Trans. Med. Imaging **29**, 598–609 (2010). https://doi.org/10.1109/TMI.2009.2022630
51. Tang, J., Alelyani, S., Liu, H.: Feature selection for classification: a review. Data Classif. Algorithm. Appl. 37–64 (2014). https://doi.org/10.1.1.409.5195
52. Vafaie, H., Imam, IIF.: Feature Selection Methods : Genetic Algorithms vs. Greedy-like Search (1994)
53. Wang, R., Tang, K.: Feature selection for maximizing the area under the ROC curve. In: 2009 IEEE International Conf Data Min Work, pp. 400–405. https://doi.org/10.1109/ICDMW.2009.25
54. Xu, J., Suzuki, K.: Max-AUC feature selection in computer-aided detection of polyps in CT colonography. Biomed. Heal. Inform. IEEE J. **18**, 585–593 (2014)
55. Zarshenas, A., Suzuki, K.: Binary coordinate ascent: an efficient optimization technique for feature subset selection for machine learning. Knowl.-Based Syst. **110**, 191–201 (2016). https://doi.org/10.1016/j.knosys.2016.07.026
56. Zhang, H.: The optimality of Naive Bayes. In: Proceedings of the Seventeenth International Florida Artificial Intelligence Research Society Conference (FLAIRS 2004), vol. 1, pp. 1–6 (2004). https://doi.org/10.1016/j.patrec.2005.12.001
57. Zhu, J., Rosset, S., Hastie, T., Tibshirani, R.: 1-norm Support Vector Machines. Nips, pp. 49–56 (2003)

Part II
Computer-Aided Detection

Automated Lung Nodule Detection Using Positron Emission Tomography/Computed Tomography

Atsushi Teramoto and Hiroshi Fujita

Abstract Lung cancer is a leading cause of death in human globally. Owing to the low survival rates among lung cancer patients, it is essential to detect and treat cancer at an early stage. In some countries, positron emission tomography (PET)/ X-ray computed tomography (CT) examination is also used for the cancer screening in addition to diagnosis and follow-up of treatment. PET/CT images provide both anatomical and functional information of the lung cancer. However, radiologists must examine a large number of these images and therefore, support tools for the localization of lung nodule are desired. This chapter highlights our recent contributions to a hybrid detection scheme of lung nodules in PET/CT images. In the CT image, a massive region is first detected using a cylindrical nodule enhancement filter (CNEF), which is a cylindrical kernel shaped by contrast enhancement filter. Subsequently, high-uptake regions detected by the PET images are merged with the region detected by the CT image. False positives (FPs) among the leading candidates are eliminated by a rule-based classifier and three support vector machines based on the characteristic features obtained from CT and PET images. Experimentally, the detection capability was evaluated using 100 cases of PET/CT images. As a result, the sensitivity in detecting candidates was 83%, with 5 FPs/case. These results indicate that the proposed hybrid method may be useful for the computer-aided detection of lung cancer in clinical practice.

A. Teramoto (✉)
Faculty of Radiological Technology, School of Health Sciences, Fujita Health University, Toyoake, Japan
e-mail: teramoto@fujita-hu.ac.jp

H. Fujita
Department of Intelligent Image Information, Division of Regeneration and Advanced Medical Sciences, Graduate School of Medicine, Gifu University, Gifu, Japan
e-mail: fujita@fjt.info.gifu-u.ac.jp

© Springer International Publishing AG 2018
K. Suzuki and Y. Chen (eds.), *Artificial Intelligence in Decision Support Systems for Diagnosis in Medical Imaging*, Intelligent Systems Reference Library 140, https://doi.org/10.1007/978-3-319-68843-5_4

1 Introduction

Statistically, in the United States, 210828 people were diagnosed with lung cancer, out of which 157423 people died in 2012 [1]. Currently, lung cancer is the leading cause of death among mankind in the United States, Europe, and many Asian countries [2]. Owing to the low survival rates among lung cancer patients, early stage detection and treatment are necessary. Conventional radiography has long been used to screen for lung cancer. However, small pulmonary nodules may remain undetected by this method because the bone and mediastinum obscure the nodules [3]. Computed tomography (CT) is also used for lung cancer screening [4]. According to the results of a national lung screening trial [5], low-dose CT scan-based screening reduces deaths by 20%, and thus is regarded as a suitable diagnostic tool for early detection of lung cancer.

Recently, in some Asian countries such as Korea and Japan, positron emission tomography (PET)/CT has also been adopted as a mass screening tool for diagnosis of cancers [6, 7]. In this combined technique, PET images provide functional information while CT images render anatomical information, making it possible to detect small pulmonary nodules with high glucose metabolism. Wever et al. have recently reported the clinical effectivity of PET/CT in detection and characterization [8]. It can be used to detect malignancy in lung nodules, and nodules at the hilum pulmonis that are difficult to identify by CT alone. Therefore, PET/CT examination can be widely used for screening in near future.

Although PET/CT is a powerful diagnostic tool for cancer, it has a primary disadvantage: it generates about 1000 slice images per scan. Since most cancer screening cases are normal, radiologists must identify a small number of abnormal lesions from a large number of images without any oversight. This can be cumbersome along with concern regarding the deterioration of diagnostic accuracy or fluctuation of results.

Here, Computer-aided detection (CADe) provides a digital output as a "second opinion" to support a radiologist's diagnosis and assist in evaluating a large number of images to identify lesions and arrive at the diagnosis. In this study, we focused on the automated detection of lung tumors, such as nodules, by using PET/CT images.

1.1 Related Works

Several researchers have developed CADe methods to detect lung nodules for CT [9–19], PET [20–22], and PET/CT [23–25]. Lee et al. proposed a method for detecting lung nodules using CT images alone based on genetic algorithms and template matching [9]. Suzuki et al. proposed the false positive reduction method for pulmonary nodule detection using massive training artificial neural network [10]. Messay et al. developed a nodule detection method that incorporates a two-dimensional local contrast enhancement filter and more than 40 characteristic features [14]. Arnaud reported the automatic detection of the major pulmonary nodules using thresholding and morphological operations [16]. Han et al. proposed fast and adaptive detection of pulmonary nodules using a hierarchical vector quantization scheme [17]. Wang et al. reviewed the imaging technique for lung diseases and automated detection systems [18]. We also have developed a fast detection method for pulmonary nodules using CNEF [19]. During the process, we found that our method was 4 to 36 times faster than the existing methods with the same or even better detection capabilities and it was equivalent to or faster than the image acquisition speed of a CT scanner. Similarly, several automated detection methods for high-uptake regions in whole-body PET images have been proposed [20–22]. Guan et al. developed an automated detection method for high uptake regions based on competition-diffusion segmentation and mode-seeking region-growing algorithms [20]. Montgomery et al. developed a method for the automated analysis of tumors using wavelet transform and statistical methods [21]. Hara et al. proposed an automated scoring system for PET scans by using a database of the distribution of the means and standard deviations of standardized uptake values (SUVs) [22]. As for automated detection schemes using PET/CT images, Cui et al. and Balangan et al. have independently proposed different automated detection schemes for lung tumors in PET images in which the lung regions were CT imaged [23, 24]. Song et al. studied the lesion detection and characterization in the lung PET/CT images by using context driven approximation; out of 158 hot-spot lesions, 157 were detected [25]. The previous methods described in the above studies detect the pulmonary nodules from CT [9–19] or PET [20–25] images alone. However, in current clinical settings, radiologists identify nodules using both PET and CT images. Therefore, CAD is enhanced when using PET/CT images to detect nodules.

1.2 Objectives

We have proposed an automated detection scheme for lung nodules using both CT and PET images. The main goal of the method is to develop a basic approach for automated detection of both malignant and benign nodules. In our recent studies, the sensitivity of the combined method was favorable compared to those obtained by independent methods using CT or PET alone [26–28]. This chapter describes the CADe scheme of lung nodules to introduce hybrid nodule detection and false positive (FP) reduction with three classifiers and assesses the detection performance on screening PET/CT images.

2 Methods

2.1 Method Overview

The summary of the method developed for lung nodule detection in PET/CT images is shown in Fig. 1. The nodule candidate regions were first detected distinctly from the given PET and CT images using specific features of each image. Subsequently, the final candidate regions were identified by the combination of the two detections followed by FP reduction.

2.2 Nodule Detection Using CT Images

Solitary nodules, including ground glass opacity (GGO), were detected in the lung region on CT images by the main procedure shown in Fig. 2, involving the following steps: segmentation of the lung region, nodule enhancement, and nodule segmentation.

2.2.1 Lung Segmentation

The first process of our CADe scheme involves automatic segmentation of the lung region from CT images in order to prevent FPs outside this region. We introduced three major conventional steps as follows: (1) extraction of an initial lung region by using thresholding based on the Hounsfield value (cut-off = − 400), (2) removal of invalid voxels outside the lung region, and (3) filling the lack of blood vessels and lung nodules using the mathematical morphology operation. Figure 3 shows images of each step in the lung segmentation.

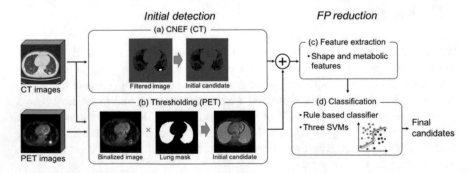

Fig. 1 Outline of the proposed detection method

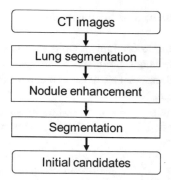

Fig. 2 Flowchart of nodule detection in CT images

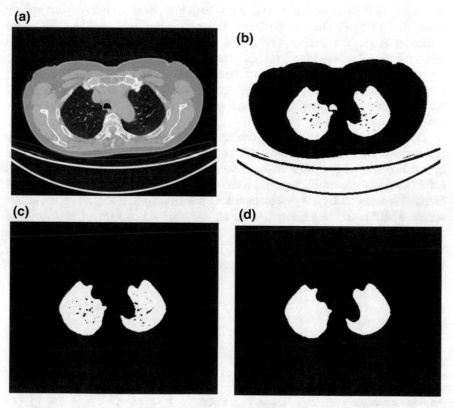

Fig. 3 Steps in the lung region segmentation. **a** Original image, **b** image after thresholding has been applied (cut-off = − 400), **c** image after removal of pixels outside the lung, and **d** final output (white pixels) of the lung region segmentation after performing mathematical morphology filter

2.2.2 Nodule Enhancement and Segmentation

This is the essential technique for lung nodule detection. However, 3D enhancement encompasses a significant number of the total calculations in the CAD scheme. Hence, we developed a fast enhancement method named as cylindrical nodule-enhancement filter (CNEF).

The CNEF has a cylindrical shape of radius r_1 and height $2r_1$ (Fig. 4). The output of the filter is calculated by the following equations,

$$c(x,y,z) = f(x,y,z) - \max_{(x_c,y_c,z_c \in K_{CNEF})} \left\{ f(x-x_c, y-y_c, z-z_c) \left| \begin{array}{ll} x_c^2 + y_c^2 \leq r_1^2 & and \quad z_c = \pm r_1 \\ x_c^2 + y_c^2 = r_1^2 & and \quad -r_1 < z_c < r_1 \end{array} \right. \right\}$$

(1)

where $f(x,y,z)$ is the input image, $c(x,y,z)$ is the output image, and K_{CNEF} is the filter kernel of the CNEF. The CNEF represents the difference between the value of the center voxel and the maximum value on the cylinder surface (sidewall, top and bottom lids). When the blood vessels penetrate the filter, the values of these two regions are identical, and the output of the filter decreases. In contrast, when there is an isolated nodule within the cylinder, only the center voxel has a high value and the output of the filter increases. Thus, the CNEF enhances the nodule selectively based on the object shape.

The cylindrical surface of CNEF can be divided into a sidewall and two lids (top and bottom). Here, the maximum value on the cylinder sidewall is equivalent to the maximum value on the circle whose radius is r_1 in a maximum intensity projection (MIP) image of slab width $2r_1$. This means that the 3D calculation for the cylinder sidewall is replaced by 2D processing using a MIP image. It should be noted that only one MIP processing is required for all the voxels in one slice. The outputs of two lids are equal to the output of the morphological filter [19] with a maximum value in the circle of radius r_1 at $z = \pm r_1$. The largest of the maximum values of the cylinder sidewall and lids is the final output of the cylinder. Therefore, the

Fig. 4 The structure of the cylindrical filter. The filter outputs the difference between the value of the pixel at the center of the cylinder around (x, y, z), $f(x, y,z)$, and the maximum pixel value on the cylinder surface

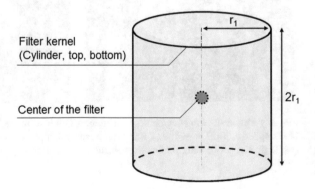

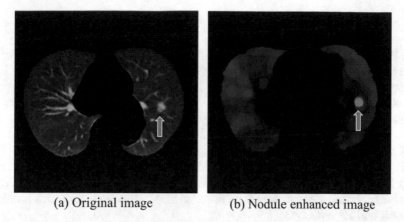

(a) Original image   (b) Nodule enhanced image

Fig. 5 Nodule enhancement with the CNEF. The arrows indicate the detected nodules

CNEF uses only three 2D images, thereby significantly reducing the number of calculations.

CNEF enhances the nodules when the size is less than that of the filter. However, if the filter size is much larger than that of the nodule, the output of CNEF may decrease because the filter kernel contacts with lung structures such as bronchus, blood vessels, and lung wall. Therefore, several filters with varied diameters (ex. diameter = 10, 20, 30 mm) are applied to each voxel; the highest filter output is automatically adopted as the final output.

The original and processed images obtained using CNEF are shown in Fig. 5. The nodule appears to have a high CT value (Fig. 4a), equivalent to those of the blood vessels. In the enhanced result (Fig. 4b), the blood vessels are suppressed, but the nodules have a selectively high CT value. Subsequent to enhanced images, the initial nodule regions are segmented by thresholding and labeling.

The advantage of this method is the detection speed. The detection performance and time of CNEF were evaluated using images from the lung image database consortium (LIDC) [29]. Sensitivity was 80% with the number of FPs/case at 4.2 and detection speed was 25–34 s per case. The detection performance of CNEF was either the same or superior to the existing methods while the time was 4–36 fold faster.

2.3   Nodule Detection in PET Images

The PET scanner produces images of the 3D distribution of systemic uptake of the intravenous radioactive tracer 2-deoxy-2-(18F) fluoro-D-glucose (FDG). High FDG uptake indicates that increased glucose metabolism, which has been proven to correlate to tumor malignancy [30–32]. Thus, this feature can be used for the characterization of tumors. However, high uptake is also observed in organs that have intrinsically high glucose metabolism (i.e., physiological uptake). CAD methods must account for FPs in PET images from the physiologic uptake of FDG.

In the present study, high-uptake regions in the chest were detected automatically as candidates on PET images. Our novel detection algorithm, shown in Fig. 6, involved following steps: transformation to SUV, detection of initial candidate regions, and FP reduction.

2.3.1   SUV Transformation

Tissue radioactivity concentration (in kBq/mL) is available from PET images, but the measurement varies with the injected dose and patient's weight. Therefore, the standardized uptake value (SUV) is calculated for each image as the ratio of measured activity to injected dose/patient body weight [33].

$$SUV = \frac{Measured\ activity[Bq/mL]}{Injected\ dose[Bq]/patient's\ weight[g]} \qquad (2)$$

2.3.2   Detection of Initial Candidates

The SUV is a semi-quantitative criterion. High SUV suggests malignancy. In the lung region, an area with maximum SUV $\geq$ 2.5 is generally suspected as

Fig. 6 Flowchart of nodule detection in PET images

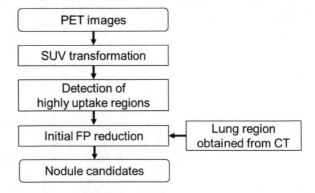

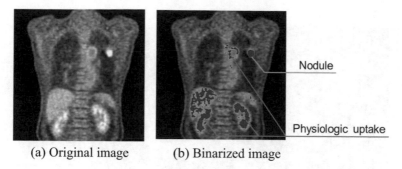

(a) Original image   (b) Binarized image

Fig. 7 Initial nodule detection in PET images. Regions with an SUV >2.0 are indicated in red [28]

malignancy [34]. Here, for initial detection of candidate nodules, thresholding and labeling were performed with SUV threshold = 2.0 to obtain a stable region with SUV $\geq$ 2.5. Figure 7 shows a result of initial nodule detection in PET images. The nodule in the left lung was detected by thresholding. However, the physiologic uptake in the myocardium, liver, and kidneys is initially mistaken for high uptake regions.

2.3.3 Initial FP Reduction

The high-uptake regions inside the lungs can be exclusively detected after extracting the lung regions, and the FPs due to physiological uptake outside the lungs are avoided. The precise extraction of the lung regions from the PET images is very difficult, even after consideration of breathing-induced transformation, because of the incomplete anatomical information provided by PET scanning. To address this, we introduced the lung regions obtained by the CT images described in the previous section. However, the size of the lungs varies depending on the degree of breathing and should be considered to avoid misdetection especially around the border of the lung. A study reports that the deviation of the position between PET and CT images was approximately 7.5 mm [35]. Therefore, the lung region in PET images was determined by performing the procedure where a dilation of 8 mm (2 pixels in the PET image) was applied to the primary lung region detected by CT images. In all the cases of PET/CT images, there were no missed nodules resulting from elimination by lung segmentation using the PET images.

High-uptake regions observed in the cardiac, and hepatic regions outside the lungs (green color) were thus eliminated (Fig. 8), leaving the single initial candidate (red color) in the left lung, which was identified as a true finding.

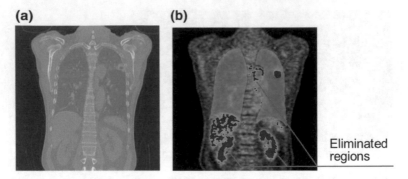

Fig. 8 Reduction of FP outside the lung. Lung regions were isolated by CT (**a**) and FP reduction was thus achieved (**b**) [28]

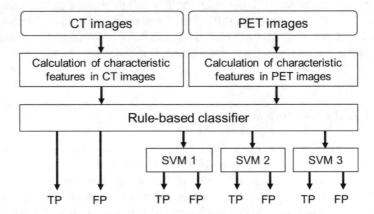

Fig. 9 FP reduction scheme using the rule-based classifier and three SVMs

2.4 Integration and False Positive Reduction

Initial candidate regions detected by CT and PET are represented as binary images, and combined by logic OR, followed by individual pixel examination. The region detected by at least one modality is treated as a nodule. Although improvement of sensitivity by combining the two modalities was expected, the increase of FPs was a challenge at the same time. There were approximately 50 FPs per case in the initial combined candidates. Therefore, FP reduction was performed using multiple characteristic features and multi-step classifiers including a rule-based classifier and three support vector machines (SVMs) [36]. The flow chart of this FP reduction method is shown in Fig. 9.

2.4.1 Calculation of Characteristic Features

For each candidate region, eight types of characteristic features are calculated using CT and PET images as follows.

(i) *Sectional area (X–Y, X–Z, and Y–Z planes)*

Cross-sectional areas are expressed as the number of pixels at the center of the nodule candidate in the X–Y, X–Z, and Y–Z planes.

(ii) *Volume*

The product of the total number of voxels inside the nodule candidate and volume of the voxel is defined as the *volume*.

(iii) *Surface area*

The contour of the nodule candidate is determined in all its slices; the product of the total number of contour voxels and area of a single plane of the voxel is defined as the *surface area*.

(iv) *CT value* (CT image only)

The CT values (max, center, standard deviation) in the nodule candidate in CT images are calculated.

(v) *SUV* (PET image only)

The SUVs (max, center, mean) in the nodule candidate in PET images are computed.

(vi) *Convergence* (CT image only)

Convergence is the characteristic value calculated from CT images to evaluate the concentration of voxel values as shown in Fig. 10. The change in CT value of each point in the original image F in the x, y and z directions was calculated as the gradient vector $\vec{G}$.

$$\vec{G} = (G_x, G_y, G_z) \tag{3}$$

$$G_x = \frac{dF}{dx}, \ G_y = \frac{dF}{dy}, \ G_z = \frac{dF}{dz} \tag{4}$$

Consequently, the inner product of the gradient vector in voxel value and the vector to the nodule center at each voxel is calculated. The summation of such inner products is then defined as the *convergence*.

$$convergence = \sum_{R} \vec{G} \cdot \vec{C} \tag{5}$$

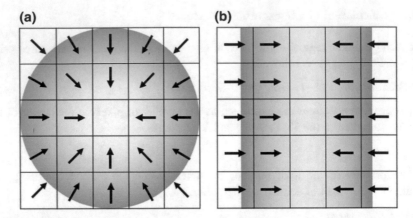

Fig. 10 Illustration of the concentration of gradient vectors in **a** massive object such as nodule and **b** line object such as blood vessel

$\vec{C}$ Vector to the nodule center at each voxel.

R Euclidean space

(vii)   *Diameter* (CT image only)

When the diameters of the nodule and blood vessel are compared in the same volume, the former has a larger value. Thus, we introduced the diameter as a characteristic shape feature. It is calculated in 3D; the minimum length of the segment, which intersects the center of a nodule candidate and has endpoints on the surface, is defined as the *diameter*.

(viii)   *Overlapping area* (CT image only)

Blood vessels exist throughout the lung region. However, nodules are usually isolated. To enhance this feature, a fixed sphere with a 30 mm diameter, is placed at the center of a nodule candidate. The ratio of the number of voxels that overlap the spherical surface and the nodule candidate and the number of voxels of the spherical surface is counted as the *overlapping area* from CT images (Fig. 11).

2.4.2   Rule-Based Classifier

Characteristic values for each nodule candidate are calculated and specified to the rule-based classifier. Obvious FPs and true positives (TPs) that can be easily classified using only one characteristic feature are identified. In general, the trouble-shooting by the SVM is simplified by eliminating the obvious false and true positives, which results in the improvement of classification performance.

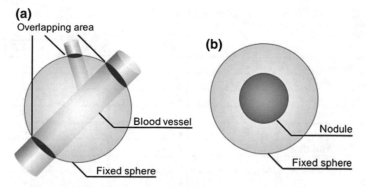

Fig. 11 Illustration for determining the overlapping area. **a** The blood vessel has a continuous structure and overlaps the fixed sphere. **b** The nodule is isolated and hence, no overlap occurs

2.4.3 SVM Classifiers

The remaining candidates were divided into three categories: (1) nodules detected in CT images, (2) nodules detected in PET images, and (3) nodules detected by both modalities. Types of characteristic features for FP reduction depended on the above categories. For example, a nodule candidate obtained by CT images alone cannot be reproduced from the PET images because of the absence of similar high-uptake segmented regions. Therefore, we introduced the three SVMs (SVM 1–3) to correspond to each category. Each SVM classifies candidates into TP and FP based on the given characteristic values.

Suitable characteristic features were granted for each SVM, as listed in Table 1. SVM 1 and SVM 2 employed characteristic features of SUV and CT values derived from undetected images, respectively. These simple features can be obtained if the center co-ordinates of the detected regions are known. Finally, candidate regions are achieved by merging the output of the three SVMs.

3 Experiments

3.1 Materials

In order to evaluate the detection ability of our scheme, 100 PET/CT images were collected. Images were acquired during a cancer-screening program at the East Nagoya Imaging Diagnosis Center (Nagoya, Japan) using a Siemens True Point Biograph 40 PET/CT scanner (Siemens). PET images with a matrix size of 168×168 pixels (voxel size, $4.0 \times 4.0 \times 2.0$ mm^3) were obtained with free breathing and CT images with a matrix size of 512×512 pixels and a voxel size of $0.97 \times 0.97 \times 2.0$ mm^3 were achieved during expiration breath-hold. These PET and CT images were aligned automatically by the PET/CT scanner.

Table 1 Characteristic features are given to the three SVMs

Characteristic features	Selected features		
	SVM 1	SVM 2	SVM 3
Features obtained from CT images			
Sectional Area (X-Y, Y-Z, X-Z plane)	✓		✓
Surface area	✓		✓
Volume	✓		✓
CT value (center, max)	✓	✓	✓
CT value (standard deviation)	✓		✓
Convergence	✓		✓
Diameter	✓		✓
Overlapping area	✓		✓
Feature obtained from PET images			
Sectional Area (X-Y, Y-Z, X-Z plane)		✓	✓
Volume		✓	✓
Surface area		✓	✓
SUV (center, max)	✓	✓	✓
SUV (mean)		✓	✓

The dataset included 79 abnormal scans with pulmonary nodules and 21 normal scans. The abnormality was defined based on either one or two modalities. Among the 79 abnormal scans, 186 nodules were detected by radiologist's standard interpretations for clinical cancer screenings. Figure 12 shows histograms of the diameters (a) and CT values (b) of nodules included from the images. The diameters of the nodules were manually measured by in-house software. The average diameter and CT value were 18 mm and 13 Hounsfield unit, respectively. This study was approved by our institutional review board, and the patient agreement was based on the assumption that all data were anonymized.

3.2   Evaluation Methods

Among 100 cases, 50 were randomly selected as the training dataset, comprising a total of 91 nodules, for the optimization of parameters for nodule detection. For an objective evaluation of the efficacy of our method for unseen cases, 50 additional PET/CT images with 95 nodules were evaluated. Regarding detection parameters for CT examinations, CNEF radius and the threshold for nodule detection were set at 15 mm and 75 mm, respectively. For the PET examinations, the cut-off value for detection and feature extraction was set as SUV = 2.0. The rule-based classifier used for FP reduction was designed according to the following conditions using the training dataset:

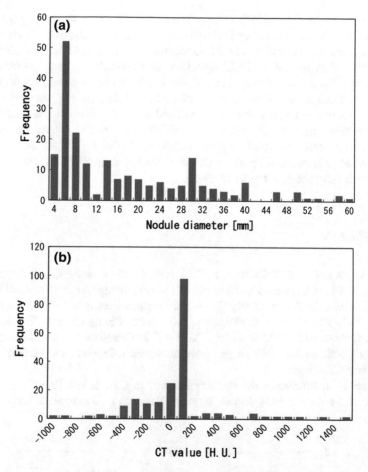

Fig. 12 Histograms of nodule diameters **a** and CT values **b** in the dataset

(a) In PET detection, candidates with SUV > 10.0 were judged as TP.
(b) In CT detection, candidates whose vector concentration value was < 0.4 were judged as FPs.
(c) In CT detection, candidates whose volume was <25 mm^3 were judged as FPs.

During this evaluation, different pairs of sensitivity and the number of FPs per case were calculated by changing the parameters (cost, gamma, and weight) for SVM, and thus the FROC (Free-response Receiver Operating Curve) was obtained. Here, sensitivity was defined as the ratio of the number of detected true nodules to the number of true nodules in the database and is expressed as a percentage. Furthermore, FROCs for CT or PET detection alone were obtained for comparing with the combined detection. The FP reduction in these detections was carried out similarly as that for the PET/CT detection, using single images. Therefore, the number of characteristic values obtained was restricted. We used one SVM, and the number of characteristic features was smaller than the number of features listed in Table 1. About 6–9 types of features calculated in the candidate regions for CT and PET detection, respectively, and a single SVM classified the candidates into TPs and FPs using these features. In order to reduce the FP for the SVMs, we introduced the LibSVM [37] and C-support vector classification as an SVM algorithm and the radial basis function as a kernel function.

3.3 Results

Figure 13 shows the FROCs for CT, PET, and combined detection. Many modern CAD systems for lung nodules have been evaluated using sensitivity with FPs/case of ~5.0. Similarly, the sensitivity for detecting nodules using only CT images in the present study was 67.0% with FP/case = 5.0. By combining CT and PET detection, sensitivity increased to 83.0% with FP/case = 5.0. Therefore, the sensitive nature of our hybrid scheme was 16% greater than that of the independent detection systems using only CT images.

Figure 14 demonstrates the nodules detected in CT images. Sample 1 shows a GGO that would not have shown high uptake on PET. Sample 2 indicates the

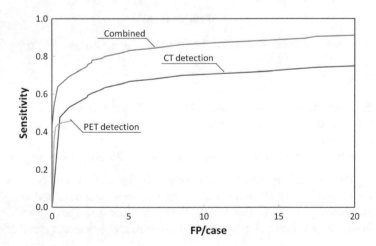

Fig. 13 FROC curves for CT, PET, and combined detection algorithms

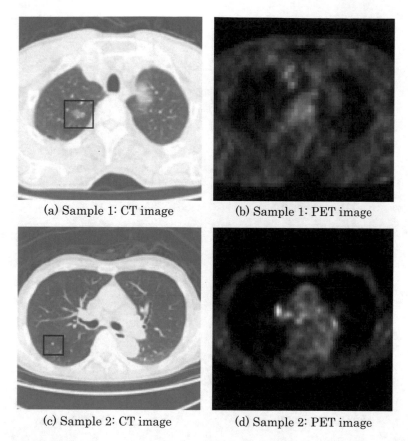

(a) Sample 1: CT image   (b) Sample 1: PET image

(c) Sample 2: CT image   (d) Sample 2: PET image

Fig. 14 Nodule detected by CT images. The boxes indicate the nodules detected by the proposed CAD algorithm [28]

detection of a calcified granuloma without metabolic activity. Figure 15 shows examples of nodules detected by the PET algorithms. When the nodule size increases, it is likely to merge with blood vessels, lung wall, and mediastinum. These types of nodules are difficult to detect in CT images using the detection algorithm for solitary nodules. Furthermore, significant increases in uptake can be accurately detected by PET. A nodule detected by both PET and CT images is shown in Fig. 16.

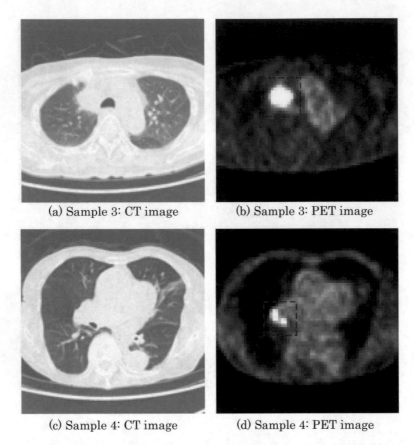

(a) Sample 3: CT image   (b) Sample 3: PET image

(c) Sample 4: CT image   (d) Sample 4: PET image

Fig. 15 Nodule detected by PET images. Dashed boxes indicate the nodules detected by the proposed CAD algorithm [28]

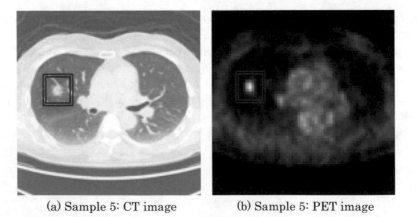

(a) Sample 5: CT image   (b) Sample 5: PET image

Fig. 16 Nodule detected by CT and PET images. Double lined boxes indicate the nodules detected by the proposed CAD method [28]

4 Discussions

Because the CAD system integrates the detection abilities of two different types of imaging modalities, the sensitivity of our hybrid scheme is higher than that of the independent detection systems using either CT or PET. The Venn diagram of the nodules detected by both CT and PET with a sensitivity of 83.0% and FPs/case = 5.0 is shown in Fig. 17. As seen in the figure, 27.4% of the nodules were detected by both CT and PET while 40.0% and 15.8% of the nodules were detected by CT and PET alone, respectively. These results indicated that the combination of CT and PET yields equivalent results.

On the other hand, out of 95 nodules present, 16 were not detected by the proposed methods. These undetected nodules are shown in Fig. 18. Most of the undetected nodules were GGOs that merged or overlapped with blood vessels or bronchi.

The detection capabilities of the proposed algorithms were dependent on the nodule size and contrast (visibility). In order to analyze the characteristics of the proposed method, we investigated the relationship between CT values of the nodules and sensitivity, as well as nodule diameter (D_n) and sensitivity.

Table 2 shows the relationship between D_n and sensitivity. Here, all the nodules in the evaluation dataset were classified into 3 categories based on their diameter: <10 mm, 10–30 mm, and > 30 mm. We observed that most nodules with diameters <10 mm were detected using CT images. These were not detectable by PET since the SUV of small nodules was decreased as a result of the partial volume effect. On the other hand, 91.3% of the nodules with a diameter of more than 30 mm were detected using PET images. CT detection performance decreased

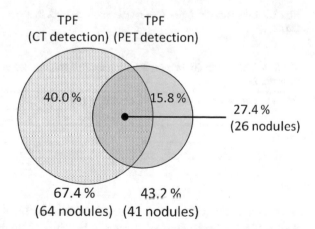

Fig. 17 Venn diagram of the nodules detected by CT and PET—27.4% of the nodules were detected by both the modalities; 40.0 and 15.8% of the nodules were detected by CT and PET, respectively

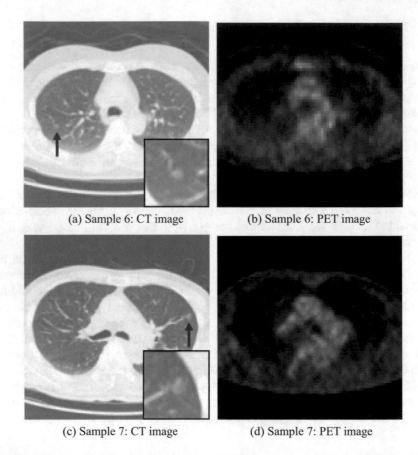

(a) Sample 6: CT image   (b) Sample 6: PET image

(c) Sample 7: CT image   (d) Sample 7: PET image

Fig. 18 Undetected nodules. The images show nodules that were missed by the CAD algorithms [28]

Table 2 The sensitivity of each detection method for nodules classified according to the nodule diameter D_n

Nodule diameter D_n [mm]	Sensitivity [%]		
	CT detection	PET detection	Combined
$D_n < 10$	77.3	4.0	78.6
$10 \leq D_n \leq 30$	76.7	66.7	86.7
$D_n > 30$	39.1	91.3	91.3

since large nodules do not have massive structure by fusing the mediastinum and chest wall while PET detection was enhanced because of significantly high uptake values.

Next, the relationship between CT values and sensitivity was investigated. We defined CT_{max} as the maximum CT value calculated inside the nodule regions identified by a radiologist. Most solid nodules havd a CT value >0, and GGO nodules have a CT value <0 [38]. Therefore, we classified the nodules into those with $CT_{max} < 0$ and $CT_{max} \geq 0$. Table 3 shows the relationship between CT values and sensitivity. The nodules with $CT_{max} \geq 0$ were associated with slightly greater CT sensitivity compared to PET and that of the combined detection improved to 91.6%. This indicated that the proposed method was successful for nodules with high CT values. The sensitivity of detection, by PET, for nodules with $CT_{max} < 0$ was 23.8%, which was much lower than that obtained with CT. Although the sensitivity of the combined result was improved to 80.6%, the detection performance was still lower than that observed for the nodules with high CT values. Detection performance for these low CT-value nodules should be improved by designing and introducing alternate detection algorithms.

In order to evaluate the bias of the image dataset, we calculated the detection performance by swapping the training and evaluation datasets. As a result, the sensitivity was 83.5% with the number of FPs/case at 4.1. This result was similar to the original result, indicating that the bias between the training and evaluation datasets was negligible.

Table 3 The sensitivity of each detection method for CT values divided into 2 ranges	CT_{max} [H.U.]	Sensitivity [%]		
		CT detection	PET detection	Combined
	$CT_{max} < 0$	73.1	23.8	80.6
	$CT_{max} \geq 0$	69.7	57.1	91.6

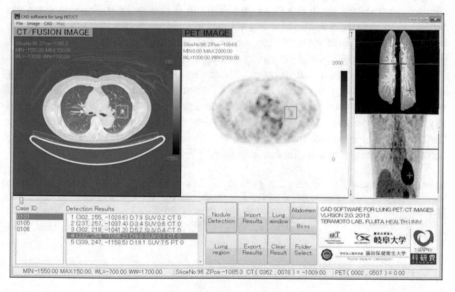

Fig. 19 CAD software. We developed an in-house software for this study. Image loading and nodule detection are fully automated. Detected positions are marked on the image

The processing time of automated detection by our CAD software (Fig. 19) was approximately 1 min/scan using a 2.8 GHz personal computer. This is much faster than the time required to read an image by the radiologist. The speed could allow further detailed examinations to be performed without delay. For example, automated nodule detection could be completed on the patient on the scanning bed, and if indicated by the automated result, high-resolution CT scan or a late-phase PET scan can be obtained immediately.

5 Conclusion

In this chapter, we described our recent study on a hybrid method of automated lung nodule detection using PET/CT images. Hitherto, the usual scheme for pulmonary nodule detection involves imaging by either CT or PET alone. The method proposed here detects lung nodules using both the anatomical information obtained by CT and the functional information obtained with PET, as well as an interpretation procedure by radiologists. CT images detect solitary nodules using CNEF that we developed previously. The PET images are binarized based on the standard uptake values (SUVs) and detection of high-uptake regions. Initial candidate nodules are identified by combining CT and PET results. FPs among the leading candidates are eliminated using a rule-based classifier and three support vector machines (SVMs) with characteristic values obtained from CT and PET images. In the present study, we evaluated this proposed method using 100 cases with PET/CT images. We found that the sensitivity of the integrated results was 83.0% with FPs/case = 5.0, and these results are much more desirable than those obtained via independent detection methods using CT or PET. In summary, the results indicate that this novel hybrid method may be useful for the detection of lung cancers, perhaps particularly in mass-screening settings.

In regard to our recent progress involving this study, we are optimizing improvements using deep learning method. We introduce the convolutional neural network (CNN), which is inspired by biological processes and specifically designed to emulate the behavior of visual systems. False positives are eliminated combining the results of the conventional FP reduction technique and CNN classifier. Thus, the detection capability will be further improved [39].

Acknowledgements The authors are grateful to Tsuneo Tamaki, Masami Nishio, Osamu Yamamuro, Katsuaki Takahashi, Toshiki Kobayashi of the Nagoya Radiological Diagnosis Foundation. This research was supported in part by a Grant-in-Aid for Scientific Research on Innovative Areas (#26108005), MEXT, Japan; in part by Tateishi Science and Technology Foundation, Japan.

References

1. Centers for disease control and prevention (2012) 1999–2012 Cancer Incidence and Mortality Data. https://www.nccd.cdc.gov/uscs/
2. Ferlay J, Shin HR, Bray F, Forman D, Mathers C and Parkin DM (2008) GLOBOCAN 2008 v2.0, cancer incidence and mortality worldwide: IARC CancerBase No. 10. https://www.globocan.iarc.fr
3. Bartjan, H., Cornelia, S., Hester, A.G., Pim, A.J., Bram, G., et al.: Screening for lung cancer with digital chest radiography: Sensitivity and number of secondary work-up CT examinations. Radiology 255(2), 629–637 (2010)
4. Sone, S., Takashima, S., Li, F., Yang, Z., Honda, T., et al.: Mass screening for lung cancer with mobile spiral computed tomography scanner. Lancet 351, 1242–1245 (1998)
5. The National lung screening trial research team: Reduced lung-cancer mortality with low-dose computed tomographic screening. N Engl J Med 365, 395–409 (2011)
6. Ide, M., Suzuki, Y.: Is whole-body FDG-PET valuable for health screening? Eur J Nucl Med Mol Imaging 32(3), 339–341 (2005)
7. Lee, J.W., Kang, K.W., Paeng, J.C., Lee, S.M., Jang, S.J., et al.: Cancer screening using 18F-FDG PET/CT in Korean asymptomatic volunteers: a preliminary report. Ann Nucl Med 23(7), 685–691 (2009)
8. Wever, W., Meylaerts, L., Ceuninck, L., Stroobants, S., Verschakelen, J.A.: Additional value of integrated PET-CT in the detection and characterization of lung metastases: correlation with CT alone and PET alone. Eur Radiol 17, 467–473 (2007)
9. Lee, Y., Hara, T., Fujita, H., Itoh, S., Ishigaki, T.: Automated detection of pulmonary nodules in helical CT images based on an improved template-matching technique. IEEE Trans Med Imaging 20(7), 595–604 (2001)
10. Suzuki K, Armato SG III, Li F, Sone S, Doi K (2003) Massive training artificial neural network (MTANN) for reduction of false positives in computerized detection of lung nodules in low-dose CT. Med Phys 30(7):1602–1617
11. McNitt-Gray, M.F.: Lung nodules and beyond: approaches, challenges and opportunities in thoracic CAD. Int Congr Ser 1268, 896–901 (2004)
12. Way, T.W., Hadjiiski, L.M., Sahiner, B., Chan, H.P., Cascade, P.N., et al.: Computer-aided diagnosis of pulmonary nodules on CT scans: segmentation and classification using 3D active contours. Med Phys 33(7), 2323–2337 (2006)
13. Li Q, Li F, Doi K (2008) Computerized detection of lung nodules in thin-section CT images by use of selective enhancement filters and an automated rule-based classifier. Acad Radiol 15(2):165–175
14. Messay, T., Hardie, R., Rogers, S.: A new computationally efficient CAD system for pulmonary nodule detection in CT imagery. Med Image Anal 14(3), 390–406 (2010)
15. Firmino, M., Morais, A.H., Mendoca, R.M., Dantas, M.R., Hekis, H.R.: Computer-aided detection system for lung cancer in computed tomography scans: Review and future prospects. Biomed Eng Online 13(41), 1–16 (2014)
16. Setio, A.A.A., Jacobs, C., Gelderblom, J., Ginneken, B.: Automatic detection of large pulmonary solid nodules in thoracic CT images. Med Phys 42(10), 5642–5653 (2015)
17. Han, H., Li, L., Han, F., Song, B., Moore, W., Liang, Z.: Fast and adaptive detection of pulmonary nodules in thoracic CT images using a hierarchical vector quantization scheme. IEEE J Biomed Health 19(2), 648–659 (2015)
18. Wang, Y X, Gong, J.S., Suzuki, K., Morcos, S.K.: Evidence-based imaging strategies for solitary pulmonary nodule. J Thorac Dis 6(7), 872–887 (2015)
19. Teramoto, A., Fujita, H.: Fast lung nodule detection in chest CT images using cylindrical nodule-enhancement filter. Int J CARS 8(2), 182–205 (2013)
20. Guan H, Kubota T, Huang X, Zhou XS, Turk M (2006) Automatic hot spot detection and segmentation in whole body FDG-PET images. In: Proceedings of IEEE International Conference on Image Processing, pp 85–88

21. Montgomery, D.W., Amira, A., Zaidi, H.: Fully automated segmentation of oncological PET volumes using a combined multiscale and statistical model. Med Phys **34**(2), 722–736 (2007)
22. Hara T, Kobayashi T, Kawai K, Zhou X, Ito S et al (2008) Automated scoring system of standard uptake value for torso FDG-PET. In: Proceedings of SPIE medical imaging 2008: computer-aided diagnosis, vol 6915, pp 691534-1– 691534-4
23. Cui Y, Zhao B, Akhurst TJ, Yan J, Schwartz LH et al (2008) CT-guided, automated detection of lung tumors on PET images. In: Proceedings of SPIE medical imaging 2008: computer-aided diagnosis, vol 6915, pp 69152 N-1– 69152 N-6
24. Ballangan C, Wang X, Eberl S, Fulham M, Feng D (2009) Automated detection and delineation of lung tumors in PET-CT volumes using a lung atlas and iterative mean-SUV threshold. In: Proceedings of SPIE medical imaging 2009: computer-aided diagnosis vol 7259, pp 72593F-1–72593F-8
25. Song, Y., Cai, W., Huang, H., Wang, X., Zhou, Y., Fulham, M., Feng, D.: Lesion detection and characterization with context driven approximation in thoracic FDG PET-CT images of NSCLC studies. IEEE Trans Med Imag **33**(2), 408–421 (2014)
26. Teramoto A, Fujita H, Tomita Y, Takahashi K, Yamamuro O et al (2011) Hybrid CAD scheme for lung nodule detection in PET/CT images. In: Proceedings of SPIE Medical Imaging 2011: computer-aided diagnosis, vol 7963, pp 7963351–796335-6
27. Teramoto A, Fujita H, Tomita Y, Takahashi K, Yamamuro O et al (2012) Pulmonary nodule detection in PET/CT images: improved approach using combined nodule detection and hybrid FP reduction. In: Proceedings of SPIE Medical Imaging 2012: computer-aided diagnosis, vol 8315, pp 83152 V-1–83152 V-6
28. Teramoto, A., Fujita, H., Takahashi, K., Yamamuro, O., Tamaki, T., Nishio, M., Kobayashi, T.: Hybrid method for the detection of pulmonary nodules using positron emission tomography/computed tomography: a preliminary study. Int. J CARS **9**, 59–69 (2014)
29. Armato III, S.G., McLennan, G., Bidaut, L., McNitt-Gray, M.F., Meyer, C.R., et al.: The Lung image database consortium (LIDC) and image database resource initiative (IDRI): A completed reference database of lung nodules on CT scans. Med Phys **38**(2), 915–931 (2011)
30. Kubota, K., Matsuzawa, T., Fujiwara, T., Ito, M., Hatazawa, J., et al.: Differential diagnosis of lung tumor with positron emission tomography: a prospective study. J Nucl Med **31**(12), 1927–1933 (1990)
31. Duhaylongsod, F.G., Lowe, V.J., Patz, E.F., Vaughn, A.L., Coleman, R.E., et al.: Detection of primary and recurrent lung cancer by means of F-18 fluorodeoxyglucose positron emission tomography. J Thorac Cardiovasc Surg **110**(1), 130–139 (1995)
32. Pauwels, E.K., Ribeiro, M.J., Stoot, J.H., McCready, V.R., Bourguignon, M., et al.: FDG accumulation and tumor biology. Nucl Med Biol **25**(4), 317–322 (1998)
33. Keyes, J.W.: SUV: standard uptake or silly useless value? J Nucl Med **36**(10), 1836–1839 (1995)
34. Lowe, V.J., Hoffman, J.M., DeLong, D.M., Patz, E.F., Coleman, R.E.: Semiquantitative and visual analysis of FDG-PET images in pulmonary abnormalities. J Nucl Med **35**(11), 1771–1776 (1994)
35. Cohade, C., Osman, M., Marshall, L.N., Wahl, R.N.: PET-CT: accuracy of PET and CT spatial registration of lung lesions. Eur J Nucl Med Mol Imaging **30**(5), 721–726 (2003)
36. Cristianini, N., Shawe-Taylor, J.: An introduction to support vector machines and other kernel-based learning methods. Cambridge University Press, Cambridge (2000)
37. Chang CC, Lin CJ LIBSVM: A library for support vector machines, Software. https://www.csie.ntu.edu.tw/~cjlin/libsvm/
38. Yamada, N., Kusumoto, M., Maeshima, A., Suzuki, K., Matsuno, Y.: Correlation of the solid part on high-resolution computed tomography with pathological scar in small lung adenocarcinomas. Jpn J Clin Oncol **37**(12), 913–917 (2007)
39. Teramoto, A., Fujita, H., Yamamuro, O., Tamaki, T.: Automated detection of pulmonary nodules in PET/CT images: ensemble false-positive reduction using a convolutional neural network technique. Med Phys **43**(6), 2821–2827 (2016)

Detecting Mammographic Masses via Image Retrieval and Discriminative Learning

Menglin Jiang, Shaoting Zhang and Dimitris N. Metaxas

Abstract During the past half century, numerous computer-aided diagnosis (CAD) approaches have been proposed to assist the detection of masses in mammograms. Most of these methods are based on either machine learning or content-based image retrieval (CBIR) techniques. Nevertheless, either category has its limitations. Learning-based methods are affected by the fact that masses have large variation in shape and size and are often indistinguishable from surrounding tissues. CBIR-based methods, on the other hand, rely heavily on radiologist-specified suspicious regions and cannot work fully automatically. To overcome the drawbacks of both kinds of methods, we introduce an automatic CAD approach that integrates image retrieval and discriminative learning. A large set of previously diagnosed mammographic masses are collected to form an exemplar database. A query mammogram is first matched with all the exemplar masses, getting a series of similarity maps. Then, these maps are subtracted by discriminatively learned thresholds to eliminate noise. At last, individual similarity maps are aggregated, and local maxima in the final map are selected as masses. For each detected mass, the most similar exemplar masses are also presented to the radiologist. Compared with learning-based methods, our approach could achieve better mass detection accuracy since it utilizes rare exemplar masses to detect "unusual" query masses. Moreover, it provides radiologists with relevant diagnosed cases as decision support. Compared with CBIR-based methods, our approach serves as a fully automated "double reading" aid without radiologists' labeling of suspicious regions. Our approach is validated on a dataset constructed from the digital database for screening mammography (DDSM), which consists of 2,021 exemplar masses, 500 mammograms containing masses and 500

M. Jiang · D. N. Metaxas
Department of Computer Science, Rutgers University, Piscataway, NJ 08854, USA
e-mail: menglin.jiang@cs.rutgers.edu

D. N. Metaxas
e mail: dnm@cs.rutgers.edu

S. Zhang (✉)
Department of Computer Science, University of North Carolina at Charlotte,
Charlotte, NC 28223, USA
e-mail: szhang16@uncc.edu, Rutgers.shaoting@gmail.com

© Springer International Publishing AG 2018
K. Suzuki and Y. Chen (eds.), *Artificial Intelligence in Decision Support Systems
for Diagnosis in Medical Imaging*, Intelligent Systems Reference Library 140,
https://doi.org/10.1007/978-3-319-68843-5_5

111

mammograms depicting healthy breasts. The proposed approach achieves high mass detection accuracy and retrieval precision, comparing favorably with traditional methods.

Keywords Mammography · Breast masses · Computer-aided diagnosis (CAD) Content-based image retrieval (CBIR) · Machine learning

1 Introduction

For years, breast cancer remains the second leading cause of cancer-related death among women [3]. Nevertheless, early diagnosis could improve the chances of recovery dramatically: the five-year relative survival rate rises from 24% when breast cancer is diagnosed at distant stage to 99% if it is diagnosed at localized stage [28]. Currently, among all the imaging techniques for breast examination, mammography is the most effective and the only widely accepted method, and it is recognized as the gold standard for breast cancer detection by American Cancer Society (ACS) [3].

The major indicators of breast cancer are masses and microcalcifications. Interpretation of these abnormalities is a great challenge due to their low prevalence [6]. Besides, radiologists are often overwhelmed by the enormous mammogram volume generated in widespread screening [61], and even experienced radiologists have substantial inter-observer and intra-observer variability in their interpretation of mammograms [69]. What's more, the detection of mammographic masses is even more difficult than that of microcalcifications, since masses vary substantially in shape, margin, size and usually have obscure boundaries [6]. Consequently, a considerable portion of retrospectively visible masses is missed by radiologists [7], and biopsies are frequently conducted on normal tissues and benign lesions [29]. It is widely recognized that double reading could remarkably improve sensitivity without increasing recall rates [8], yet it might be unaffordable in many underserved areas due to limited manpower.

Computer-aided diagnosis (CAD) provides a cost-effective alternative to double reading. It is observed that CAD-assisted single reading could achieve a performance comparable to double reading [14, 25]. Since the 1960s, numerous CAD approaches have been proposed to facilitate mammographic mass diagnosis [84]. Most of them are based on either machine learning or content-based image retrieval (CBIR) techniques. Generally speaking, learning-based approaches first segment a query mammogram into several regions, then extract certain features from these regions, and finally classify each region as mass or normal tissue using the extracted features and pre-trained classifiers [13, 20, 24, 57, 61, 72]. However, it is very difficult for classifiers to model all the training masses, therefore they are likely to miss query masses of "uncommon" appearances or sizes [57]. Besides, their performance may be affected by the obscure boundaries of masses [72], since many of them need to perform image segmentation before mass detection.

During the past decade, CBIR techniques have gained their popularity among CAD methods for mammograms as well as other medical images. CBIR addresses the problem of searching query images from an image database using visual content inherent in the images [16, 41, 43, 64, 70], as opposed to text-based image retrieval (TBIR) that utilizes manually annotated keywords. Typically, certain visual characteristics referred to as features are extracted from database images and usually organized in an index structure. Then for each user-specified query image, the same feature is extracted, and similarities between query feature and database features are calculated with the aid of index. At last, those database images with highest similarities, referred to as retrieval set, are presented to the user.

Mammograms are expected to be an ideal application of CBIR techniques [19, 52], since they depict a limited number of objects and have standard interpretation schemes, such as the breast imaging reporting and data system (BI-RADS) [17]. Specifically, CBIR-based CAD methods first prompt radiologists to label a region of interest (ROI) in the query case, then compare it with database ROIs extracted from previously diagnosed cases, and finally return the most similar cases along with the likelihood of a mass in the query case [35, 52, 61, 72]. Such approaches have several advantages over learning-based methods. First of all, they could detect "unusual" masses as long as there are several similar database ROIs. Second, the obscure mass boundary problem is eliminated, since no segmentation is required. Third, they provide radiologists with relevant diagnosed cases as valuable decision support for diagnosis of new cases. Last but not least, they can also help improve the performance of picture archiving and communication systems (PACS) and facilitate radiologist training. Especially, the recent progress of scalable CBIR techniques has been a catalyst for the increase of such CAD systems [31, 32, 38]. Nevertheless, CBIR-based CAD methods are semi-automatic and rely heavily on radiologist-specified ROIs. A nonrepresentative region, e.g. a normal region in a malignant mammogram, will lead to wrong diagnosis.

To overcome the aforementioned drawbacks of both learning-based and CBIR-based CAD methods, we introduce a novel approach that combines image retrieval with discriminative learning [33], which is illustrated in Fig. 1. In particular, a large database of exemplar masses is constructed, and a query mammogram is matched with each exemplar to compute a series of similarity maps and similarity scores [66, 67]. A similarity map describes the probabilities of a mass centered at each pixel in the query mammogram. Second, the similarity maps and scores are subtracted by discriminatively learned thresholds to remove non-mass regions. Finally, individual similarity maps are summed up, and masses are detected by simply choosing local maxima in the aggregated map. For each detected mass, the exemplar masses with highest similarity scores, denoted as support masses, are also returned to radiologists. Our approach has several advantages over traditional learning-based methods. First, it could detect "unusual" masses as long as there are several similar exemplars in the database. Second, the obscure mass boundary problem is eliminated, since no segmentation is required. Third, our method returns not only a detection result but also support masses, which are helpful to the interpretation of current case. The presented approach is also superior to CBIR-based methods regarding that it does not need artificial labeling of suspicious regions. Therefore it provides radiologists with "double reading" aid automatically.

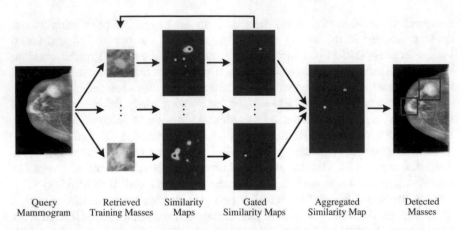

| Query
Mammogram | Retrieved
Training Masses | Similarity
Maps | Gated
Similarity Maps | Aggregated
Similarity Map | Detected
Masses |

Fig. 1 Overview of our mass detection approach based on image retrieval and discriminative learning [33]

The rest of this chapter is organized as follows. Section 2 reviews some relevant works on both learning-based and CBIR-based CAD methods. Section 3 describes our mass detection approach. Section 4 presents the experimental results. Finally, Sect. 5 draws a conclusion and discusses potential directions for future work.

2 Related Work

In this section, we first review some learning-based CAD methods designed for mammographic masses. Then, we summarize some CBIR-based CAD methods for mammograms and other medical images.

2.1 Learning-Based CAD Methods

Learning-based CAD methods typically first segment a mammogram into suspicious regions, and then classify each region using certain features and pre-trained classifiers. The key techniques here are to design appropriate features and to choose proper classifiers. A lot of features and classifiers have been investigated in the literature. For example, Chan et al. [12] used eight texture features derived from spatial grey level dependence (SGLD) matrices and a linear discriminant analysis (LDA) classifier to distinguish masses from normal tissues. For the same purpose, Sahiner et al. [65] adopted three SGLD and four gray-level difference statistics (GLDS) texture features and a convolution neural network (CNN) classifier. Wei et al. [83] developed a CAD system for full field digital mammograms (FFDM). In their system, suspicious regions are first identified using gradient field analysis with gray level information. Then, each region is classified using morphological and SGLD texture features and a LDA classifier with simplex optimization. This method was extended to the so-called "dual" system in [81]. Specifically, the dual system incorporates two CAD systems, which are optimized for "average" masses and "subtle" masses respectively, and fuses the decision scores from their LDA classifiers with an artificial neural network (ANN). A fully automated CAD system was presented in [5]. After identifying suspicious regions in the whole mammogram via an edge-based segmentation algorithm, the system classifies the regions with eight gray-tone independent texture features and an ANN classifier. In [51], suspicious regions are first segmented based on the analysis of iso-intensity contour groups, then oriented flow-field textural information and LDA are exploited to determine whether each region is mass or normal tissue. Detected masses are further classified as malignant or benign lesions using five texture features based on gray-level co-occurrence matrices and logistic regression. Li et al. [36] proposed a CAD method for FFDM images. A query mammogram is first decomposed with directional wavelet transform and represented at two scales. At either scale, suspicious regions are first separated from normal tissue through adaptive segmentation, and then classified using intensity and morphological features along with a competitive classification strategy [37]. Detection results from both scales are combined to generate the final result. In [95], fractal dimension analysis and multiresolution Markov random field (MMRF) segmentation are implemented to localize and segment suspicious regions, which are then classified using intensity and morphological features and binary decision tree.

A few automatic feature selection approaches were presented for mammographic mass detection. For instance, Melendez et al. [48] proposed two techniques, namely feature maxima propagation and local feature selection, to solve the problems of maxima misalignment and different maxima spread during feature vector construction. Tan et al. [71] presented a fast feature selection method named sequential floating forward selection (SFFS) for an ANN-based CAD system.

CAD systems have been criticised for generating excessive false positives. Many approaches aim at solving this problem. For example, in [23], Bayesian template matching is first carried out to identify suspicious regions, then two-dimensional principal components analysis (PCA) is adopted to classify these regions as masses or normal tissues. In [42], local binary patterns (LBP) and a support vector machine (SVM) classifier are employed to distinguish true masses from suspicious normal tissues. Similarly, texture features extracted from ranklet images and multiscale spatial Weber law descriptors, along with SVM classifiers, are utilized in [30, 46] respectively.

As another improvement, some CAD methods fuse two ipsilateral views of mammograms following clinical experience. To this end, Paquerault et al. [59] proposed a geometrical model to match objects in two views. For each pair of corresponding objects, textural and morphological features are extracted and merged together, then LDA is employed to classify the object pair as mass or normal tissue. The same idea was adopted in [21], which first matches suspicious objects in two views and then classifies each object pair using multiple features and an ANN classifier. In [93], a single-image-based CAD is first applied to two views independently, then mass candidates in two views are matched using geometric information, finally morpho-logical and density features along with an ANN classifier are utilized to classify each object pair. Similarly, Wei et al. [82] improved the dual system developed in [81] using view fusion. Mass candidates detected in two views by the dual system are matched using region registration, cross correlation and similarity analysis, and a decision score is computed for each pair of object. Many other learning-based CAD methods are elaborated in the review papers [13, 20, 24, 57, 61, 72].

2.2 CBIR-Based CAD Methods

The past two decades have witnessed many CBIR-based mammographic CAD meth-ods. For example, in [75, 76], template matching based on information-theoretic similarity measures is utilized to retrieve mammographic ROIs, and similarity scores between the query ROI and its best matches are used to determine whether it con-tains a mass. This approach was accelerated by restricting the template matching to those exemplar ROIs that are similar in entropy value to the query ROI [74]. Alto et al. [2] adopted features related to texture, shape and edge sharpness to search for similar mammographic masses. For the same purpose, Tao et al. [73] fused inten-sity, texture and shape features during distance calculation to achieve better retrieval precision. In order to search for similar malignant masses, Zheng et al. [94] first let radiologists rate the margin spiculation of the query ROI, and then searched from the exemplar ROIs with similar levels of spiculation using morphological and intensity-related features. This work was further improved by removing poorly effective ROIs from the exemplar database [60]. Several works tried to find mammographic masses with similar BI-RADS characteristics [17], such as shape, margin and pathology.For example, Wei et al. [80] combined intensity, shape and texture features using adap-tive weights, and exploited user interaction to optimize retrieval set. Narváez et al. [54] fused shape and texture features from two views (CC and MLO) together, and used the retrieved masses to annotate the query mass. In their improved work [53], a mass ROI is first curvelet transformed and then characterized by its marginal curvelet subband distribution.

Recently, CAD methods began to adopt scalable CBIR techniques in order to better manage the rapidly growing mammographic data. For example, in [32], scale-invariant feature transform (SIFT) [44] features are extracted from a query ROI and searched in a vocabulary tree, which stores all the quantized SIFT features extracted from the exemplar database. The retrieved exemplar ROIs are then used to deter-mine whether the query ROI contains a mass. As one of the most scalable CBIR approaches, the vocabulary tree framework could retrieve from millions of images in real time. Liu et al. [38] introduced hashing-based scalable retrieval to diagno-sis of mammographic masses. Specifically, anchor graph hashing (AGH) [40] is employed to compress two features, i.e. quantized SIFT and a global feature named GIST [56], into compact binary codes, and similarity search is performed in Ham-ming space.

CBIR techniques have also been applied to other mammographic lesions as well as other medical images and videos. For instance, El-Naqa et al. [19] adopted shape features to retrieve similar microcalcification clusters (MCCs) in mammograms, and they proposed a learning scheme to predict the similarity scores rated by radiologists so that the retrieved MCCs are consistent with human perception. Zhang et al. [88–92] employed hashing-based retrieval techniques for diagnosis of histopathological images. In particular, they employed kernel-based supervised hashing (KSH) [39] for efficient retrieval of histopathological images [89]. Subsequently, Zhang et al. [88] adopted a query specific re-ranking algorithm [86, 87] to consolidate the results of KSH and exhaustive search for better retrieval precision and diagnostic accuracy. They also integrated multiple features in AGH [40] through affinity aggregation [92]. In their latest works [90, 91], cells in histopathological images are first extracted and then retrieved using a hashing method with content-aware weights, and the retrieval results are used to determine the pathology of individual cells and the whole images. Cai et al. [10] employed a physiological kinetic feature to retrieve relevant positron emission tomography (PET) images of human brains. Their method was further extended to deal with four-dimensional dynamic PET images, which are first segmented into volumes of interest (VOI's) and then retrieved using visual, functional, and textual features [34]. In [1], computed tomography (CT) images of chest are first classified to a certain disease category, and then searched for similar images using features corresponding to that disease, which are automatically chosen from 125 features related to intensity, texture, and geometric properties. Similarly, a subset of more than 300 features related to intensity, texture, morphology and spatial relationship is selected to retrieve images of lymphoma cells [47]. Several methods adopted the "bag of words" (BoW) framework [68] to quantize local features like SIFT. For instance, André et al. [4] represented each endomicroscopy video as a BoW of "dense" SIFT features, which are derived from dense grids instead of difference of Gaussians (DoG) space. Similarly, in [26], a 2D medical image is described using a BoW of SIFT features derived from superpixels. Some other CBIR-based CAD methods are investigated in [35, 52, 61, 72].

3 Mass Detection via Retrieval and Learning

In this section, we first introduce the similarity matching between a query mammogram and exemplar masses, then present the refinement of similarity maps based on discriminative learning, and finally describe how to detect masses using these similarity maps. The overview of our approach is shown in Fig. 1.

3.1 Local Feature Voting-Based Mass Retrieval

Our approach builds upon the "bag of words" (BoW) framework [11, 32, 66–68], which describes an image with a series of quantized local features. The local feature we choose here is SIFT [44]. SIFT has been successfully applied to medical image retrieval and analysis [11, 32], owing to its excellent robustness and discriminability.

During offline stage, a large set of SIFT features extracted from a separate database are used to train a visual vocabulary (VOC) through k-means clustering. After that, SIFT features are extracted from exemplar database D, then quantized using this VOC. Each SIFT feature is represented by the ID of its nearest visual word (cluster center), and an exemplar mass is characterized by all the quantized SIFT features along with their locations. During online stage, given a mammogram q in the query set Q, SIFT features are extracted and quantized using the same VOC. Following [66, 67], each exemplar d is matched with q to calculate a similarity score $sim(q, d)$ and a similarity map $S(q, d)$, where $S(q, d)[x, y]$ indicates the similarity between a region of q centered at (x, y) and d.

Formally speaking, q is represented as a BoW, $q = \{v_i^q\}_{i=1}^m$, where v_i^q denotes its ith quantized feature. Similarly, d is represented as $d = \{v_j^d\}_{j=1}^n$. Supposing d is transformed to $d_{\alpha,s}$ after rotation α and scale s, and $d_{\alpha,s}$ matches a region in q denoted as $q_{\alpha,s}$, then their features should match with each other and have similar locations relative to their centers. For a given pair of matched features $v_i^q = v_j^d = v$, the center of $q_{\alpha,s}$, denoted as c_i^q, can be localized based on the locations of v_i^q and v_j^d:

$$l_{ci}^q = l_{vi}^q - s \cdot R \cdot l_{vj}^d, \quad R = \begin{bmatrix} \cos\alpha & -\sin\alpha \\ \sin\alpha & \cos\alpha \end{bmatrix}, \tag{1}$$

where l_{vj}^d is the location of v_j^d relative to the center of d, α and s are transformation parameters, l_{vi}^q and l_{ci}^q are the absolute locations of v_i^q and c_i^q respectively.

After localizing c_i^q, v_i^q casts its vote. To resist gentle nonrigid deformation, v_i^q votes in favor of not only c_i^q but also c_i^q's neighbors. c_i^q earns a full vote, and each neighbor gains a vote shrinked by a Gaussian weight:

$$S(q, d_{\alpha,s})[x_{ci}^q + \delta x, y_{ci}^q + \delta y] + = \frac{idf^2(v)}{tf(v, q) \cdot tf(v, d)} \cdot \exp\left(-\frac{\delta x^2 + \delta y^2}{\sigma^2}\right), \tag{2}$$

where $(x_{ci}^q, y_{ci}^q) = l_{ci}^q$ is the location of c_i^q, $(\delta x, \delta y)$ is the deviation from c_i^q to its neighbor and satisfies $\delta x^2 + \delta y^2 \leq r^2$, $tf(v, q)$ and $tf(v, d)$ are the term frequencies (TFs) of v in q and d respectively, and $idf(v)$ is the inverse document frequency (IDF) of v. TF-IDF [62, 85] is widely adopted in BoW-based CBIR methods. It reflects the importance of a visual word to an image in a collection of images. The vote score in Eq. (2) is defined based on the observation that visual words occurring rarely in the whole database (with high IDF) are more informative, and visual words occurring frequently in a single mammogram (with high TF) are less informative.

The cumulative votes of all matched pairs generate a similarity map $S\left(q, d_{\alpha,s}\right)$. The center of $q_{\alpha,s}$ is localized by finding the maximum value in $S\left(q, d_{\alpha,s}\right)$. This value represents the similarity between q and $d_{\alpha,s}$, and is denoted as $sim\left(q, d_{\alpha,s}\right)$. For the robustness to rotation and scale transformations, d is *virtually* transformed using every combination of 8 α (from 0 to $7\pi/4$) and 8 s (from $1/2$ to 2). Among all the 64 similarity maps, the one with highest similarity score is selected. The chosen similarity map and score serve as the similarity map and score between q and d, which are referred to as $S\left(q, d\right)$ and $sim\left(q, d\right)$ respectively:

$$sim\left(q, d\right) = \max_{\alpha,s} \max_{x,y} S\left(q, d_{\alpha,s}\right)[x, y] .$$ (3)

Let (x^*, y^*) and (α^*, s^*) be the parameters that maximize Eq. (3), then the query mass is localized at (x^*, y^*). Calculation of $S\left(q, d_{\alpha,s}\right)$ and $sim\left(q, d_{\alpha,s}\right)$ is illustrated in Fig. 2.

The above image retrieval approach has several advantages. First, it performs mass retrieval and localization simultaneously. Second, it is robust to translation, rotation and scale transformations of masses. Last, without resort to sliding window-based scanning, our approach is computationally efficient.

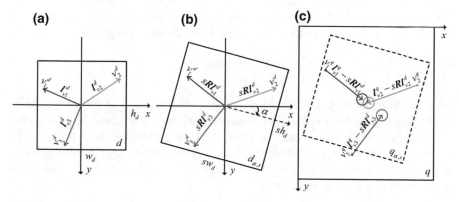

Fig. 2 Illustration of local feature voting-based similarity measure. **a** An exemplar mass d. **b** d is virtually transformed to $d_{\alpha,s}$ using parameters (α, s). **c** A query mammogram q with three features v_1^q, v_2^q and v_3^q matched with v_1^d, v_2^d and v_3^d respectively. v_1^q and v_2^q vote for nearby centers, whereas v_3^q is a noise and votes for a wrong center. $q_{\alpha,s}$ is localized by finding the maximum value in $S\left(q, d_{\alpha,s}\right)$. It is worthwhile to point out that only one pair of (α, s) is used here, whereas 64 pairs are used in practice. Also note that a mammogram commonly reaches thousands of pixels along each direction, much larger than the scale in this illustration indicates

3.2 Learning Similarity Thresholds

With the quantization of local features for fast retrieval, their discriminative power is weakened. Therefore some non-mass regions may receive high similarity scores, as shown in the third column of Fig. 1. To solve this problem, following [67], we subtract a similarity score $sim(q, d)$ by a pre-trained threshold θ_d:

$$\overline{sim}(q,d) = \begin{cases} sim(q,d) - \theta_d & \text{if } sim(q,d) > \theta_d \\ 0 & \text{otherwise} \end{cases}, \tag{4}$$

where $\overline{sim}(q, d)$ denotes the gated similarity score between q and d.

After applying the thresholds, only those exemplars with positive similarity scores are kept. For each remaining exemplar d, its similarity map $S(q, d)$ is also gated, resulting in $\bar{S}(q, d)$:

$$\bar{S}(q,d)[x,y] = \begin{cases} S(q,d)[x,y] - \theta_d & \text{if } S(q,d)[x,y] > \theta_d \\ 0 & \text{otherwise} \end{cases}. \tag{5}$$

As demonstrated in the fourth column of Fig. 1, most noise in the similarity maps could be successfully eliminated.

In order to learn all the thresholds, a group of mammograms depicting healthy breasts are collected to form a negative query set $\tilde{Q}$. For each exemplar d, its threshold is chosen as the maximum similarity score between d and any negative query $\tilde{q} \in \tilde{Q}$:

$$\theta_d = \max_{\tilde{q} \in \tilde{Q}} sim(\tilde{q}, d) . \tag{6}$$

It is worth pointing out that the above threshold scheme can be interpreted as naive Bayes classification [67]. Each gated similarity score $\overline{sim}(q, d)$ is regarded as the output of a simple classifier, where a positive score indicates a mass. The threshold θ_d learned in Eq. (6) satisfies the constraint that no negative query $\tilde{q} \in \tilde{Q}$ is mistaken for a positive one by d. In the meantime, it maximizes the likelihood that a positive query is correctly detected.

3.3 Detection of Masses

After obtaining all the exemplars with positive similarity scores $\overline{sim}(q, d)$, we sum up their similarity maps $\bar{S}(q, d)$ to calculate the final similarity map of q, denoted as $\hat{S}(q)$:

$$\hat{S}(q) = \sum_{d\,:\,sim(q,d)>0} \bar{S}(q,d). \tag{7}$$

Then, non-maximum suppression is exploited to find the local maxima in $\hat{S}(q)$, and masses are asserted around these maxima points. Finally, each mass is localized based on its support masses. Let (x^*, y^*) be the center of an asserted mass, the individual similarity maps $\bar{S}(q,d)$ contributing to $\hat{S}(q)\left[x^*, y^*\right]$ can be identified. Remember that in Sect. 3.1, the mass region is localized when calculating $S(q,d)$. The final mass region is determined as the per-component median of the regions corresponding to all support masses. An example is provided in the fifth and sixth columns of Fig. 1.

It is noteworthy that during the above detection and localization process, the support masses for each query mass are also found. These exemplars, along with their diagnosed pathologies, can be displayed to the radiologists. Such clinical evidence is a by-product of our method.

4 Experiments

This section validates our CAD approach for mammographic masses. First, the dataset employed in our experiments is described. Then, the presented method is evaluated on mass detection task. Finally, its mass retrieval performance is discussed.

4.1 Dataset

Our dataset is constructed from the digital database for screening mammography (DDSM) [27, 77], which is currently the largest public mammogram database. DDSM is comprised of 2,604 cases, and every case consists of four views, i.e. LEFT-CC, LEFT-MLO, RIGHT-CC and RIGHT-MLO. Masses in this DDSM have diverse shapes, sizes, margins, breast densities as well as patients' races and ages, and are associated with annotations labeled by experienced radiologists.

To build our dataset, mammograms are first mapped from grey level to optical density according to DDSM's instructions [77] to eliminate visual difference caused by different scanners. Second, normalized mammograms are processed for better visual quality using inversion, breast segmentation, and contrast enhancement. Third, 2,021 ROIs centered at masses are extracted to form an exemplar database D. Finally, 500 mammograms containing masses are randomly selected as query set Q. Besides, 500 mammograms depicting healthy breasts compose a negative query set $\tilde{Q}$, which is utilized to train the similarity thresholds. D, Q and $\tilde{Q}$ are randomly selected from different cases to avoid positive bias. This process is demonstrated in Fig. 3.

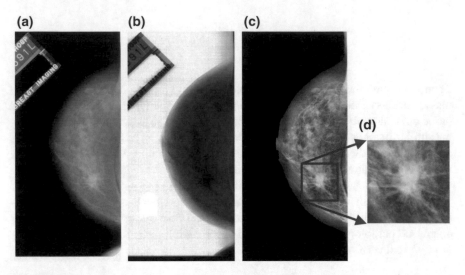

Fig. 3 Preprocessing of mammograms and extraction of exemplar masses. **a** Original mammogram in grey level format. **b** Normalized mammogram in optical density format. **c** Visually enhanced mammogram. **d** An exemplar mass annotated by experienced radiologists

4.2 Mass Detection Performance

We first measure the mass detection accuracy of the presented approach. Three methods are implemented for comparison. The first two methods adopt a cascade of boosted classifiers [79]. This framework and its variations obtain good results in mammographic lesion detection [9, 55, 58]. The first method employs the same Haar feature as in [9, 79], and the second one utilizes histogram of oriented gradient (HOG) [15] to better describe mass appearance and shape. HOG and its variations demonstrate encouraging performance in the latest works on mammographic mass detection and segmentation [49, 50]. The last comparison method [78] is based on Iris filter and back-propagation neural network classifier. It achieves best performance among seven mass detection systems in a quantitative comparison [57]. All the comparison methods are trained on the masses in D and regions randomly extracted from the healthy mammograms in $\tilde{Q}$, which are used as positive and negative training samples respectively. These methods are denoted as "B+Haar" (boosted cascade of Haar), "B+HOG" (boosted cascade of HOG), and "NN" (neural network).

All the methods are evaluated using receiver operating characteristic (ROC) curve and ROC area index A_z. The results are shown in Fig. 4. Our approach outperforms all the comparison methods: it achieves an A_z score of 0.89, whereas the A_z scores of other methods are 0.80, 0.85, and 0.83 respectively. Detailed results show that the comparison methods miss many "uncommon" query masses, which is expected since classifiers can hardly recognize minority features extracted from the exemplar database. On the contrary, our approach could precisely detect and localize these

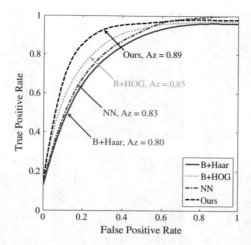

Fig. 4 ROC and A_z scores of the evaluated methods

masses as long as there are a few similar exemplar masses. An example can be found in Fig. 5. The query mammogram contains a malignant mass of great size, lobulated shape and microlobulated margin. There are only several similar masses in the exemplar database, which cannot be modeled by classifiers. Consequently, the comparison methods fail to detect this query mass. Nevertheless, these exemplar masses are sufficient for our approach to find the query mass.

It is worth mentioning that a considerable portion of false positives is caused by the visual similarity between malignant masses and normal regions with bright cores and spiculated boundaries. A possible solution is to filter out these regions through an additional mass validation step [67]. In particular, a series of annotated mammograms depicting either healthy or abnormal breasts should be collected to make up a validation database V. Then, an asserted mass q is matched with each validation mammogram using the same similarity measure explained in Sect. 3.1. A true positive is expected to discover some masses in V, while a false positive is likely to find normal tissues or localize masses inaccurately. Therefore a validation score can be calculated for q based on how much its retrieved regions overlap with the annotated mass regions in V. q is reported only if it has a high validation score.

4.3 Mass Retrieval Performance

Studies show that biopsy and other follow-up examinations are frequently carried out on benign masses [29], which causes unnecessary trouble to the patients. Considering this fact, it is preferable that CAD methods not only distinguish masses from normal tissues, but also discriminate between malignant and benign masses. To this

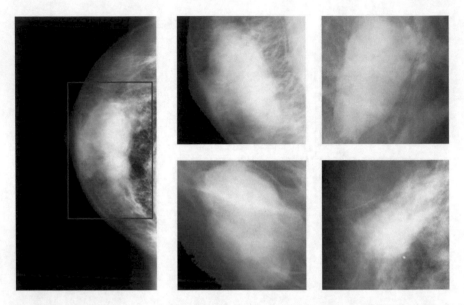

Fig. 5 A query mammogram (left) and its top four support masses retrieved by our approach (right). The query contains a huge malignant mass (cancer) with lobulated shape and microlobulated margin. The proposed approach successfully finds exemplar masses of similar sizes, shapes, and margins. Based on these masses, it accurately detects the query mass

Table 1 Retrieval precision at different values of k (number of retrieved masses)

k	TM (%)	FC (%)	BoW (%)	Ours (%)
1	72.4	82.6	78.5	**84.4**
5	70.3	83.3	77.8	**85.5**
20	71.7	81.4	78.0	**85.1**

end, we examine whether the retrieved support masses have the same pathology as that of the query mass.

Three methods are compared. The first one, presented in [75], performs a template matching between query mass and each exemplar mass based on normalized mutual information. The second approach, presented in [2], characterizes each mass with concatenated features related to texture, shape and edge sharpness, and returns the exemplar masses with nearest Euclidean distances. The last method, similar to [4, 26], represents each mass with a SIFT BoW histogram and measures their χ^2 distance. These approaches are referred to as "TM" (template matching), "FC" (feature concatenation), and "BoW".

The evaluation measure adopted here is "retrieval precision", the most widely used metric in image retrieval. In our context, precision is defined as the percentage of retrieved support masses that have the same malignant/benign pathology as that of the query mass. Overall the precision score changes slightly as k increases from

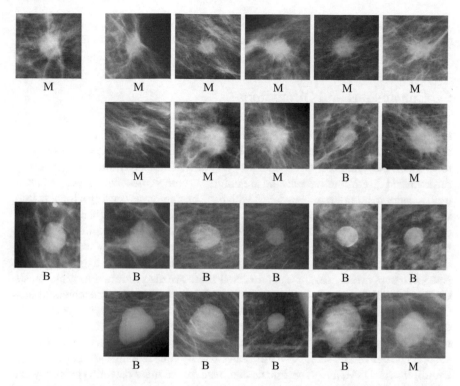

Fig. 6 Two masses in query mammograms (left) and their top 10 similar exemplar masses returned by our approach (right). For each mass, its pathology is shown below. "M" stands for "malignant", and "B" denotes "benign"

1 to 20, where k denotes the number of retrieved support masses. The precision scores at $k = 1$, 5, and 20 are summarized in Table 1. In addition, two examples are provided in Fig. 6 for visual evaluation. The results show that our approach surpasses all the comparison methods. Especially, it outperforms "BoW", which employs the same feature but utilizes a different similarity measure. The results demonstrate the efficacy of our retrieval method. In particular, a match between a query feature and a training feature assures that the two local patches, from where the SIFT features are extracted, have similar appearances. Besides, Hough voting guarantees that two matched objects have similar shapes and sizes. Consequently, our retrieval step could find exemplar masses which are similar in local appearance and global shape to the query mass. It is observed that shape and margin are strongly correlated to pathology of masses: malignant masses usually have spiculated and irregular shapes along with rough and blurry boundaries, whereas benign masses often have round and regular shapes along with smooth and well-circumscribed boundaries [17]. Of course, there do exist masses with atypical shapes and boundaries, which may explain the irrelevant exemplar masses returned by our method. Nevertheless, in summary, these

visually and semantically similar support masses along with their associated diagnostic reports could contribute to diagnosis of the query mammogram.

5 Conclusions and Discussions

During the past decades, a large number of CAD approaches have been presented to assist mammographic mass detection, which are based on machine learning or CBIR techniques. Nevertheless, either category has its limitations. In this chapter, image retrieval and discriminative learning are unified to complement each other. In particular, a query mammogram is matched with each exemplar mass using a local feature voting scheme, achieving mass retrieval and localization simultaneously. Then, discriminatively learned thresholds are employed to prune non-mass regions, which can be regarded as naive Bayes classification. Finally, gated similarity maps are accumulated, and masses are detected by finding local maxima in the aggregated map. Retrieved support masses for each detected mass are also returned to radiologists. Compared with learning—based CAD methods, the proposed approach could handle unusual masses by using a large exemplar database. In addition, it gets rid of the obscure mass boundary problem, and provides radiologists with relevant diagnosed cases. Compared with CBIR-based methods, it doesn't rely on radiologist-labeled suspicious regions and serves as a fully automated double reading aid. A large dataset is built from DDSM, and experiments demonstrate the mass detection accuracy and retrieval precision of our method.

Further endeavors will be devoted to extending our approach to handle mass segmentation and classification. In addition to mass retrieval and detection, mass segmentation and classification have also been widely investigated [13, 20, 57]. However, most existing methods address these four tasks in isolation, rather than handle them together. It is believed that related medical image analysis tasks should be considered jointly, since they are intrinsically relevant [18, 22, 45]. For example, mass detection is usually the first step of mass segmentation, which further fosters mass classification since boundary-related features are strongly correlated to pathology of masses [17].

In response, we propose a joint framework to tackle mammographic mass retrieval, detection, segmentation, and classification, which is illustrated in Fig. 7. Specifically, the mass retrieval and detection steps are the same as in Sect. 3. For each detected mass in the query mammogram, its contour is computed via segmentation transfer [63], which learns shape and appearance priors from its most similar exemplar masses. Each query mass is also classified into benign or malignant pathology according to its support masses and margin-related characteristics. In the end, for each query mass, our approach provides radiologists with a bounding box, pixel-level contour, pathology, and the most similar diagnosed cases, serving as a comprehensive double reading aid.

Our four-in-one joint framework has several advantages over traditional methods designed for individual tasks. First of all, it realizes full benefits of exemplar masses

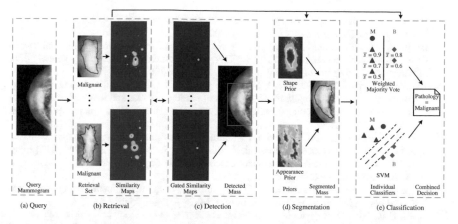

Fig. 7 Overview of our four-in-one mass diagnosis approach. The mass detection stage works on the retrieval result, and refines it in return. Segmentation is carried out based on the retrieval result and detected bounding box. Using the retrieval result and margin-related features, the query mass is classified

(especially their segmentation) and its own intermediate results, which promotes the performance on all the tasks. Especially, by learning from similar exemplar masses instead of all of them, our method could achieve better results on detection, segmentation, and classification. Second, this approach has better robustness and overall efficiency, as it only needs to carry out the modules shared by different tasks once, such as feature extraction. Last but not least, the joint framework could help researchers to gain new insights into medical image analysis by identifying the key parts that run through the major research branches [18].

References

1. Aisen, A.M., Broderick, L.S., Winer-Muram, H., Brodley, C.E., Kak, A.C., Pavlopoulou, C., Dy, J., Shyu, C.R., Marchiori, A.: Automated storage and retrieval of thin-section CT images to assist diagnosis: system description and preliminary assessment. Radiology **228**(1), 265–270 (2003)
2. Alto, H., Rangayyan, R.M., Desautels, J.E.L.: Content-based retrieval and analysis of mammographic masses. J. Electron. Imaging **14**(2), 023016–17 (2005)
3. American Cancer Society: Breast Cancer Facts and Figures 2013–2014. American Cancer Society, Atlanta, GA, USA (2013)
4. André, B., Vercauteren, T., Buchner, A.M., Wallace, M.B., Ayache, N.: Learning semantic and visual similarity for endomicroscopy video retrieval. IEEE Trans. Med. Imaging **31**(6), 1276–1288 (2012)
5. Bellotti, R., De Carlo, F., Tangaro, S., Gargano, G., Maggipinto, G., Castellano, M., Massafra, R., Cascio, D., Fauci, F., Magro, R., Raso, G., Lauria, A., Forni, G., Bagnasco, S., Cerello, P., Zanon, E., Cheran, S.C., Lopez Torres, E., Bottigli, U., Masala, G.L., Oliva, P., Retico, A., Fantacci, M.E., Cataldo, R., De Mitri, I., De Nunzio, G.: A completely automated CAD system for mass detection in a large mammographic database. Med. Phys. **33**(8), 3066–3075 (2006)

6. Birdwell, R.L.: The preponderance of evidence supports computer-aided detection for screening mammography. Radiology **253**(1), 9–16 (2009)
7. Birdwell, R.L., Ikeda, D.M., O'Shaughnessy, K.F., Sickles, E.A.: Mammographic characteristics of 115 missed cancers later detected with screening mammography and the potential utility of computer-aided detection. Radiology **219**(1), 192–202 (2001)
8. Blanks, R.G., Wallis, M.G., Moss, S.M.: A comparison of cancer detection rates achieved by breast cancer screening programmes by number of readers, for one and two view mammography: results from the UK national health service breast screening programme. J. Med. Screen. **5**(4), 195–201 (1998)
9. Bria, A., Karssemeijer, N., Tortorella, F.: Learning from unbalanced data: A cascade-based approach for detecting clustered microcalcifications. Med. Image Anal. **18**(2), 241–252 (2014)
10. Cai, W., Feng, D.D., Fulton, R.R.: Content-based retrieval of dynamic PET functional images. IEEE Trans. Inf. Technol. Biomed. **4**(2), 152–158 (2000)
11. Caicedo, J.C., Cruz, A., González, F.A.: Histopathology image classification using bag of features and kernel functions. In: Proceedings of AIME, pp. 126–135 (2009)
12. Chan, H.P., Wei, D., Helvie, M.A., Sahiner, B., Adler, D.D., Goodsitt, M.M., Petrick, N.: Computer-aided classification of mammographic masses and normal tissue: linear discriminant analysis in texture feature space. Phys. Med. Biol. **40**(5), 857–876 (1995)
13. Cheng, H.D., Shi, X.J., Min, R., Hu, L.M., Cai, X.P., Du, H.N.: Approaches for automated detection and classification of masses in mammograms. Pattern Recognit. **39**(4), 646–668 (2006)
14. Ciatto, S., Del Turco, M.R., Risso, G., Catarzi, S., Bonardi, R., Viterbo, V., Gnutti, P., Guglielmoni, B., Pinelli, L., Pandiscia, A., Navarra, F., Lauria, A., Palmiero, R., Indovina, P.L.: Comparison of standard reading and computer aided detection (CAD) on a national proficiency test of screening mammography. Eur. J. Radiol. **45**(2), 135–138 (2003)
15. Dalal, N., Triggs, B.: Histograms of oriented gradients for human detection. In: Proceedings of IEEE CVPR, pp. 886–893 (2005)
16. Datta, R., Joshi, D., Li, J., Wang, J.Z.: Image retrieval: ideas, influences, and trends of the new age. ACM Comput. Surv. **40**(2) (2008)
17. D'Orsi, C.J., Sickles, E.A., Mendelson, E.B., Morris, E.A., et al.: ACR BI-RADS Atlas, Breast Imaging Reporting And Data System, 5th edn. American College of Radiology, Reston, VA, USA (2013)
18. Duncan, J.S., Ayache, N.: Medical image analysis: progress over two decades and the challenges ahead. IEEE Trans. Pattern Anal. Mach. Intell. **22**(1), 85–106 (2000)
19. El-Naqa, I., Yang, Y., Galatsanos, N.P., Nishikawa, R.M., Wernick, M.N.: A similarity learning approach to content-based image retrieval: application to digital mammography. IEEE Trans. Med. Imaging **23**(10), 1233–1244 (2004)
20. Elter, M., Horsch, A.: CADx of mammographic masses and clustered microcalcifications: a review. Med. Phys. **36**(6), 2052–2068 (2009)
21. van Engeland, S., Karssemeijer, N.: Combining two mammographic projections in a computer aided mass detection method. Med. Phys. **34**(3), 898–905 (2007)
22. Eslami, A., Karamalis, A., Katouzian, A., Navab, N.: Segmentation by retrieval with guided random walks: application to left ventricle segmentation in MRI. Med. Image Anal. **17**(2), 236–253 (2013)
23. Freixenet, J., Oliver, A., Martí, R., Lladó, X., Pont, J., Pérez, E., Denton, E.R.E., Zwiggelaar, R.: Eigendetection of masses considering false positive reduction and breast density information. Med. Phys. **35**(5), 1840–1853 (2008)
24. Ganesan, K., Acharya, U.R., Chua, C.K., Min, L.C., Abraham, K.T., Ng, K.H.: Computer-aided breast cancer detection using mammograms: a review. IEEE Rev. Biomed. Eng. **6**, 77–98 (2013)
25. Gromet, M.: Comparison of computer-aided detection to double reading of screening mammograms: review of 231,221 mammograms. Am. J. Roentgenol. **190**(4), 854–859 (2008)
26. Haas, S., Donner, R., Burner, A., Holzer, M., Langs, G.: Superpixel-based interest points for effective bags of visual words medical image retrieval. In: Proceedings MCBR-CDS, pp. 58–68 (2011)

27. Heath, M., Bowyer, K., Kopans, D., Kegelmeyer Jr, W.P., Moore, R., Chang, K., Munishku-maran, S.: Current status of the digital database for screening mammography. In: Digital Mammography, pp. 457–460. Springer (1998)
28. Howlader, N., Noone, A.M., Krapcho, M., Garshell, J., Neyman, N., Altekruse, S.F., Kosary, C.L., Yu, M., Ruhl, J., Tatalovich, Z., Cho, H., Mariotto, A., Lewis, D.R., Chen, H.S., Feuer, E.J., Cronin, K.A.: SEER cancer statistics review, 1975-2010. National Cancer Institute (2013)
29. Hubbard, R.A., Kerlikowske, K., Flowers, C.I., Yankaskas, B.C., Zhu, W., Miglioretti, D.L.: Cumulative probability of false-positive recall or biopsy recommendation after 10 years of screening mammography: a cohort study. Ann. Intern. Med. **155**(8), 481–492 (2011)
30. Hussain, M.: False-positive reduction in mammography using multiscale spatial Weber law descriptor and support vector machines. Neural Comput. Appl. **25**(1), 83–93 (2014)
31. Jiang, M., Zhang, S., Huang, J., Yang, L., Metaxas, D.N.: Joint kernel-based supervised hashing for scalable histopathological image analysis. In: Proceedings of International Conference on MICCAI, vol. 3, pp. 366–373 (2015)
32. Jiang, M., Zhang, S., Li, H., Metaxas, D.N.: Computer-aided diagnosis of mammographic masses using scalable image retrieval. IEEE Trans. Biomed. Eng. **62**(2), 783–792 (2015)
33. Jiang, M., Zhang, S., Metaxas, D.N.: Detection of mammographic masses by content-based image retrieval. In: Proceedings of International Workshop on MLMI, pp. 33–41 (2014)
34. Kim, J., Cai, W., Feng, D.D., Wu, H.: A new way for multidimensional medical data management: Volume of interest (VOI)-based retrieval of medical images with visual and functional features. IEEE Trans. Inf. Technol. Biomed. **10**(3), 598–607 (2006)
35. Kumar, A., Kim, J., Cai, W., Fulham, M., Feng, D.: Content-based medical image retrieval: a survey of applications to multidimensional and multimodality data. J. Digit. Imaging **26**(6), 1025–1039 (2013)
36. Li, L., Clark, R.A., Thomas, J.A.: Computer-aided diagnosis of masses with full-field digital mammography. Acad. Radiol. **9**(1), 4–12 (2002)
37. Li, L., Zheng, Y., Zhang, L., Clark, R.A.: False-positive reduction in CAD mass detection using a competitive classification strategy. Med. Phys. **28**(2), 250–258 (2001)
38. Liu, J., Zhang, S., Liu, W., Zhang, X., Metaxas, D.N.: Scalable mammogram retrieval using anchor graph hashing. In: Proceedings of ISBI, pp. 898–901. IEEE (2014)
39. Liu, W., Wang, J., Ji, R., Jiang, Y., Chang, S.: Supervised hashing with kernels. In: Proceedings of CVPR, pp. 2074–2081. IEEE (2012)
40. Liu, W., Wang, J., Kumar, S., Chang, S.: Hashing with graphs. In: Proceedings of ICML, pp. 1–8 (2011)
41. Liu, Y., Zhang, D., Lu, G., Ma, W.Y.: A survey of content-based image retrieval with high-level semantics. Pattern Recognit. **40**(1), 262–282 (2007)
42. Lladó, X., Oliver, A., Freixenet, J., Martí, R., Martí, J.: A textural approach for mass false positive reduction in mammography. Comput. Med. Imaging Graph. **33**(6), 415–422 (2009)
43. Long, F., Zhang, H., Feng, D.D.: Fundamentals of content-based image retrieval. In: Multimedia Information Retrieval and Management, pp. 1–26. Springer (2003)
44. Lowe, D.G.: Distinctive image features from scale-invariant keypoints. Int. J. Comput. Vis. **60**(2), 91–110 (2004)
45. Lu, C., Chelikani, S., Jaffray, D.A., Milosevic, M.F., Staib, L.H., Duncan, J.S.: Simultaneous nonrigid registration, segmentation, and tumor detection in MRI guided cervical cancer radiation therapy. IEEE Trans. Med. Imaging **31**(6), 1213–1227 (2012)
46. Masotti, M., Lanconelli, N., Campanini, R.: Computer-aided mass detection in mammography: false positive reduction via gray-scale invariant ranklet texture features. Med. Phys. **36**(2), 311–316 (2009)
47. Mattie, M.E., Staib, L.H., Stratmann, E., Tagare, H.D., Duncan, J.S., Miller, P.L.: Pathmaster: content-based cell image retrieval using automated feature extraction. J. Am. Med. Inform. Assoc. **7**(4), 404–415 (2000)
48. Melendez, J., Sánchez, C.I., van Ginneken, B., Karssemeijer, N.: Improving mass candidate detection in mammograms via feature maxima propagation and local feature selection. Med. Phys. **41**(8), 081904–1–11 (2014)

49. Molinara, M., Marrocco, C., Tortorella, F.: A boosting-based approach to refine the segmentation of masses in mammography. In: Proceedings of International Conference on ICIAP, pp. 572–580 (2013)
50. Moura, D.C., Guevara-López, M.Á.: An evaluation of image descriptors combined with clinical data for breast cancer diagnosis. Int. J. Comput. Assist. Radiol. Surg. **8**(4), 561–574 (2013)
51. Mudigonda, N.R., Rangayyan, R.M., Desautels, J.E.L.: Detection of breast masses in mammograms by density slicing and texture flow-field analysis. IEEE Trans. Med. Imaging **20**(12), 1215–1227 (2001)
52. Müller, H., Michoux, N., Bandon, D., Geissbühler, A.: A review of content-based image retrieval systems in medical applications - clinical benefits and future directions. Int. J. Med. Inform. **73**(1), 1–23 (2004)
53. Narváez, F., Díaz, G., Gómez, F., Romero, E.: A content-based retrieval of mammographic masses using a curvelet descriptor. In: Proceedings of SPIE Medical Imaging 2012: Computer-Aided Diagnosis, vol. 8315, pp. 83150A–83150A–7 (2012)
54. Narváez, F., Díaz, G., Romero, E.: Multi-view information fusion for automatic BI-RADS description of mammographic masses. In: Proceedings of SPIE Medical Imaging 2011: Computer-Aided Diagnosis, vol. 7963, pp. 79630A–79630A–7 (2011)
55. Nemoto, M., Shimizu, A., Kobatake, H., Takeo, H., Nawano, S.: Study on cascade classification in abnormal shadow detection for mammograms. Digital Mammography, 324–331 (2006)
56. Oliva, A., Torralba, A.: Modeling the shape of the scene: a holistic representation of the spatial envelope. Int. J. Comput. Vis. **42**(3), 145–175 (2001)
57. Oliver, A., Freixenet, J., Martí, J., Pérez, E., Pont, J., Denton, E.R.E., Zwiggelaar, R.: A review of automatic mass detection and segmentation in mammographic images. Med. Image Anal. **14**(2), 87–110 (2010)
58. Oliver, A., Torrent, A., Lladó, X., Tortajada, M., Tortajada, L., Sentís, M., Freixenet, J., Zwiggelaar, R.: Automatic microcalcification and cluster detection for digital and digitised mammograms. Knowl. Based Syst. **28**, 68–75 (2012)
59. Paquerault, S., Petrick, N., Chan, H.P., Sahiner, B., Helvie, M.A.: Improvement of computerized mass detection on mammograms: fusion of two-view information. Med. Phys. **29**(2), 238–247 (2002)
60. Park, S.C., Sukthankar, R., Mummert, L., Satyanarayanan, M., Zheng, B.: Optimization of reference library used in content-based medical image retrieval scheme. Med. Phys. **34**(11), 4331–4339 (2007)
61. Rangayyan, R.M., Ayres, F.J., Leo Desautels, J.E.: A review of computer-aided diagnosis of breast cancer: toward the detection of subtle signs. J. Franklin Inst. **344**, 312–348 (2007)
62. Robertson, S.: Understanding inverse document frequency: on theoretical arguments for IDF. J. Doc. **60**(5), 503–520 (2004)
63. Rosenfeld, A., Weinshall, D.: Extracting foreground masks towards object recognition. In: Proceedings of IEEE ICCV, pp. 1371–1378 (2011)
64. Rui, Y., Huang, T.S., Chang, S.F.: Image retrieval: current techniques, promising directions, and open issues. J. Vis. Commun. Image Represent. **10**(1), 39–62 (1999)
65. Sahiner, B., Chan, H.P., Petrick, N., Wei, D., Helvie, M.A., Adler, D.D., Goodsitt, M.M.: Classification of mass and normal breast tissue: a convolution neural network classifier with spatial domain and texture images. IEEE Trans. Med. Imaging **15**(5), 598–610 (1996)
66. Shen, X., Lin, Z., Brandt, J., Avidan, S., Wu, Y.: Object retrieval and localization with spatially-constrained similarity measure and k-nn re-ranking. In: Proceedings of IEEE CVPR, pp. 3013–3020 (2012)
67. Shen, X., Lin, Z., Brandt, J., Wu, Y.: Detecting and aligning faces by image retrieval. In: Proceedings of IEEE CVPR, pp. 3460–3467 (2013)
68. Sivic, J., Zisserman, A.: Video google: a text retrieval approach to object matching in videos. In: Proceedings of IEEE ICCV, pp. 1470–1477 (2003)
69. Skaane, P., Engedal, K., Skjennald, A.: Interobserver variation in the interpretation of breast imaging. Acta Radiol. **38**(4), 497–502 (1997)

70. Smeulders, A.W.M., Worring, M., Santini, S., Gupta, A., Jain, R.: Content-based image retrieval at the end of the early years. IEEE Trans. Pattern Anal. Mach. Intell. **22**(12), 1349–1380 (2000)
71. Tan, M., Pu, J., Zheng, B.: A new and fast image feature selection method for developing an optimal mammographic mass detection scheme. Med. Phys. **41**(8), 081906–1–12 (2014)
72. Tang, J., Rangayyan, R.M., Xu, J., El Naqa, I., Yang, Y.: Computer-aided detection and diagnosis of breast cancer with mammography: recent advances. IEEE Trans. Inf. Technol. Biomed. **13**(2), 236–251 (2009)
73. Tao, Y., Lo, S.C.B., Freedman, M.T., Xuan, J.: A preliminary study of content-based mammographic masses retrieval. In: Proceedings of SPIE Medical Imaging 2007: Computer-Aided Diagnosis, vol. 6514, pp. 65141Z–1–12 (2007)
74. Tourassi, G.D., Harrawood, B., Singh, S., Lo, J.Y.: Information-theoretic CAD system in mammography: entropy-based indexing for computational efficiency and robust performance. Med. Phys. **34**(8), 3193–3204 (2007)
75. Tourassi, G.D., Harrawood, B., Singh, S., Lo, J.Y., Floyd, C.E.: Evaluation of information-theoretic similarity measures for content-based retrieval and detection of masses in mammograms. Med. Phys. **34**(1), 140–150 (2007)
76. Tourassi, G.D., Vargas-Voracek, R., Catarious Jr., D.M., Floyd Jr., C.E.: Computer-assisted detection of mammographic masses: a template matching scheme based on mutual information. Med. Phys. **30**(8), 2123–2130 (2003)
77. University of South Florida: USF digital mammography home page (2001). http://marathon.csee.usf.edu/Mammography/Database.html
78. Varela, C., Tahoces, P.G., Méndez, A.J., Souto, M., Vidal, J.J.: Computerized detection of breast masses in digitized mammograms. Comput. Biol. Med. **37**(2), 214–226 (2007)
79. Viola, P.A., Jones, M.J.: Rapid object detection using a boosted cascade of simple features. In: Proceedings of IEEE CVPR, pp. I–511–518 (2001)
80. Wei, C.H., Li, Y., Huang, P.J.: Mammogram retrieval through machine learning within BI-RADS standards. J. Biomed. Inform. **44**(4), 607–614 (2011)
81. Wei, J., Chan, H.P., Sahiner, B., Hadjiiski, L.M., Helvie, M.A., Roubidoux, M.A., Zhou, C., Ge, J.: Dual system approach to computer-aided detection of breast masses on mammograms. Med. Phys. **33**(11), 4157–4168 (2006)
82. Wei, J., Chan, H.P., Sahiner, B., Zhou, C., Hadjiiski, L.M., Roubidoux, M.A., Helvie, M.A.: Computer-aided detection of breast masses on mammograms: dual system approach with two-view analysis. Med. Phys. **36**(10), 4451–4460 (2009)
83. Wei, J., Sahiner, B., Hadjiiski, L.M., Chan, H.P., Petrick, N., Helvie, M.A., Roubidoux, M.A., Ge, J., Zhou, C.: Computer-aided detection of breast masses on full field digital mammograms. Med. Phys. **32**(9), 2827–2838 (2005)
84. Winsberg, F., Elkin, M., Macy, J., Bordaz, V., Weymouth, W.: Detection of radiographic abnormalities in mammograms by means of optical scanning and computer analysis. Radiology **89**(2), 211–215 (1967)
85. Wu, H.C., Luk, R.W.P., Wong, K.F., Kwok, K.L.: Interpreting TF-IDF term weights as making relevance decisions. ACM Trans. Inf. Syst. **26**(3), 13:1–37 (2008)
86. Zhang, S., Huang, J., Li, H., Metaxas, D.N.: Automatic image annotation and retrieval using group sparsity. IEEE Trans. Syst. Man Cybern. B Cybern. **42**(3), 838–849 (2012)
87. Zhang, S., Yang, M., Cour, T., Yu, K., Metaxas, D.N.: Query specific rank fusion for image retrieval. IEEE Trans. Pattern Anal. Mach. Intell. **37**(4), 803–815 (2015)
88. Zhang, X., Dou, H., Ju, T., Xu, J., Zhang, S.: Fusing heterogeneous features from stacked sparse autoencoder for histopathological image analysis. IEEE J. Biomed. Health Inform. **20**(5), 1377–1383 (2016)
89. Zhang, X., Liu, W., Dundar, M., Badve, S., Zhang, S.: Towards large-scale histopathological image analysis: hashing-based image retrieval. IEEE Trans. Med. Imaging **34**(2), 496–506 (2015)
90. Zhang, X., Su, H., Yang, L., Zhang, S.: Fine-grained histopathological image analysis via robust segmentation and large-scale retrieval. In: Proceedings of IEEE CVPR, pp. 5361–5368 (2015)

91. Zhang, X., Xing, F., Su, H., Yang, L., Zhang, S.: High-throughput histopathological image analysis via robust cell segmentation and hashing. Med. Image Anal. **26**(1), 306–315 (2015)
92. Zhang, X., Yang, L., Liu, W., Su, H., Zhang, S.: Mining histopathological images via composite hashing and online learning. In: Proceedings of MICCAI, vol. 2, pp. 479–486 (2014)
93. Zheng, B., Leader, J.K., Abrams, G.S., Lu, A.H., Wallace, L.P., Maitz, G.S., Gur, D.: Multiview-based computer-aided detection scheme for breast masses. Med. Phys. **33**(9), 3135–3143 (2006)
94. Zheng, B., Lu, A., Hardesty, L.A., Sumkin, J.H., Hakim, C.M., Ganott, M.A., Gur, D.: A method to improve visual similarity of breast masses for an interactive computer-aided diagnosis environment. Med. Phys. **33**(1), 111–117 (2006)
95. Zheng, L., Chan, A.K.: An artificial intelligent algorithm for tumor detection in screening mammogram. IEEE Trans. Med. Imaging **20**(7), 559–567 (2001)

Part III
Computer-Aided Diagnosis

High-Order Statistics of Micro-Texton for HEp-2 Staining Pattern Classification

Xian-Hua Han and Yen-Wei Chen

Abstract This study addresses the classification problem of the HEp-2 cell using indirect immunofluorescent (IIF) image analysis, which can indicate the presence of autoimmune diseases by finding antibodies in the patient serum. Generally, the method used for IIF analysis remains subjective, and depends too heavily on the experience and expertise of the physician. Recently, studies have shown that it is possible to identify the cell patterns using IIF image analysis and machine learning techniques. However, it still has large gap in recognition rates to the physical experts' one. This paper explores an approach in which the discriminative features of HEp-2 cell images in IIF are extracted and then, the patterns of the HEp-2 cell are identified using machine learning techniques. This study aims to realize a method for extracting highly-discriminant features from HEp-2 cell images by exploring a robust local descriptor inspired by Weber's law. The investigated local descriptor is based on the fact that human perception for distinguishing a pattern depends not only on the absolute intensity of the stimulus but also on the relative variance of the stimulus. Therefore, we firstly transform the original stimulus (the images in our study) into a differential excitation-domain according to Weber's law, and then explore a local patch, also called as micro-Texton, in the transformed domain as Weber local descriptor. Furthermore, we propose to employ a parametric probability process to model the Weber local descriptors, and extract the higher-order statistics to the model parameters for image representation. The proposed strategy can adaptively characterize the Weber local descriptor space using generative probability model, and then learn the parameters for better fitting the training space, which would lead to more discriminant representation for HEp-2 cell images. The simple linear support vector

X.-H. Han (✉)
Graduate School of Science and Technology for Innovation, Yamaguchi University,
1677-1 Yoshida, Yamaguchi City, Yamaguchi 753-8511, Japan
e-mail: hanxhua@yamaguchi-u.ac.jp

Y.-W. Chen
Ritsumeikan University, 1-1-1, NojiHigashi, Kusatsu, Shiga 525-8577, Japan
e-mail: chen@is.ritsumei.ac.jp

Y.-W. Chen
College of Science and Technology, Zhejiang University, Hangzhou, China

© Springer International Publishing AG 2018
K. Suzuki and Y. Chen (eds.), *Artificial Intelligence in Decision Support Systems for Diagnosis in Medical Imaging*, Intelligent Systems Reference Library 140,
https://doi.org/10.1007/978-3-319-68843-5_6

machine is used for cell pattern identification because of its low computational cost, in particular for large-scale datasets. Experiments using the open HEp-2 cell dataset used in the ICIP2013 contest validate that the proposed strategy can achieve a much better performance than the widely used local binary pattern (LBP) histogram and its extensions, Rotation Invariant Co-occurrence LBP (RICLBP) and Pairwise Rotation Invariant Co-occurrence LBP (PRICoLBP), and that the achieved recognition error rate is even very significantly below the observed intra-laboratory variability.

1 Introduction

Indirect Immunofluorescence (IIF) is widely utilized as a diagnostic tool via image analysis, which can reveal the presence of autoimmune diseases by finding antibodies in the patient serum. In IIF, the human larynx carcinoma (HEp-2) substrate, which bonds with serum antibodies, thus forming a molecular complex, is applied, and recognition of the HEp-2 cell pattern can then be used to identify antinuclear autoantibodies (ANA). Since it is effective for diagnosing autoimmune diseases [1, 2], the demand for applying IIF image analysis in diagnostic tests is increasing. However, the practical image analysis method for IIF still remains subjective, which not only need a highly specialized and experienced technician or physician to achieve acceptable diagnostic results, but also too much of the physician's time. Furthermore, because the physician is provided with insufficient quantitative information and the IIF images differ according to the different illumination conditions and reading systems, there exists an almost 10% variance in the results of the simple task of positive/negative intensity recognition, and a more than 20% variance in the classification of the staining pattern [3]. Motivated by this fact, recent research efforts have been directed toward the development of a computer-aided-diagnosis (CAD) system for supporting the IIF diagnostic procedure, which focus mainly on image acquisition [4, 5], segmentation [6–8], fluorescence intensity classification [9], and staining cell pattern recognition [8, 10–14]. In this study, we explore primarily the identification of the HEp-2 staining cell pattern in IIF images using the progressive techniques developed in the computer vision and machine learning fields. Several attempts to achieve automatic recognition of the HEp-2 staining pattern have been made. Perner et al. [8] proposed extracting the texture and statistics features for cell image representation, and combined this with a decision tree model for HEp-2 cell image classification. This approach can achieve an approximately 75% recognition rate. Soda and Iannello [12] investigated a multiple expert system (MES) in which an ensemble of classifiers was combined in a fusion way to label the patterns of single cells. In their study, the wavelet method was used to extract features and select the effective statistics and spectral measurements from those that were extracted. However, research in the field of IIF image analysis is still in its early stages, and there is still great potential for improving the performance of the HEp-2 staining cell recognition further. In addition, although several approaches have been proposed, they have usually been developed and tested on different private datasets under varying conditions, such as image acquisition according to different criteria, different staining patterns, and so on. Therefore, it is difficult to compare the effectiveness of different approaches because they were evaluated over different datasets.

In this study, we aim to achieve automatic recognition of six HEp-2 staining patterns in an open HEp-2 dataset, which was recently released for the second HEp-2 cells classification contest at ICIP2013. In the first HEp-2 cells classification contest, which took place at ICIP2012, it was shown that the local binary pattern (LBP) and its extended versions, such as Rotation Invariant Co-occurrence LBP (RICLBP) [15] for cell image representation, can achieve a promising HEp-2 cell classification performance [3]. In addition, in the second HEp-2 cells classification contest at ICIP2013 it was proved that the combination of another extended LBP version, Pairwise Rotation Invariant Co-occurrence LBP (PRICoLBP) [16], and Bag-of-Features (BOF) [17] with a Sift descriptor [18] achieves the best recognition results. LBP [19–21] characterizes each 3×3 local patch (microstructure) into a binary series by comparing the surrounding pixel intensity with that of the center one, which sets the bit of a surrounding pixel as 1 if its intensity is larger than the center one; otherwise as 0. Then, we can obtain an 8-bit binary series from a 0-255 LBP value for each focused pixel (the center pixel). The image representation can be extracted as the histogram of the LBP value in a cell image. However, the LBP value retains the information only when the surrounding pixel intensity is greater than that of the center one, and then, the quantitative difference between them is lost as a result of the binary coding in LBP. Therefore, it is possible for quite different local structures (patches) to be represented as the same LBP value, which means the LBP is very limited in terms of representing the local structure given the fixed approximate quantization of the feature space as a binary pattern. In addition, local binary pattern (local structure) distribution is commonly represented using a histogram, and hence, is restricted to the use of low-order statistics. In contrast to these previous works, in our work we aims to realize a method for extracting highly-discriminant features from HEp-2 cell images by exploring a robust local descriptor inspired by Weber's law. The investigated local descriptor is based on the fact that human perception for distinguishing a pattern depends not only on the absolute intensity of the stimulus but also on the relative variance of the stimulus. Therefore, we firstly transform the original stimulus (the images in our study) into a differential excitation-domain according to Weber's law, and then explore a local patch, also called as micro-Texton, in the transformed domain as Weber local descriptor (WLD). Furthermore, we propose characterizing the Weber local descriptor of HEp-2 cell images adaptively as a Gaussian mixture model (GMM) [22, 23], and we explore the WLD high-order statistics for cell image representation. Within the assumed model, we can achieve data-driven partitioning of the WLD space using parametric mixture models with parameters learned using training data to represent the distribution of the WLD extracted from an image. The extracted weighted histogram (distribution) of the local descriptor (here, WLD) [24], which is widely used as image representation for generic image classification, represents the mean probabilities of all the WLDs belonging to the previously learned models, and includes only low-order statistics, which can be called 0th-order statistics. Furthermore, in order to represent the image more efficiently, we explore the high-order statistics of the WLD in the learned model, which are the deviation (gradient) statistics of the mean and variance parameters of GMM and also can be called the first and second statistics. The concatenated vector of the simple histogram and the deviation statistics in the learned model is used for image representation. Therefore, the coding of vectors is intrinsically adapted to the recognition task, and the computations involved remain very simple despite their strength. Using the high-order coded vector of adaptive WLD space, we simply apply a linear SVM [25], instead of the nonlinear one widely used for classification to achieve acceptable results, for HEp-2 cell recognition. The flowchart of our proposed strategy is shown in Fig. 1.

Our primary contributions are four-fold: (1) exploring a simple, yet powerful local descriptor, called Weber local descriptor, for a local structure representation, which is inspired by a psychological law: Weber's law, called as Weber local descriptors (WLD) (2) the characterization of the WLD as a GMM, which can adaptively achieve data-driven partitioning of WLD space, is examined; (3) a method for extracting not only low-order (distribution of the WLD) but also high-order statistics (gradient of the mean and variance of the learned GMM) for image representation, which is significantly more discriminant for classification, is described; (4) Experimental validation that the proposed high-order statistics can greatly improve the recognition performance as compared with the conventional LBP and its extensions, RICLBP and PRICoLBP representation, is presented. Experimental results for the open HEp-2 cell dataset used at the ICIP2013 contest show that the variability of the recognition performance achieved by our proposed strategy is even significantly less than the observed intra-laboratory variability for both positive and intermediate intensity

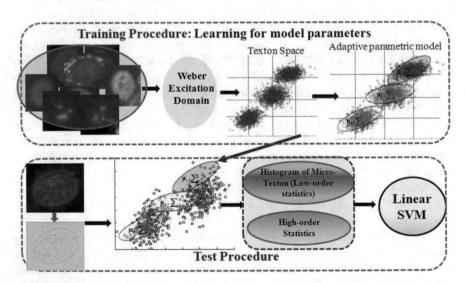

Fig. 1 Proposed adaptive WLD space model for HEp-2 cell image recognition. The upper row shows the learning procedure for the model parameters in GMM. The lower row shows the extraction of image features based on the learned GMM model and HEp-2 staining pattern recognition

cell types. Our proposed extraction framework of image representation is shown in Fig. 1.

The paper is organized as follows. In Sect. 2, medical context used in our experiments is described. Section 3 introduces the basic micro-Texton space for local structure representation inspired by Weber's law, and the characterized WLD space modeled with mixture Gaussian. Section 4 describes the underlying principle of high-order statistics of the parameter models, which is also called a fisher kernel, and the implementation of the coded vector in the learned adaptive WLD space. Experimental results and conclusions are given in Sects. 5 and 6, respectively.

2 Medical Context

In ANA tests, the HEp-2 substrateis, in general, applied, and both fluorescence intensity and staining pattern need to be classified, which is a challenging task that affects the reliability of IIF diagnosis. For classifying fluorescent intensity, the guidelines established by the Center for Disease Control and Prevention in Atlanta, Georgia (CDC) [26] suggest semi-quantitative scoring be performed independently by two physician IIF experts. The score ranges from 0 to 4+ according to the intensity: negative (0), very subdued fluorescence (1+), defined pattern but diminished fluorescence (2+), less brilliant green (3+), and brilliant green or maximal fluorescence (4+). The values are relative to the intensity of a negative and a positive control. The cell with positive intensity allows the physician to check the correctness of the preparation process, whereas that with negative intensity represents the auto-fluorescence level of the slide under examination. To reduce the variability of multiple readings, Rigon et al. [27] recently proposed classifying the fluorescence intensity into three classes, named negative, intermediate, and positive, by statistically analyzing the variability between several physicians' fluorescence intensity classification.

The open ICIP2013 HEp-2 dataset includes two intensity types of HEp-2 cells, intermediate and positive, and the purpose of the research is to recognize the staining pattern given the intensity types (intermediate or positive). The studied staining patterns primarily include six classes:

(1) Homogeneous: characterized by a diffuse staining of the interphase nuclei and staining of the chromatin of mitotic cells;
(2) Speckled: characterized by a granular nuclear staining of the interphase cell nuclei, which then consists of fine and coarse speckled patterns;
(3) Nucleolar: characterized by clustered large granules in the nucleoli of interphase cells that tend toward homogeneity, with fewer than six granules per cell;
(4) Centromere: characterized by several discrete speckles (~40–60) distributed throughout the interphase nuclei and characteristically found in the condensed nuclear chromatin during mitosis as a bar of closely associated speckles;

(5) Golgi: also called the Golgi apparatus, is one of the first organelles to be discovered and observed in detail. It is composed of stacks of membrane-bound structures known as cisternae;

(6) NuMem: Abbreviated from nuclear membrane, characterized as a fluorescent ring around the cell nucleus and are produced by anti-gp210 and anti-p62 antibodies.

In the open ICIP2013 HEp-2 cell dataset, there are more than 10000 images, each showing a single cell, which were obtained from 83 training IIF images by cropping the bounding box of the cell. The detailed information about the different staining patterns is shown in Table 1, and some example images for all six staining patterns of the positive and intermediate intensity types are shown in Fig. 2. Using the provided HEp-2 cell images and their corresponding patterns, we can extract the features that are effective for image representation, and learn a classifier (or a mapping function) using the extracted features of cell images and the corresponding staining patterns. Using the constructed classifier (the mapping function), the staining pattern can automatically be predicted given any HEp-2 cell image. In the classification procedure, the method used to extract the discriminant feature for cell image representation has a significant effect on the recognition performance. Next, we describe in detail the feature extraction strategy for cell image representation.

Table 1 Cell image number for different staining patterns and different intensity types

	Homogeneous	Speckled	Nucleolar	Centromere	NuMem	Golgi
Positive	1087	1457	934	1387	943	347
Intermediate	1407	1374	1664	1364	1265	377

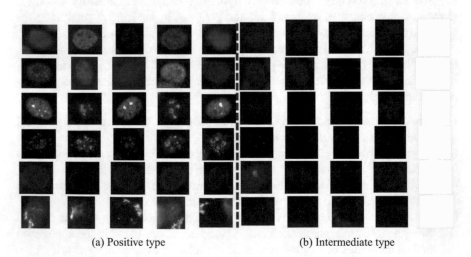

(a) Positive type   (b) Intermediate type

Fig. 2 Example images of six HEp-2 staining patterns of both positive and intermediate intensity types. **a** Positive intensity type; **b** intermediate intensity type

3 Micro-Structure Representation in Differential Excitation Domain

Studies in the computer vision field have shown that texture analysis can be implemented on the processed images and the statistics of microstructures by using the learned distribution of filter bank (a number of filters or wavelets) responses [28–30]. Recent research [31, 32] showed that it is possible to discriminate between textures using pixel neighborhoods as small as a 3 × 3 pixel region. Awate etc. [33] explored nonparametric neighborhood statistics and manifested promising performance for texture segmentation. Pietikinen et al. [32, 34] showed that despite the global structure of the textures, very good discrimination can be achieved by exploiting the distributions of such pixel neighborhoods. Therefore, the exploitation of these microstructures for representing images in the distributions of local descriptors has gained much attention and has led to state-of-the-art performances [33–36] for different classification and segmentation problems in computer vision. The system proposed by Foggia et al. [14] and the recognition system submitted in [3] for HEp-2 staining patterns achieved an improved recognition performance. In these studies, the statistics of microstructures (local binary pattern-LBP) was also investigated, and it was proved that it is possible to recognize the HEp-2 staining patterns automatically. However, these methods suffer from several important limitations, such as the use of fixed quantization of the input vector for pruning volumes in the feature space, and the restricted use of low-order statistics with a feature histogram. In addition, the general local descriptors are extracted from the original (raw) image space, and then there exist some gaps to the perception excitation-domain of human being. Therefore, this section explores micro-structure representation in a differential excitation domain, which would adaptively be transformed according to human perception process inspired by Weber's law. Next, we first introduce the basic local-structure representation using local binary pattern and the adaptively normalized differential vector between the surrounding pixels and the center one based on Weber's law, called the Weber local descriptor (WLD), and then, adaptively characterize the WLD space as a parametric probability process using a GMM.

3.1 Local Binary Pattern

The local binary pattern operator is an image operator that transforms an image into an array of integer labels describing the small-scale appearance of the image. These labels or their statistics, most commonly the histogram, are then used for further image analysis. Given an image $\mathbf{I}$, let us denote the ith pixel intensity I_i at (x_i, y_i) and its surrounding pixel intensities in a 3 × 3 region by I_i^j ($j = 0, 1, \ldots, 7$). The LBP operator sets the threshold of the difference between I_i and I_i^j as 0 or 1 (binary), and the 8 binary numbers are combined as a decimal number for labeling the i_{th} pixel. Figure 3 shows a specific example of extracting the LBP value of a focused pixel.

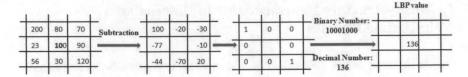

Fig. 3 Example of the basic LBP operator

The derived binary numbers are called Local Binary Patterns or LBP codes. Mathematically, the resulting LBP of the ith pixel at (x_i, y_i) can be expressed in decimal form as

$$LBP(x_i, y_i) = \sum_{j=0}^{7} T(I_i^j - I_i)2^j \qquad (1)$$

where the function $T(z)$ is a threshold function, defined as

$$T(z) = \begin{cases} 1 \text{ if } z \geq 0 \\ 0 \text{ if } z < 0 \end{cases} \qquad (2)$$

By the definition above, the LBP operator is invariant to the monotonic gray-scale transformations, which preserves the pixel intensity order in local neighborhoods. The histogram of LBP labels can be exploited as a texture descriptor. In addition, in some works, the general LBP was extended to Co-occurrence of LBP (CoLBP) [37] and the improved LBP, Pairwise Rotation Invariant Co-occurrence LBP (PRI-CoLBP) [16] for integrating the relation between different local patterns, which yield more promising performances than the conventional LBP. However, LBP code and its extended versions quantize each different intensity between the surrounding pixels and the center one into only two intensity levels, 0 or 1, which means that it is possible to code two very different local structures into one and the same LBP value, and two similar local structures into very different LBP values, as shown in Fig. 4. Therefore, the LBP operator and its extensions are very limited for representing the local structures of images, and thus, the formed histogram of the global image also is not sufficiently discriminatory for image classification purposes.

3.2 Weber Local Descriptors

Weber's law: Ernst Heinrich Weber, an experimental psychologist in the 19th century, approached the study of the human response to a physical stimulus in a quantitative fashion, and observed that the ratio of the increment threshold to the background intensity is a constant [38]. This observation shows that the just-noticeable difference between two stimuli is proportional to the magnitude of the stimuli, which is well-known as Weber's law and can be formulated as:

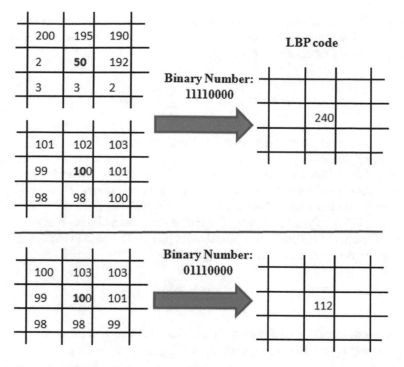

Fig. 4 Examples of LBP codes for two very different local structures, and two similar local structures

$$\frac{\triangle I}{I} = a \qquad (3)$$

where $\triangle I$ denotes the increment threshold (just noticeable difference for discrimination) and I denotes the initial stimulus intensity; a is known as the *weber fraction*, which indicates that the proportion on the left hand of the equation remains constant in spite of variance in I. Simply speaking, Weber's Law states that the size of the just noticeable difference (JND) is a constant proportion (a times) of the original stimulus value, which is the minimum amount that stimulus intensity must be changed in order to produce a noticeable variation in sensory experience.

Weber local descriptor: Weber's law states that the just noticeable difference (JND) is a constant proportion of the original stimulus magnitude, which corresponds to the perception excitation domain of human being. Thus this part describes how to transform the original (raw) image domain into a differential excitation domain, which would be suitable to human perception response, and then presents how to construct the local structure representation in the excitation domain. In order to transform the original image domain to the differential excitation domain of human perception, we use the intensity differences between its neighbors and a current (focused) pixel as the incremental threshold (changes) of it. Through this way, we aim to find the salient variations within an image, which can simulate the pattern perception of human beings. Firstly we calculate the difference between a current pixel and its neighbors using a filter s_0:

$$\triangle I_c = \sum_{i=0}^{p-1}(\triangle I_c^i) = \sum_{i=0}^{p-1}(I_c^i - I_c) \tag{4}$$

where I_c denotes the stimulus magnitude at position x_c, and I_c^i $(i = 0, 1, \ldots, p-1)$ is the ith neighbor of I_c, p is the number of neighbors. As stated in Weber's law, the ratio of the difference to the stimulus (intensity) of the current position would be directly affected if the human perception is activated or excitable. If we consider that the stimulus is also a filtered version from the original image domain with a filter which also has the size of 3×3 with 1 in the center point and 0 in other points. The output of stimulus is actually the original input image. The ratio of the difference to the stimulus is expressed as the following formula:

$$H_{ratio}(x_c) = \frac{\triangle I_c}{I_c} \tag{5}$$

In order to calculate the differential excitation of the current pixel $\xi(x_c)$, denoted as v_c, we employ the arctangent function on H_{ratio} as the following:

$$v_c = \xi(x_c) = \arctan[H_{ratio}(x_c)] = \arctan[\frac{\triangle I_c}{I_c}]$$

$$= \arctan[\sum_{i=0}^{p-1}\frac{(I_c^i - I_c)}{I_c}] \tag{6}$$

The procedure for transforming the original image domain to the differential excitation domain is shown in Fig. 5. It is obvious that the differential excitation $\xi(x_c)$ has a

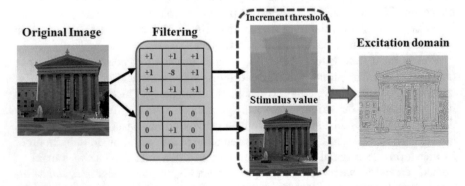

Fig. 5 Illustration of transforming the original image domain to the differential excitation domain

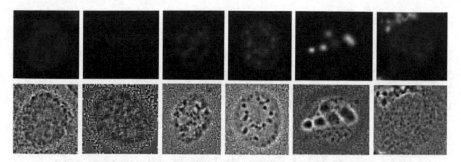

Fig. 6 Image samples in original image (up) and transformed excitation domains (down)

magnitude region $[-\frac{\pi}{2}, \frac{\pi}{2}]$, which can be directly applied for local pattern extraction in the excitation-domain and thus preserves more discrimination than only with the absolute value of $\xi(x_c)$. Intuitively, positive value of $\xi(x_c)$ simulates the case that the surroundings are lighter than the current pixel, and contrastively negative value of $\xi(x_c)$ simulates the one that the surroundings are darker than the current pixel. Some image examples from ICIP2013 HEp-2 competition datasets and their corresponding transformed excitation images are show in Fig. 6, which signifies some detected saliency patterns in the transformed excitation domain.

After transforming the original image domain to the differential excitation domain, we work with all possible $l \times l$, (l can be $3, 5, \ldots$, and so on) neighborhoods for micro structure representation, called Weber local descriptor: WLD, in the excitation image, i.e., $\mathbf{v}^c = \{v_c, v_c^1, v_c^2, \ldots, v_c^{l*l-1}\}$ where v_c is the the excitation magnitude of the center pixel and the rest are those of its ($l \times l - 1$)-neighbors. This WLD representation can capture the main salience pattern, which would activate human perception, and then will be much more discriminant for image representation. How to aggregate the large amount of micro-structure vector into a compact and discriminant vector for image representation would affect on the post-performance for image classification applications. The general approach [26] is to reduce the $l \times l$ local structure into a much lower-dimensional histogram vector, and then concatenate all local vectors from an image for the image representation. However, in order to achieve not so-high dimensional vectors, the divided local regions (structures) have to be constrained to a limited and fixed number for all processed images, and then, sometimes the size ($l \times l$) of local structures has to be set as large value for compact representation, which thus cannot preserve locality. Motivated by the works on image feature extraction in generic image classification that aggregate local descriptor extracted from original image domain into histogram such as BOF, LBP and so on, We propose to exploit the distribution $p(\mathbf{v}^c|\mathbf{I})$ of these WLD, for a given image, to represent the image. The following subsection gives the adaptive modeling of the proposed WLD.

4   Extraction of Image Representation for HEp-2 Cell

In this section, we aim to extract the discriminate features of HEp-2 cell images. We propose to exploit the distribution $p(\mathbf{v}^c|\mathbf{I})$ of the previous explored WLD, for a given HEp-2 image, to represent the image. The following subsection gives the adaptive modeling of the proposed WLD.

4.1   The Adaptive WLD Space Modeled by Mixture Gaussian

Let's denote the WLD space samples as $\mathbf{X} = [\mathbf{x}_1, \mathbf{x}_2, \ldots, \mathbf{x}_T]$, with $\mathbf{x}_i \in \mathbf{R}^D$ and T being sample number, which are randomly selected from training images. In order to easily visualize, we take the first elements of the WLD space samples $\mathbf{X}$, and form the samples $\mathbf{X}^1$ of one-dimensional variable. By statistically analyzing the one-dimensional samples $\mathbf{X}^1$, the histogram shown in Fig. 7 is calculated, from which we can observe that there are multiple peaks (called as multimodal) in the histogram probability plot. As explored in the works [39, 40], the variable given the samples $\mathbf{X}^1$, which have a multi-modal histogram, can be modeled as a Gaussian mixture model (GMM). By assuming an independent and identical distribution among the elements of $\mathbf{x}_t$, the WLD space samples also can be modeled as the probability distribution like a multi-dimensional mixture model of Gaussian (GMM). With the assumed GMM model, we can formulate WLD sample space $\mathbf{X}$ as

Fig. 7 The histogram probability of one element of WLD samples

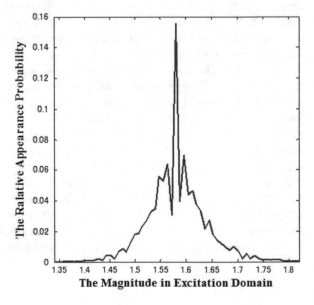

$$P(\mathbf{X}|\lambda) = \sum_{k=1}^{K} w_k N(\mathbf{X}|\mu_k, \Sigma_k)$$

$$= \sum_{k=1}^{K} w_k \frac{1}{(2\pi)^{\frac{D}{2}} |\Sigma_k|^{\frac{1}{2}}} exp\{-\frac{1}{2}(\mathbf{X} - \mu_k)^T \Sigma_k^{-1}(\mathbf{X} - \mu_k)\} \tag{7}$$

where λ are the parameters for formulating the probability function, in the Gaussian mixture model with K-components, denoted $\lambda = \{w_k, \mu_k, \Sigma_k, k = 1, \dots, K\}$. w_k, μ_k, Σ_k are the mixture weight, mean vector and covariance matrix of Gaussian k, respectively.

Given the training WLD space samples, we can adaptively learn the prior parameters $\lambda = \{w_k, \mu_k, \Sigma_k, k = 1, \dots, K\}$ of GMM using Expectation maximization (EM) strategy [24, 41] in the following three steps.

Step 1: Take initial guesses for the parameters $\lambda = \{w_k, \mu_k, \Sigma_k, k = 1, \dots, K\}$

Step 2 (Expectation Step): compute the responsibilities (posterior probability for each training samples):

$$\gamma_{t,k} = \frac{w_k P(k|\mathbf{x}_t, \lambda)}{\sum_{k=1}^{K} w_k P(k|\mathbf{x}_t, \lambda)}$$

$$= \frac{w_k \frac{1}{(2\pi)^{\frac{D}{2}} |\Sigma_k|^{\frac{1}{2}}} exp\{-\frac{1}{2}(\mathbf{x}_t - \mu_k)^T \Sigma_k^{-1}(\mathbf{x}_t - \mu_k)\}}{\sum_{k=1}^{K} w_k \frac{1}{(2\pi)^{\frac{D}{2}} |\Sigma_k|^{\frac{1}{2}}} exp\{-\frac{1}{2}(\mathbf{x}_t - \mu_k)^T \Sigma_k^{-1}(\mathbf{x}_t - \mu_k)\}} \tag{8}$$

Step 3 (Maximization Step): compute the weighted means and variances:

$$\mu_k = \frac{\sum_{t=1}^{T} \gamma_{t,k} \mathbf{x}_t}{\sum_{t=1}^{T} \gamma_{t,k}} \tag{9}$$

$$\Sigma_k = \frac{\sum_{t=1}^{T} \gamma_{t,k} \mathbf{x}_t^2}{\sum_{t=1}^{T} \gamma_{t,k}} - \mu_k^2 \tag{10}$$

and then the mixture weight (the mixing probability):

$$w_k = \frac{1}{T} \sum_{t=1}^{T} \gamma_{t,k} \tag{11}$$

The expectation and maximization steps are repeated until reaching a predefined iteration number or satisfying the objective function. Then we can achieve the parameters $\lambda = \{w_k, \mu_k, \Sigma_k, k = 1, \dots, K\}$ in GMM for fitting the training WLD samples. Figure 8 shows the simple uniformly quantization and the fitted model using GMM on a two-dimensional data (50000 samples), which are the first two elements of the

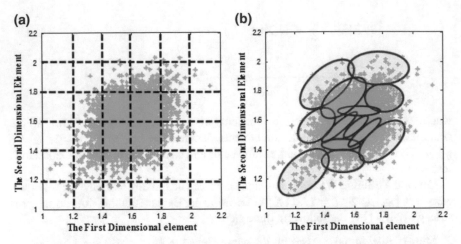

Fig. 8 The modeled space of a two-dimensional data. **a** The uniformly quantization space with dot line; **b** the adaptively learned space with the generative probability model (GMM)

WLD samples from the HEp-2 cell dataset. We observe from Fig. 8 that some quantized regions in the uniform quantization, the partitions of which are represented by the dashed line, contain almost no samples, and more than half (23) of the 36 regions are ineffective for representing the samples. However, the components of the parametric GMM, adaptively learned from the sample space, intensively locate the massed sample regions, and the variation regions of the 13 components of the learned GMM cover more than 99.9% samples (49950 out of 50000 samples). Thus we can easily conclude that the learned parameter of GMM in Fig. 8b can better model the input space samples than the uniformly quantization shown in Fig. 8a. Further, we implement uniformly quantization and the data-driven GMM model on the randomly selected WLD samples from 100 food images and 100 HEp-2 cell image, which are used for validating our proposed framework in the following experiment section, respectively. In our experiments, we set l as 3, and then produce 8-dimensional WLD space. For uniformly quantization, even only using binary quantization of each element in the 8-dimensional WLD samples will result in $2^8 = 256$ patterns, and the ternary quantization obtains $3^8 = 6561$. With GMM model, we can freely set the Gaussian component number such as $32, 64, 128 \ldots$. For comparison, we compute the 256 representative patterns of the binary (uniformly) quantization, which is the mean of the WLD sample belonging to each distinct pattern index, and use the means of GMM model as the representative patterns. The reconstruction errors for all WLD samples to their assigned representative patterns are calculated using different models: binary quantization (BQ: 256 patterns) and GMM (32, 64,128 models), and the histogram probabilities with different reconstruction errors are shown in Fig. 9a and b for the WLD samples of food and HEp-2 cell images, respectively. From Fig. 9 we observe that the probabilities with small error even using small number of Gaussian components are higher than those with larger bin quantization (BQ256), and

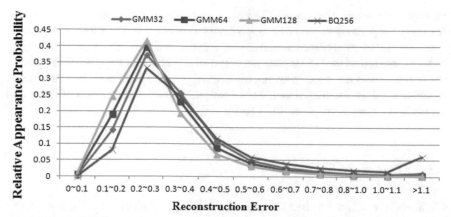

(a) The probability of reconstruction errors of WLD samples for HEp-2 cell imagess

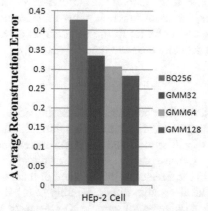

(b) The average reconstruction errors

Fig. 9 The reconstruction errors of WLD samples from HEp-2 cell images

otherwise the probabilities with larger error using GMM are lower than BQ256 for both types of images. Figure 9c gives the average reconstruction errors of different models (BQ:256; GMM:32, 64, 128), and manifests the average errors using GMM are lower than the binary quantization.

5 High-Order Statistics of Adaptive WLD Model

In the above section, the GMM is used for modeling training WLD space samples, which are randomly selected from all possible appearing pattern images in a specific application. Therefore the learned model parameters are generic to WLD space from all types of images. For the WLD samples of a given image, the GMM with the learned prior parameters would have some deviations from it. Therefore, it is possible to use the distribution of the learned model, and the deviations to the first and second order parameters of the WLD space samples as the features for the given image. Next, we will describe the underlying principle of high-order statistics from parametric models, which is also named as fisher kernel, and the implementation of the coded vector in the learned adaptive WLD space.

5.1 The Fisher Kernel

Let $\mathbf{X} = \{\mathbf{x}_t, t = 1, \ldots, T\}$ be a T observations (samples) with $\mathbf{x}_t \in R^D$, and let $P_\lambda(\mathbf{X})$ be a probability density function, which models the generative process of elements in R^D. $\lambda = [\lambda_1, \lambda_2, \ldots, \lambda_L]^T \in R^L$ denotes the parameter vector in the generative model of $P_\lambda(\mathbf{X})$. In statistics, the score function, which represents the deviation direction of the model parameters for better fitting the data, is given by the gradient of the log-likelihood of the data based on the model [42, 43];

$$\mathbf{G}_\lambda^{\mathbf{X}} = \triangle_\lambda \log P_\lambda(\mathbf{X}) \tag{12}$$

This gradient can describe the contribution of the individual parameters to the generative process. With the given data set $\mathbf{X}$, it also describes how the parameters of the generative model P_λ should be modified to fit them better, and then can be considered as a specific property (representative features) of the given data set. Regardless of the samples number of the dataset $\mathbf{X}$, the gradient of the log-likelihood of the generative probability model always has dimensionality L: $\mathbf{G}_\lambda^{\mathbf{X}} \in R^L$. Therefore, the score function transforms a variable length sample $\mathbf{X}$ into a fixed length vector, whose size is only dependent on the number of parameters in the generative model.

From the theory of information geometry [44], a parametric family of distributions $\mathbf{P} = \{P_\lambda, \lambda \in \Lambda\}$ can be regarded as a Riemanninan manifold $\mathbf{M}_\Lambda$ with a local metric given by the Fisher information Matrix (FIM) $\mathbf{F}_\lambda \in R^{L \times L}$:

$$\mathbf{F}_\lambda = E_{\mathbf{X} \sim P_\lambda}[\mathbf{G}_\lambda^{\mathbf{X}^T} \mathbf{G}_\lambda^{\mathbf{X}}] \tag{13}$$

For measuring the similarity between two sample sets $\mathbf{X}$ and $\mathbf{Y}$, the fisher kernel (FK) is proposed [45] as the following formulation according to the above observation:

$$\mathbf{K}_{FK}(\mathbf{X}, \mathbf{Y}) = \mathbf{G}_\lambda^{\mathbf{X}^T} \mathbf{F}_\lambda^{-1} \mathbf{G}_\lambda^{\mathbf{Y}} \tag{14}$$

From Eq. (13), it is obvious that $\mathbf{F}_\lambda$ is positive semi-definite, and its inverse has similar property. Using the Cholesky decomposition $\mathbf{F}_\lambda^{-1} = \check{\mathbf{F}}_\lambda^T \check{\mathbf{F}}_\lambda$, the fisher kernel in Eq. (14) can be rewritten explicitly as a dot-product:

$$\mathbf{K}_{FK}(\mathbf{X}, \mathbf{Y}) = \{\check{\mathbf{G}}_\lambda^\mathbf{X}\}^T \check{\mathbf{G}}_\lambda^\mathbf{Y} \tag{15}$$

with

$$\check{\mathbf{G}}_\lambda^\mathbf{X} = \check{\mathbf{F}}_\lambda \mathbf{G}_\lambda^\mathbf{X} = \check{\mathbf{F}}_\lambda \nabla_\lambda \log P_\lambda(\mathbf{X}) \tag{16}$$

This normalized gradient vector is also called as the Fisher Vector (FV) of the data set $\mathbf{X}$. The dimensionality of the FV $\check{\mathbf{G}}_\lambda^\mathbf{X}$ is equal to that of the gradient vector $\mathbf{G}_\lambda^\mathbf{X}$. If utility of the fisher kernel $\mathbf{K}_{FK}$ as the kernel machine in a discriminative classification model, which is inherently non-linear, would be equivalent to a linear kernel machine with $\check{\mathbf{G}}_\lambda^\mathbf{X}$ as feature vector. Therefore, the benefit of the explicit formulation with $\check{\mathbf{G}}_\lambda^\mathbf{X}$ as feature vector is that, a linear classifier can be used very efficiently.

5.2   Coded Vector with Higher Order Statistics

As we introduced in Sect. 5, we model the WLD space of processed images as GMM, and learn the adaptive parameters $\lambda = w_k, \mu_k, \Sigma_k, k = 1, \dots, K$ of a generative probability model $P(\mathbf{X}|\lambda) = \sum_{k=1}^K w_k N(\mathbf{X}|\mu_k, \Sigma_k)$ using the randomly selected WLD samples from all types of images in a specific application. Each Gaussian represents a representative word of the WLD prototypes (vocabulary): w_k encodes the relative frequency of WLD word k, μ_k the mean of the WLD word and Σ_k the variation around the mean. Given WLD samples $\mathbf{X} = \{\mathbf{x}_t, t = 1, \dots, T\}$ of any image, we will try to modify the generative model learned from training images to better fit it, which means to extract the gradient of generative model to the parameter $\lambda = w_k, \mu_k, \Sigma_k, k = 1, \dots, K$. For convenient computation, we assume that the weights are subject to the constraint:

$$\sum_{k=1}^K w_k = 1 \tag{17}$$

and with D-dimensional WLD space, we assume the covariance matrix is diagonal, denoted as $\Sigma_k = diag(\Sigma_k)$.

   Given any WLD sample $\mathbf{x}_t$ in the dataset $\mathbf{X}$ of an image, the occupancy probability to the kth Gaussian can be formulated as:

$$\gamma_t(k) = \frac{w_k P(k|\mathbf{x}_t, \lambda)}{\sum_{k=1}^K w_k P(k|\mathbf{x}_t, \lambda)} \tag{18}$$

In order to avoid enforcing explicitly the constraints in Eq. (17), we take a new relative parameter α_k to adopt soft-max formalism for defining w_k Then

$$w_k = \frac{exp(\alpha_k)}{\sum_{j=1}^K exp(\alpha_j)} \tag{19}$$

After re-parametrization using α_k, the straightforward deducing of the gradient to the parameter $\lambda = \alpha_k, \mu_k, \Sigma_k, k = 1, \ldots, K$ can be formulated as:

$$\frac{\partial P(\mathbf{X}|\lambda)}{\partial \alpha_k} = \sum_{t=1}^{T} [\gamma_t(k) - w_k], \tag{20}$$

$$\frac{\partial P(\mathbf{X}|\lambda)}{\partial \mu_k^d} = \sum_{t=1}^{T} \gamma_t(k) [\frac{x_t^d - \mu_k^d}{(\sigma_k^d)^2}], \tag{21}$$

$$\frac{\partial P(\mathbf{X}|\lambda)}{\partial \sigma_k^d} = \sum_{t=1}^{T} \gamma_t(k) [\frac{(x_t^d - \mu_k^d)^2}{(\sigma_k^d)^3} - \frac{1}{\sigma_k^d}], \tag{22}$$

where the superscript d denotes the dth dimension of the input vector $\mathbf{x}_t$. The final fisher vector is just the concatenation of the partial derivative with respect to all the parameters.

After obtaining the gradients, the remaining question is how to compute the diagonal of the Fisher information matrix $\mathbf{F}$. Let us denote the diagonal element of $\mathbf{F}$ to the parameters α_k, μ_k^d, and σ_k^d as $f_{\alpha_k}, f_{\mu_k^d}$ and $f_{\sigma_k^d}$, the approximation can be formulated as:

$$f_{\alpha_k} = T w_k, \tag{23}$$

$$f_{\mu_k^d} = \frac{T w_k}{(\sigma_k^d)^2}, \tag{24}$$

$$f_{\sigma_k^d} = \frac{2 T w_k}{(\sigma_k^d)^2}, \tag{25}$$

Then the normalized Fisher vector can be computed by multiplying the gradients and the root inverse of the corresponding Fisher elements for each sample as the following:

$$\check{G}_{\alpha_k}^{\mathbf{X}} = \frac{1}{\sqrt{w_k}} \sum_{t=1}^{T} [\gamma_t(k) - w_k], \tag{26}$$

$$\check{G}_{\mu_k^d}^{\mathbf{X}} = \frac{1}{\sqrt{w_k}} \sum_{t=1}^{T} \gamma_t(k) [\frac{x_t^d - \mu_k^d}{\sigma_k^d}], \tag{27}$$

$$\check{G}_{\sigma_k^d}^{\mathbf{X}} = \frac{1}{\sqrt{w_k}} \sum_{t=1}^{T} \gamma_t(k) \frac{1}{\sqrt{2}} [\frac{(x_t^d - \mu_k^d)^2}{(\sigma_k^d)^2} - 1], \tag{28}$$

The final Fisher vector is the concatenation of the gradient $\check{G}^{X}_{\alpha}$, $\check{G}^{X}_{\mu^{d}_{k}}$ and $\check{G}^{X}_{\sigma^{d}_{k}}$ for all $d = 1, 2, \ldots, D$ dimension of input feature (WLD) vector and $k = 1, 2, \ldots, K$ Gaussian components, and then is of dimension $(2D + 1)K$.

To avoid the dependence on the sample size, we normalize the resulted Fisher vector by the sample (WLD) size extracted from any given image as the following:

$$\check{\mathbf{G}}^{X}_{\lambda} = \frac{1}{T}\check{\mathbf{G}}^{X}_{\lambda} \tag{29}$$

With the Fisher vector for an image representation, we can use a linear classifier such as a linear support vector machine (SVM), for acceptable recognition performance.

6 Experiments

Using HEp-2 cell images of two types of intensity (Intermediate and Positive), we validated the recognition performance achieved by applying our proposed framework with local descriptors in raw image and the transformed excitation domain, respectively, the conventional local binary pattern (LBP) and its extended versions, RICLBP [15] and the recently developed PRICoLBP [16], which have been proven to yield the best recognition performance for the cell dataset [3]. In the open HEp-2 cell database, each pattern has a different number of available cell images, as shown in Table 1. It can be seen that the 'Golgi' pattern has much fewer available cell images than the other patterns. Thus, in our experiment, we randomly selected 600 cell images from the 5 patterns, excluding 'Golgi' and 300 from 'Golgi' as training images, and the remainder were used as testing images for both 'Positive' and 'Intermediate' intensity types. The linear SVM was used as the classifier because of its effectiveness as compared with other classifiers, such as K-nearest neighbor, and its efficiency as compared with a nonlinear SVM, which requires much more time to classify a sample. In addition, for LBP and its extended RICLBP and PRICoLBP histograms, we pre-processed them using the square root operation for classification with a linear SVM:

$$\mathbf{P}' = [p'_1, p'_2, \ldots, p'_L] = [\sqrt{p_1}, \sqrt{p_2}, \ldots, \sqrt{p_L}] \tag{30}$$

where $\mathbf{P} = [p_1, p_2, \ldots, p_L]$ is the raw histogram of LBP or PRICoLBP with dimension L, and $\mathbf{P}'$ is the normalized feature for linear SVM. It has been shown that pre-processing of the LBP, RICLBP, or PRICoLBP histogram in a linear classification model is equivalent to applying a nonlinear kernel, the Helinger kernel, for the raw histogram, and is expected to produce more promising results with the efficient linear SVM. In PRICoLBP, we used different radii (1 or 2) of neighbors and different template numbers (1 or 2: two configurations, a or b), denoted as PRICoLBP_r1t1, PRICoLBP_r1t2a, PRICoLBP_r1t2b, PRICoLBP_r2t1, PRICoLBP_r2t2a, and PRICoLBP_r2t2b, respectively, for feature extraction. Our proposed strategy using

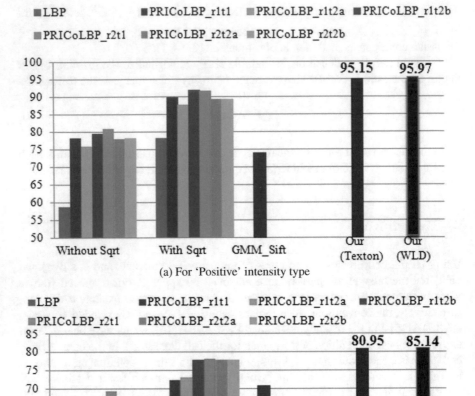

(a) For 'Positive' intensity type

(b) For 'Intermediate' intensity type

Fig. 10 Comparison of recognition performances of our proposed strategy and the state-of-the-art methods

the microt-texton and the local descriptor, SIFT [17, 18] (instead of texton, called 'GMM_Sift'), which is widely used for generic object recognition in computer vision, was combined with linear SVM without any pre-processing for cell pattern recognition.

The above procedure was repeated 20 times, and the final results are the average recognition performance of the 20 runs, calculated as the percentages of properly classified cell images for all test samples. The comparitive recognition rates for both

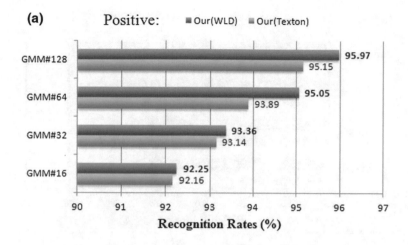

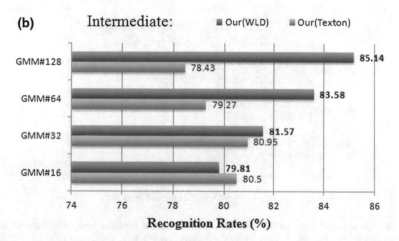

Fig. 11 The compared results with different numbers of GMM components using the micro-structures (3 × 3) in raw image and transformed excitation domains for classifying different HEp-2 cell patterns. **a** For the 'Intermediate' type dataset; **b** for the 'Intermediate' type dataset

'Positive' and 'Intermediate' intensity types using the non-sqrt or sqrt LBP, PRI-CoLBP (denoted as 'Without Sqrt' and 'With Sqrt') with different parameters, and the proposed strategy with the local patch (3 × 3) in raw image and the transformed excitation domain (called as Texton and WLD, respectively) or the widely used SIFT descriptor (denoted as 'GMM_Sift') are shown in Fig. 10. It can be clearly seen that our proposed strategy can outperform LBP, RICLBP, and PRICoLBP with different parameters and the modeling strategy of 'Sift' descriptors for both 'Positive' and 'Intermediate' intensity types.

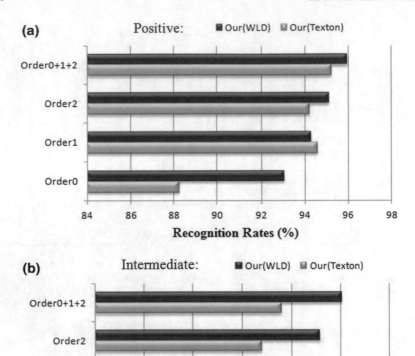

Fig. 12 The compared results with different orders of GMM statistics using the micro-structures (3×3) in raw image and transformed excitation domains for classifying different HEp-2 cell patterns. **a** For the 'Intermediate' type dataset; **b** for the 'Intermediate' type dataset

In the following, we show the effect of the GMM component number (K described in Sect. 3). As the GMM component number increases, the vector length increases proportionally. Although lower numbers of components lead to a compact representation, larger numbers usually lead to better quantization of the space and hence representation that are more discriminant. The average recognition rates for the two types of HEp-2 dataset are shown in Fig. 11 with different numbers of components. Using 3×3 local patch in raw and excitation domain, we observe that the performance for the 'Positive' intensity type increases with the number of components, and can achieve an average rate of 95.5% with 128 components and 92.95% with 16 components, which is much better than the intra-laboratory rate. However, for the 'Intermediate' intensity type, the proposed strategy with only a lower number

Table 2 The confusion matrix for classifying different HEp-2 cell patterns in the 'Positive' and 'Intermediate' type dataset using our proposed strategy with texton size 3×3

(a) Confusion matrix for Positive intensity type

%	Homogeneous	Speckled	Nucleolar	Centromere	NuMem	Golgi
Homogeneous	**96.42**	1.54	0.10	0	1.57	0.37
Speckled	5.06	**93.61**	0.06	0.54	0.65	0.082
Nucleolar	0.54	0.84	**94.97**	1.60	0.07	1.98
Centromere	0.28	1.65	1.52	**96.07**	0	0.47
NuMem	3.25	0.35	0	0	**96.36**	0.04
Golgi	1.38	3.62	5.21	0.53	1.70	**87.55**

(b) Confusion matrix for Intermediate intensity type

	Homogeneous	Speckled	Nucleolar	Centromere	NuMem	Golgi
Homogeneous	**78.81**	8.55	5.20	0.87	5.33	1.24
Speckled	6.46	**78.55**	7.88	2.58	3.88	0.65
Nucleolar	3.67	7.61	**76.97**	0.75	5.17	5.82
Centromere	0.52	1.31	2.23	**95.41**	0.26	0.26
NuMem	7.07	3.16	6.91	0.15	**81.20**	0.50
Golgi	5.19	5.19	12.99	5.19	1.30	**70.13**

of components, 32 in 3×3 micro-texton, can achieve the best performance rate, 80.95%, which decreases slightly (by 1–2%) when the number is increased to 64 and 128. One possible reason for this phenomenon is that the intensity magnitude is very low in the 'Intermediate' type, which leads to a lower signal-to-noise ratio (SNR). If we increase the component number in GMM for modeling the micro-texton, it is possible that some components model only the noise information, which results in a decrease in the performance as the number of components increases. Next, the effectiveness of the statistics with different orders (the 0th, the first and second orders) is validated by the recognition performances for 'Positive' and 'Intermediate' intensity types shown in Fig. 12, where it can be seen that the concatenated vector of all statistics can achieve the best results for both types ('Positive' type with 128 Gaussian components; 'Intermediate' with 32 Gaussian components). In addition, it can clearly be seen that our proposed strategy even with only low-order statistics (0th-order, denoted by 'order0') can markedly improve the recognition rates of HEp-2 cell patterns as compared to the LBP histogram, and achieves better or comparable results with only one-order statistics as compared to RICLBP and PRICoLBP features. Figure 12 demonstrates that high-order are more discriminant than low-order statistics, and the concatenation of all, which will be used for the following experiments, can achieve the best recognition rates. Table 2a and b are the confusion tables of the detailed information for cell recognized patterns shown in Table 2a and b for 'Positive' and 'Intermediate' types, respectively. The tables show that the recognition rates for the 5 HEp-2 cell patterns, excluding 'Golgi' can achieve a better than 95% performance rate for the 'Positive', and more than 75% performance for 'Intermediate' type.

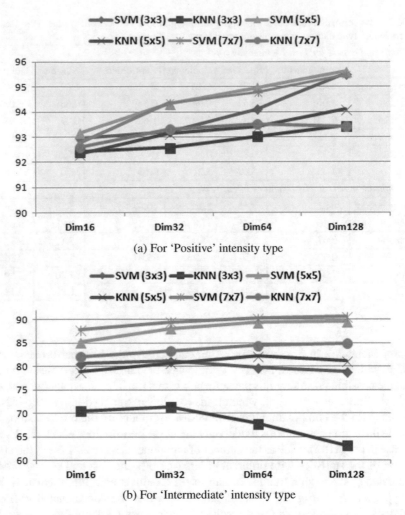

(a) For 'Positive' intensity type

(b) For 'Intermediate' intensity type

Fig. 13 The compared recognition rates of the proposed strategy using different classification methods and different number of GMM components over HEp-2 cell datasets

Further, we vary the texton size (i.e., from 3×3 to 5×5, 7×7) for extracting the high-order statistics, and conducted HEp-2 staining pattern recognition under the same experimental conditions. The comparative results are also shown in Fig. 13 for both 'Positive' and 'Intermediate' types. It is obvious that the using of larger size exton for 'Positive' type only has tiny improvement (i.e., less than 0.5 % for most cases), and most recognition accuracies with 7×7 exton even have little decreasing compared to the ones of 5×5 texton. However, for 'Intermediate' type, the performances with larger size extons can manifest a great improvement compared to 3×3 Texton; the recognition accuracies with 5×5, 7×7 sizes and 128 Gaussian components can reach 89.56 and 90.62% from about 80% with 3×3 texton.

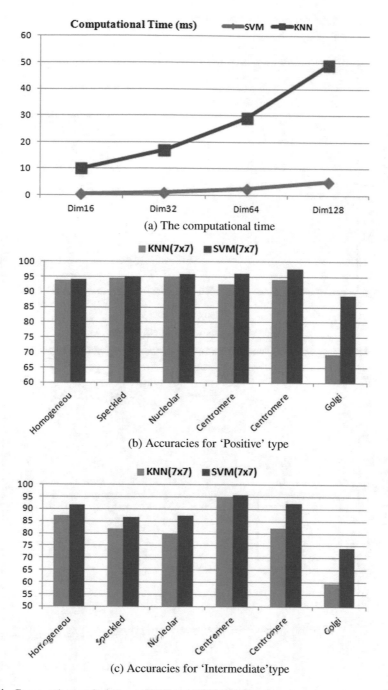

(a) The computational time

(b) Accuracies for 'Positive' type

(c) Accuracies for 'Intermediate'type

Fig. 14 Comparative results between KNN and SVM classifiers

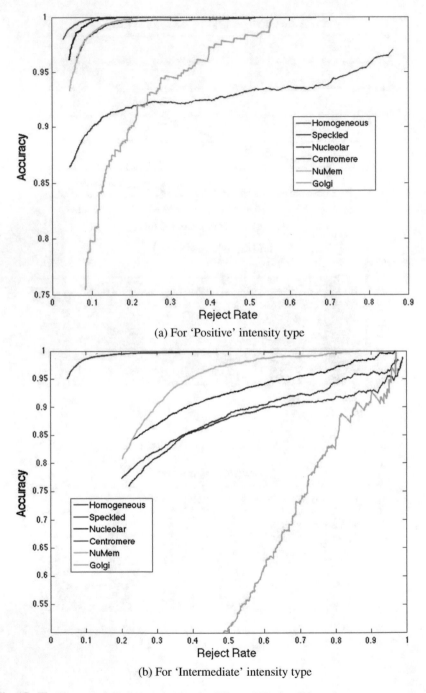

(a) For 'Positive' intensity type

(b) For 'Intermediate' intensity type

Fig. 15 The 'Accuracy'-'Reject rate' curve for different HEp-2 staining patterns

In addition, the recognition performances with K-nearest neighborhood (KNN) are also given in Fig. 13 for comparison, which show much lower accuracies than SVM classifier. However, since KNN classifier needs to calculate the distance with all samples in database, it is time-consuming; our used linear SVM can be more efficient after learning the classification model in training procedure. The compared computational time is shown in Fig. 14a, and the compared recognition rates for each staining pattern with KNN and SVM classifiers using 7×7 texton are given in Fig. 14b and c for 'Positive' and 'Intermediate' types, respectively.

To explore the confidence score of each sample to be classified as different HEp-2 cell patterns, we plotted the 'Reject rate'-'Accuracy' curves for all HEp-2 patterns. For example, there are N test samples in total, of which N_1 samples belong to the ith HEp-2 pattern. With our learned system, there exist M samples that are classified as the ith HEp-2 pattern, of which M_1 samples are correctly classified. The 'Accuracy' (Acc) and 'Reject rate' (RR) for the ith HEp-2 pattern can be calculated as

$$Acc = \frac{M_1}{M}; RR = \frac{N - M_1}{N} \tag{31}$$

The 'Reject rate'-'Accuracy' curves for all patterns are shown in Fig. 15a and b, respectively, for the 'Positive' and 'Intermediate' intensity types. For the Speckled, Nucleolar, Centromere, and NuMem patterns, the accuracy rate reaches almost 100% with only 10% 'Reject rates', and the other patterns also have a greater than 80% accuracy rate with only 20% 'Reject rates' in the 'Positive' intensity type. A greater than 75% accuracy rate with 20% 'Reject rates' can be achieved for five patterns, excluding 'Golgi' in the 'Intermediate' intensity type, which also proves the effectiveness of our proposed strategy for HEp-2 staining pattern recognition.

7   Conclusion

In this paper, we proposed an approach for classifying HEp-2 staining cells automatically using IIF image analysis, which can indicate the presence of autoimmune diseases by finding antibodies in the patient serum. Studies on HEp-2 cell pattern recognition have shown that LBP and its extension version, RICLBP, PRICoLBP for image representation, can produce promising classification accuracy rates. However, there is still a lot of room for improvement. We know that LBP only quantizes a local patch (microstructure) into a binary series by comparing the surrounding pixel intensity with that of the center pixel, and the quantitative difference is then lost as a result of the binary coding in LBP. Therefore, it is possible that very different local structures (patch) will be represented by the same LBP value, which means the LBP is very limited in terms of representing the local structure given the fixed approximate quantization of the feature space as binary patterns. In addition, in general, local binary pattern (local structure) distributions are represented by histograms, and hence, are restricted to the use of low-order statistics. This study realized a method for extracting highly-discriminant features from HEp-2 cell images by exploring a robust local descriptor inspired by Weber's law. The investigated local descriptor is based on the fact that human perception for distinguishing a pattern depends not only on the absolute intensity of the stimulus but also on the relative variance of the stimulus. Therefore, we firstly transform the original stimulus (the images in our study) into a differential excitation-domain according to Weber's law, and then explore a local patch, also called as micro-Texton, in the transformed domain as Weber local descriptor. Furthermore, we propose to employ a parametric probability process to model the Weber local descriptors, and extract the higher-order statistics to the model parameters for image representation. The proposed strategy can adaptively characterize the Weber local descriptor space using generative probability model, and then learn the parameters for better fitting the training space, which would lead to more discriminant representation for HEp-2 cell images. Furthermore, we also extract the higher-order statistics for the model parameters, which is more discriminant for image representation and can be combined with a linear classifier (such as a linear SVM). Experiments using the open HEp-2 cell dataset of the ICIP2013 contest validated that the proposed strategy can achieve a much better performance than the widely used local binary pattern (LBP) and its extensions, RICLBP, PRI-CoLBP for image representation, and the achieved recognition error rate was even very significantly below the observed intra-laboratory variability.

Acknowledgements This work was supported in part by the Grant-in Aid for Scientific Research from the Japanese MEXT under the Grant No. 15K00253, 15H01130, 16H01436 and 26330212 and in part by the MEXT Support Program for the Strategic Research Foundation at Private Universities (2013–2017).

References

1. Conrad, K., Schoessler, W., Hiepe, F., Fritzler, M.J.: Autoantibodies in Systemic Autoimmune Diseases. Pabst Science Publishers (2002)
2. Conrad, K., Humbel, R.L., Meurer, M., Shoenfeld, Y.: Autoantigens and Autoantibodies: Diagnostic Tools and Clues to Understanding Autoimmunity. Pabst Science Publishers (2000)
3. Foggia, P., Percannella, G., Soda, P., Vento, M.: Benchmarking HEp-2 cells classification methods. IEEE Trans. Med. Imaging (2013)
4. Hiemann, R., Hilger, N., Sack, U., Weigert, M.: Objective quality evaluation of fluorescence images to optimize automatic image acquisition. Cytometry Part A **69**(3), 182–184 (2006)
5. Soda, P., Rigon, A., Afeltra, A., Iannello, G.: Automatic acquisition of immunofluorescence images: algorithms and evaluation. In: 19th IEEE International Symposium on Computer Based Medical Systems, pp. 386–390 (2006)
6. Huang, Y.-L., Chung, C.-W., Hsieh, T.-Y., Jao, Y.-L.: Outline detection for the HEp-2 cells in indirect immunofluorescence images using watershed segmentatio. In: IEEE International Conference on Sensor Networks, Ubiquitous and Trustworthy Computing, pp. 423–427 (2008)
7. Huang, Y.-L., Jao, Y.-L., Hsieh, T.-Y., Chung, C.-W.: Adaptive automatic segmentation of HEp-2 cells in indirect immunofluorescence images. In: IEEE International Conference on Sensor Networks, Ubiquitous and Trustworthy Computing, pp. 418–422 (2008)
8. Perner, P., Perner, H., Muller, B.: Mining knowledge for HEp-2 cell image classification. J. Artif. Intell. Med. **26**, 161–173 (2002)

9. Soda, P., Iannello, G., Vento, M.: A multiple experts system for classifying fluorescence intensity in antinuclear autoantibodies analysis. Pattern Anal. Appl. **12**(3), 215–226 (2009)
10. Hiemann, R., Buttner, T., Krieger, T., Roggenbuck, D., Sack, U., Conrad, K.: Challenges of automated screening and differentiation of non-organ specific autoantibodies on hep-2 cells. Autoimmun. Rev. **9**(1), 17–22 (2009)
11. Hiemann, R., Buttner, T., Krieger, T., Roggenbuck, D., Sack, U., Conrad, K.: Automatic analysis of immunofluorescence patterns of HEp-2 cells. Ann. NY Acad. Sci. **1109**(1), 358–371 (2007)
12. Soda, P., Iannello, G.: Aggregation of classifiers for staining pattern recognition in antinuclear autoantibodies analysis. IEEE Trans. Inf. Technol. Biomed. **13**(3), 322–329 (2009)
13. Sack, U., Knoechner, S., Warschkau, H., Pigla, U., Emmrich, F., Kamprad, M.: Computer-assisted classification of HEp-2 immunofluorescence patterns in autoimmune diagnostics. Autoimmun. Rev. **2**, 298–304 (2003)
14. Foggia, P., Percannella, G., Soda, P., Vento, M.: Early experiences in mitotic cells recognition on HEp-2 slides. In: IEEE 23rd International Symposium on Computer-Based Medical Systems (CBMS), pp. 38–43 (2010)
15. Nosaka, R., Fukui, K.: HEp-2 cell classification using rotation invariant co-occurrence among local binary patterns. Pattern Recogn. (2013)
16. Qi, X.B., Xiao, R., Zhang, L., Guo, J.: Pairwise rotation invariant co-occurrence local binary pattern. In: 12th European conference on computer vision (ECCV2012) (2012)
17. Lazebnik, S., Schmid, C., Ponce, J.: Beyond bags of features: spatial pyramid matching for recognizing natural scene categories. In: CVPR, pp. 2169–2178 (2006)
18. Lowe, D.: Distinctive image features from scale-invariant keypoints. Int. J. Comput. Vis. **60**(2), 91–110 (2004)
19. He, D.C., Wang, L.: Texture unit, texture spectrum, and texture analysis. IEEE Trans. Geosci. Rem. Sens. **28**, 509–512 (1990)
20. Wang, X.Y., Han, T.X., Yan, S.: An HOG-LBP human detector with partial occlusion handling. In: ICCV (2009)
21. Zhao, G., Pietikainen, M.: Local binary pattern descriptors for dynamic texture recognition. Pattern Recogn. 211–214 (2006)
22. Dinov, I.D.: Expectation Maximization and Mixture Modeling Tutorial, California Digital Library, Statistics Online Computational Resource (2008)
23. Christopher, B.: Pattern Recognition and Machine Learning. Springer, New York
24. Dempster, A.P., Laird, N.M., Rubin, D.B.: Maximum likelihood from incomplete data via the EM algorithm. J. R. Stat. Soc. Ser. B **39**(1), 1–38 (1997)
25. Cristianini, N., Shawe-Taylor, J.: An Introduction to Support Vector Machines and other Kernel-Based Learning Methods. Cambridge University Press (2000)
26. Center for Disease Control: Quality assurance for the indirect immunofluorescence test for autoantibodies to nuclear antigen (IF-ANA): approved guideline, NCCLS I/LA2-A, vol. 16, no. 11 (1996)
27. Rigon, A., Soda, P., Zennaro, D., Iannello, G., Afeltra, A.: Indirect immunofluorescence in autoimmune diseases: assessment of digital images for diagnostic purpose. Cytometry B (Clin. Cytometry) **72**(3), 472–477 (2007)
28. Leung, T.J., Malik, J.: Representing and recognizing the visual appearance of materials using three-dimensional textons. IJCV **43**, 29–44 (2001)
29. Pothos, V.K., Theoharatos, C., Zygouris, E., Economou, G.: Distributional-based texture classification using non-parametric statistics. Pattern Anal. Appl. **11**(2), 117–129 (2008)
30. Han, S.D., Tao, W.B., Wu, X.L.: Texture segmentation using independent-scale component-wise Riemannian-covariance Gaussian mixture model in KL measure based multi-scale non-linear structure tensor space. Pattern Recogn. **44**(3), 503–518 (2011)
31. Varma, M., Zisserman, A.: Texture classification: are filter banks necessary. In: CVPR (2003)
32. Pietikinen, M., Hadid, A., Zhao, G., Ahonen, T.: Computer Vision Using Local Binary Patterns. Springer (2011)

33. Awate, S.P., Tasdizen, T., Whitaker, R.T.: Unsupervised texture segmentation with nonpara-metric neighborhood statistics. In: European Conference on Computer Vision, pp. 497–507 (2006)
34. Ahonen, T., Hadid, A., Pietikainen, M.: Face description with local binary patterns: application to face recognition. PAMI, vol. 28 (2006)
35. Tan, X., Triggs, B.: Enhanced local texture feature sets for face recognition under difficult lighting conditions. TIP **19**, 1635–1650 (2010)
36. Chen, J., Shan, S., He, C., Zhao, G., Pietikainen, M., Chen, X., Gao, W.: WLD: a robust local image descriptor. PAMI **32**, 1705–1720 (2010)
37. Louis, W., Plataniotis, K.N.: Co-occurrence of local binary patterns features for frontal face detection in surveillance applications. EURASIP J. Image Video Process. (2011)
38. Shen, J. (Jackie), Jung, Y.-M.: Weberized Mumford–Shah model with Bose-Einstein photon noise. In: IJCV, vol. 53, no. 3, pp. 331–358 (2006)
39. Chang, J.-H., Fan, K.-C., Chang, Yang-Lang: Multi-modal Gray-level histogram modeling and Decomposition. Neural, Parallel Sci. Comput. **20**, 203–216 (2002)
40. Aitnouri, E., Wang, S., Ziou, D.: Estimation of multi-modal histogram's pdf Using a mix-ture model. In: Proceedings of IEEE International Conference on Computer Vision, no. 7, pp. 103–118 (1999)
41. Xu, L., Jordan, M.I.: On convergence properties of the EM algorithm for gaussian mixtures. Neural Comput. **9**(1), 129–151 (1996)
42. Aran, O., Akarun, L.: A multi-class classification strategy for Fisher scores: application to signer independent sign language recognition. Pattern Recogn. **43**(5), 1776–1788 (2010)
43. Dick, U., Kersting, K.: Fisher kernels for relational data. In: ECML 2006: 17th European con-ference on machine learning, vol. 4212, pp. 114–125 (2006)
44. Amari, S., Nagaoka, H.: Methods of Information Geometry, Translations of Mathematical Monographs, vol. 191. Oxford University Press (2000)
45. Jaakkola, T., Haussler, D.: Exploiting generative models in discriminative classifiers. In: NIPS1998 (1998)

Intelligent Diagnosis of Breast Cancer Based on Quantitative B-Mode and Elastography Features

Chung-Ming Lo and Ruey-Feng Chang

Early breast cancer diagnosis improves prognosis of patients. However, the reviewing of image ultrasound is operator-dependent. Computer-aided diagnosis (CAD) systems as the helper for radiologists were proposed to reduce oversight error and increase cancer diagnosis rate. In this chapter, three CAD systems focusing on quantitative B-mode texture, elasticity analysis, and the combination of both B-mode and elasticity features are presented. Firstly, 69 cases assessed as Breast Imaging Reporting and Data System (BI-RADS) category 3 by the radiologists were used to evaluate the CAD system with intensity-invariant texture analysis. Secondly, 31 malignant and 57 benign tumors were used to evaluate the performance of 18 shear-wave elastography (SWE) features extracted from tumor and peri-tumor area. SWE image within region of interest (ROI) was expressed in RGB color histogram and represented by mean, variance, skewness, and kurtosis. Thirdly, 45 malignant and 45 benign tumors were used to evaluate the integration of B-mode features and strain features. Tumor region was mapped on elastography image from segmented tumor contour in the corresponding B-mode image. By utilizing fuzzy c-means clustering, the elastography image was converted to image with only white, gray, and black. Strain features extracted from black cluster were combined with B-mode features for tumor classification. As a result, the area under

C.-M. Lo
Graduate Institute of Biomedical Informatics, College of Medical Science and Technology, Taipei Medical University, Taipei, Taiwan
e-mail: buddylo@tmu.edu.tw

R.-F. Chang (✉)
Department of Computer Science and Information Engineering, National Taiwan University, Taipei, Taiwan
e-mail: rfchang@csie.ntu.edu.tw

R.-F. Chang
Graduate Institute of Biomedical Electronics and Bioinformatics, National Taiwan University, Taipei, Taiwan

© Springer International Publishing AG 2018
K. Suzuki and Y. Chen (eds.), *Artificial Intelligence in Decision Support Systems for Diagnosis in Medical Imaging*, Intelligent Systems Reference Library 140, https://doi.org/10.1007/978-3-319-68843-5_7

the receiver operating characteristic curve (Az) for mass texture and speckles textures were 0.58 and 0.56 without intensity-invariant transformation, 0.83 and 0.80 with intensity-invariant transformation. The extracted SWE features achieve an accuracy of 81% on tumor classification. By combining the SWE features with BI-RADS assessment, Az improved from 0.77 to 0.89. The strain features extracted from black cluster (stiff tissue) achieved an accuracy of 80%, a sensitivity of 80%, a specificity of 80% and a normalized Az of 0.84. Az was significantly improved to 0.93 with the combination of B-mode features. In conclusion, malignant tumor detection rate can be significantly improved with all three methodologies of (1) intensity-invariant transformed- tumor textures analysis, (2) SWE features, and (3) quantified strain features combined with B-mode features.

1 Introduction

Breast cancer is the second most common cause of cancer-related death for women in US [1]. Most of the breast cancer patients were asymptomatic at early stages. Confirmed diagnoses at early stages increase survival rates [2]. Mammography screening was shown to reduce breast cancer deaths by early detection [3–5]. However, mammograms are difficult to interpret in dense breast. Bilateral screening ultrasound was evaluated as a feasible screening tool and the result shows promises [6]. Multiple studies indicated the addition of breast ultrasonography to mammography increases cancer detection rate [7–9]. Hence, ultrasonography was gradually established as a secondary diagnostic tool in breast cancer due to its good presentation of soft tissue.

In order to standardize the breast image finding terminology and assessment structure of diagnosis, the American College of Radiology (ACR) developed Breast Imaging Reporting and Data System (BI-RADS) lexicon for mammography, ultrasound and MRI of the breast [10]. Each kind of breast image was assigned to a categorical score of 0–6 according to image characteristics. The score represents the likelihood of malignancy. It corresponds to respective clinical recommendations. Image of BI-RADS category 2 (benign) showed characteristics of benign changes, and it will not be biopsied. BI-RADS category 4 (suspicious abnormality) is assigned to image with identifiable lesion and biopsy will be carried out. In between these two categories, BI-RADS category 3 (probably benign) is in the clinical decision gray zone. Typical findings in this category are non-palpable microcalcification cluster, non-calcified solid nodules and other focal finding. There is no absolute recommendation for biopsy. However, there is a 2% likelihood of malignancy [11]. A 6 month follow up period is usually recommended.

To create a standardized image reading helper, CAD scheme was proposed as a second reader and showed to improve the clinician's performance in histological classification [12]. In the previous works, the methodologies of building CAD systems were developed for breast cancer diagnosis [13–15]. Intensity-invariant ranklet transformed the automated delineated mass region into coefficients for further tumor texture analysis on BI-RADS 3 cases assessed by the radiologists [13]. By referring to the same tumor area on B-mode and elastography, shear-wave elastography (SWE) image features were extracted to efficiently calculate the stiffness levels of tumor tissues compared to surrounding normal tissues [15]. The meaningful clinical stain features were then quantified in the CAD system and combined with Radiologists' assessment via B-mode features to achieve the improvement of Az [14]. The detailed methodologies are described in the following sections.

2 Intensity-Invariant B-Mode Texture Analysis for BI-RADS 3

The algorithm of the proposed CAD system is shown in Fig. 1. Firstly, tumor contour segmentation was performed as an automatic step. The area enclosed by segmentation was defined as tumor area. Secondly, a separately ranklet-transformed image was overlapping with tumor area and speckle detection area. Hence, tumor texture and speckle texture can be extracted from this intensity-invariant image.

2.1 Patients and Data Acquisition

This is a radiologist-blinded retrospective study involving 69 breast ultrasound BI-RADS category 3 cases included 21 malignant and 48 benign cases. All

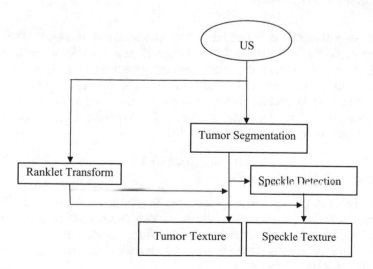

Fig. 1 Flowchart of the proposed CAD system

ultrasound data were either collected by ATL HDI 3000 (Phillips, Bothell, WA, USA) or Medison Voluson 530 scanner (Kretz Technik, Zipf, Austra) over a 2 year period. The histology results from biopsy of the 21 malignant lesions were invasive ductal carcinoma (IDC) grade 2 in 6 cases and grade 3 in 15 cases. The lesion size ranges from 1.2 to 4.7 cm with mean of 2.7 cm. The 48 benign lesions consist of 34 fibroadenomas (FA), 13 fibrocystic changes (FCCs) and 1 papilloma. Lesion size ranges from 1.4 to 4.3 cm with mean of 2.6 cm. Patient's age differences between malignant (28–84 years old, mean = 47.2 years old) and benign groups (20–53 years old, mean = 39.9 years old) were statistically significant (p-value = 0.001). Fifteen lesions were palpable, and 54 lesions are not palpable. Because these US images were acquired from different scanners, settings, and time slots, the ultrasonography setting on brightness or contrast was not fixed.

2.2 Tumor Segmentation

In order to reduce operator-dependency, tumor contour was automatically delineated by the level-set segmentation method [16]. Firstly, sigmoid filter was applied to enhance image contrast and bring out tumor with weak edges. Secondly, the image was processed by gradient magnitude filter to generate a gradient image with magnitude in both horizontal and vertical directions. Thirdly, the level-set function acquired tumor contour by the alternation of topology through gray-scale gradient as differential equation criterion.

2.3 Speckle Detection

Speckle patterns are the result of interference by scatterers in tissues. These scatterers could be ducts or glands. Speckle appears granular with heterogeneity on B-mode image. Moon et al. proposed speckles features on B-mode images are as reliable as morphology features for breast tumor classification [17, 18]. To optimize the process of speckle feature extraction, the gray-scale level 0–255 pixels B-mode was extended to an intensity image with exponential distribution with mean-to-standard deviation (SD) ratio of 1.0.

$$I(x, y) = 10^{B(x, y)/B_0} \tag{1}$$

$I(x, y)$ represents intensity with exponential distribution. $B(x, y)$ is the B-mode gray-scale value and is normalized by B_0, which corresponds to transducer frequency [19]. Speckle pixels are detected via a sliding window of the size of 5 with the allowance of 0.8–1.2 mean-to-standard deviation distributions in intensity image. The criterion is defined as

$$W_{mean}(x,y) = \sum_{i=-a}^{a} \sum_{j=-a}^{a} I(x+i, y+j)/(2a+1)^2 \qquad (2)$$

$$W_{mSD}(x,y) = \frac{W_{mean}(x,y)}{\sqrt{\sum_{i=-a}^{a} \sum_{j=-a}^{a} (I(x+i, y+j) - W_{mean}(x,y))^2}} \qquad (3)$$

W_{mean} represents the average of intensity within a 5-by-5 window. a is equal to 2, the denominator in W_{mean} represents the 5-by-5 window size. W_{mSD} represents the mean-to-standard deviation distribution tolerable range of 0.8–1.2 within the 5-by-5 window. Any speckle pixel that satisfies W_{mSD} is placed on speckle map.

2.4 Ranklet Transform

Texture analysis is an important tool for biometric pattern recognition. With respect to US images, texture is echogenicity or echo pattern under the context of B-mode image. Texture feature in the tumor and peri-tumor area are used for tumor characterization [18, 20], differentiating malignant and benign lesions. However, texture analysis is system dependent. Different ultrasonography system settings and scanners result in different performances in tumor classification. This imposes variation on tissue characteristics.

To solve the issue of gray-scale variation among various ultrasound system settings and scanners, previous studies extracted invariant texture features from the ranklet-transformed ROI for tumor detection and diagnosis [21, 22]. Instead of dealing directly with gray-scale value, it works with the relative order of the gray-scale intensities. Under ranklet transform, the gray-scale distribution of the image does not impose variation in detection and diagnosis based on image texture. A comparison of the tumor shape and echogenicity under intensity variations can be used to show the consistency of ranklet-transformed image. In Fig. 2, the tumor shape observed from the original, contrast enhanced, gamma-corrected, and histogram equalized images were independent of intensity variation and can be recognized easily. However, texture feature is highly dependent on factors that affect gray-scale distribution as it is shown by huge variation on the illustration in Fig. 2.

Ranklet transform is non-parametric, orientation-selective, and multi-resolution, [21]. Given the N number of pixels in the image, the intensity value of pixels is substituted by the relative order of brightness. Secondly, the image with N pixels is geometrically split into half forming two groups (X and Y) according to vertical, horizontal, or diagonal conformation. These three orientations of two groups are based on Haar transform support. Now, X and Y groups are consisted of pixel intensity rank. Next, compare the relative intensity order of pixels in X and Y to identify which subset is brighter than the other. Taking vertical conformation for

	Original	Contrast Enhancement	Gamma Correction	Histogram Equalization

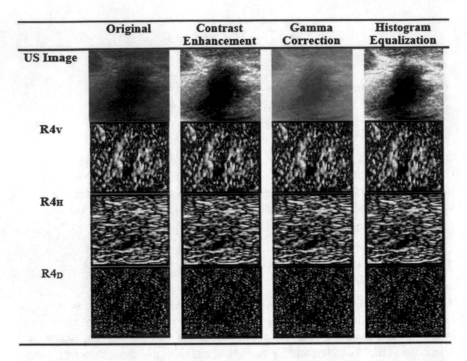

Fig. 2 Ranklet images of the original ultrasound image and processed images (contrast enhancement, gamma correction, histogram equalization)

example. If Yv is brighter than Xv, the derived ranklet transform coefficient R_O is a positive value, and a negative value, vice versa.

$$R_o = \frac{\sum_{p \in Y_o} \pi(p) - C/4(C/2+1)}{C^2/8} - 1, O = V, H, D \tag{4}$$

If a crop contains C pixels, $C/2 \times C/2 = C^2/4$ comparisons are required. $\pi(p)$ represents relative pixel ranks. Ranklet transform also takes multi-resolution into account. The resolutions of 2, 4, and 8 for an 8-by-8 image generate 49, 25, and 1 crops. For each of resolution, the transform was also applied to generate different ranklet transform coefficient R_O. Figure 2 illustrates the ranklet transform images with the resolution of 4, the orientation of vertical, horizontal, and diagonal. From the figure, the transformed results from original US image and processed images (contrast enhancement, gamma correction, histogram equalization) are more consistent on the texture. In the experiment, the minimum resolution to extract meaningful features was 2 pixels and the maximum resolution was 32 pixels. It is limited by the size of acquired tumors.

Ranklet transform was demonstrated to be a useful function for consistent texture. After transformation, gray-level co-occurrence matrix (GLCM) as a second-order statistical texture was utilized to extract texture features through the spatial relationship of pixels [23]. The matrix element $P = [p(i, j|d, \theta)]$ presents the frequencies of two adjacent pixels at d pixels and a direction θ, one with gray-scale i and another with gray-scale j. In this study, distance d is set to 1 and four offset directions, $\theta = 0°, 45°, 90°, 135°$, were pursued. The proposed GLCM textures features is defined as the following:

$$Energy = \sum_i \sum_j p(i,j|d,\theta)^2 \tag{5}$$

$$Entropy = -\sum_i \sum_j p(i,j|d,\theta)\log(p(i,j|d,\theta)) \tag{6}$$

$$Correlation = \frac{\sum_i \sum_j (i-\mu_x)(j-\mu_y)p(i,j|d,\theta)}{\sigma_x \sigma_y} \tag{7}$$

$$Local\ Homogeneity = \sum_i \sum_j \frac{1}{1+(i-j)^2}p(i,j|d,\theta) \tag{8}$$

$$Inertia = \sum_i \sum_j (i-j)^2 p(i,j|d,\theta) \tag{9}$$

$$Cluster\ Shade = \sum_i \sum_j (i+j-\mu_x-\mu_y)^3 p(i,j|d,\theta) \tag{10}$$

$$Cluster\ Prominence = \sum_i \sum_j (i+j-\mu_x-\mu_y)^4 p(i,j|d,\theta) \tag{11}$$

$$Haralick's\ Correlation = \frac{\sum_i \sum_j (i \cdot j)p(i,j|d,\theta) - \mu_x\mu_y}{\sigma_x \sigma_y} \tag{12}$$

where μ_x and μ_y are mean. σ_x and σ_y are standard deviation of the marginal distributions of $p(i, j|d, \theta)$.

$$\mu_x = \sum_i i \sum_j p(i,j|d,\theta), \mu_y = \sum_j j \sum_i p(i,j|d,\theta) \tag{13}$$

$$\sigma_x^2 = \sum_i (i-\mu_x)^2 \sum_j p(i,j|d,\theta), \sigma_y^2 = \sum_j (j-\mu_y)^2 \sum_i p(i,j|d,\theta) \tag{14}$$

The tumor texture and speckle texture were developed from GLCM features, of which was extracted from ranklet transform image of five resolutions and three orientations. Altogether, there were 240 features for each texture and speckle features (3 orientations × 5 resolutions × 8 GLCM-derived features × 2 average or standard deviation).

2.5   Statistical Analysis

Each feature was evaluated individually to understand how well it distinguishes malignant from benign lesions. Kolmogorov-Smirnov test was utilized to determine the distribution of each feature was either normal or non-normal. Student's t-test was used on normal features and Mann-Whitney U-test for non-normal features. p-values <0.05 was regarded as statistical significance. Features belong to either tumor texture or speckles texture we evaluated as a set in binary logistic regression with backward stepwise elimination. The feature set was chosen with the minimum error rate. Leave-one-out cross validation was performed by the selected features where each time one case is left out for testing while the remaining are training set. All cases were tested by accordingly.

Prediction is compared with biopsy-proven result for each case. Accuracy, sensitivity, specificity, positive predictive value (PPV), and negative predictive value (NPV) were calculated. Chi-Square test was utilized to compare the performance of two feature sets. ROC curve was drawn to demonstrate the trade-off between sensitivity and specificity. Area under the ROC curve (Az) was compared with z-test in ROCKIT software (Metz, University of Chicago, Chicago, IL, USA). Other tests were performed on SPSS software (version 16 for Windows; SPSS, Chicago, IL, USA).

2.6   Result and Discussion

In the total 240 features each, 186 tumor textures and 181 speckle textures were normally distributed. There were 46 and 35 tumor texture and speckles textures statistical significance by comparison of malignant and benign group. The most commonly selected features were from *R32H*, resolution of 32 pixels and horizontal orientation. The selected from *R32H* were entropy average, correlation standard deviation, cluster prominence standard deviation, and Haralick correlation average.

Without ranklet transformation, tumor texture and speckles texture performed poorly with only 60% correct diagnosis. Ranklet transform significantly improves the accuracy and sensitivity of tumor texture. Accuracy and sensitivity of tumor texture features improved from 58% (40/69) and 38% (8/21) with original texture features to 80% (55/69) and 76% (16/21) with ranklet transformation, respectively. The same trend was also observed in speckles features. Accuracy and sensitivity of speckles features were improved from 71% (15/21) and 33% (7/21) with original texture features to 83% (57/69) and 62% (43/69) with ranklet transformation. No significant difference for the specificities of both tumor texture and speckle texture with or without ranklet transformation. The positive predictive value of both tumor texture and speckle texture were also significantly improved with ranklet transformation. Most importantly, Az of tumor texture and speckle texture were significantly improved (p-value = 0.0009 and 0.02, respectively).

The ACR BI-RADS ultrasound descriptors were incorporated into CAD system to investigate the mass morphology in B-mode image [24]. These tumor morphologies were proven reliable in differentiating benign and malignant breast masses [25]. They were already implemented in CAD for tumor classification with promising result, especially with BI-RADS category 3 [26]. Features associated with morphology were good predictor. However, texture features were not because they were affected by gray-scale distribution.

In order to improve the texture feature analysis, ranklet transform was used to convert grayscale images and make the texture features invariant to intensity variation. Ranklet transform is feasible for texture analysis. It should be considered for the cases with the goal of intensity invariant texture analysis. Ranklet transformation was performed prior to tumor texture and speckle texture extraction. When using selected features from ranklet transform to classify BI-RADS category 3 biopsy-proven cases, Az values showed a striking improvement from 0.56–0.58 to 0.80–0.83. Previous studies were performed on tumor texture [24] and speckle texture [18] analysis. But, the possibility of different scanner settings and models was not explored. In this study, it was shown that ranklet transformed texture features were independent of different scanner settings and models. The extracted intensity-invariant speckle textures were effective on tumor classification indicating that the same methodology could also be applied to discrete pixels. Detection and analysis of speckle features can also be performed on ROI rather than tumor contour [17, 18].

In previous study using ranklet transformation in breast tumor classification, Az value range of 0.90–0.94 was achieved [22]. A lower Az value of 0.83 was achieved in study. Nonetheless, only BI-RADS category 3 cases were used. It is a gray zone for clinical diagnosis that imposes challenges to establish a correct diagnosis. The improvement of Az by utilization of ranklet transformation is much greater than in this study. Az value in the study is significantly improved from 0.58 to 0.83 whereas the improvement the previous study from 0.81 to 0.90.

3 Quantization of Multichannel Distributions in Color Shear-Wave Imaging

Palpation is in the first line of detection for breast cancer. Tissue stiffness is a very important part of clinical examination. This kind of examination inspired the development of elastography. It is an image modality that captures elasticity information and presents it in a single image [20] or cine loop [27]. With external compression (stress, σ), the elasticity or stiffness of tissues is represented by deformation (strain, ε). Elasticity can be describe in Young's modulus, $E = \sigma/\varepsilon$. It has become a part of the breast assessment in the BI-RADS Ultrasonography fifth edition. Mass deformation was visually inspected under operator-induced compression on ultrasonography transducer. However, the result by this procedure is non-reproducible and operator-dependent [28]. To overcome this problem, shear-wave elastography (SWE) was developed [29]. Instead of using mechanical compression, acoustic radiation force is induced automatically and the propagation of wave on tissue is captured through the same ultrasound transducer. The SWE images displays shear-wave propagation though tissue in kilopascals (kPa) with a RGB color map. Performance of SWE was investigated with the use of BI-RADS B-mode features. BI-RADS assessment of B-mode features and SWE together are extremely sensitive for malignancy detection [30]. The addition of SWE features improved specificity without compromising sensitivity [28, 31]. More unnecessary biopsy can be avoided with the consideration of SWE features. Nonetheless, the assessment of SWE images is a qualitative and inspector-dependent. In order to design a more efficient way of reading SWE images and eliminate possible human error, a CAD system was proposed by automating the feature extraction from multichannel distributions of SWE images [15].

3.1 Patients and Data Acquisition

88 biopsy-proven cases used in this study were with histology classification of 57 benign and 31 malignant. They came from 81 patients who had both conventional B-mode and elastography examination. The age range for patients with benign tumor was 26–77 years old (mean ± standard deviation = 50 ± 11), and 30–76 years old (mean ± standard deviation = 54 ± 13) for patients with malignant tumor. The pathology classifications of benign tumors were 25 fibrocystic change, 22 fibroadenomas, and 10 papillomas. For malignant tumors, 27 were invasive ductal carcinomas (IDC), 1 was invasive lobular carcinoma (ILC), and 3 were ductal carcinoma in situ (DCIS). The tumor size ranges were 1.42 ± 1.20 and 1.51 ± 0.76 cm for benign and malignant tumors. Radiologists were blinded to patient's medical history and tumor pathology report when categorizing tumor by BI-RADS assessment. There were 2 (2%) tumors in BI-RADS 2 (benign), 17 (19%) in BI-RADS 3 (probably benign), 52 (59%) in BI-RADS 4 (suspicious abnormality), and 17 (19%) in BI-RADS 5 (highly suggestive of malignancy).

B-mode and elastography images were acquired by Aixplorer ultrasound system (SuperSonic Image, Les Jardins de la Duranne, Aix en Provence, France) with a 5–14 MHz linear broadband transducer (SL15-4). B-mode image was used to identify the location of mass. The ROI including the tumor and peri-tumor areas were defined to generate SWE image. Elasticity is presented with Young's modulus. The default maximum elasticity in the color display for all cases was 180 kPa (7.7 m/s).

3.2   Shear-Wave Elastography (SWE) Features

In the following sections, the quantification and extraction of SWE features are explained in detail. SWE features came from histogram distribution in individual or multiple color channels of the color map. Spatial correlation was also referred in the formulation of elasticity features.

3.2.1   Single-Channel Features

Examples of SWE image with corresponding RGB histograms of benign and malignant breast tumors are shown in Fig. 3. Benign tumor and the peri-tumor area are soft and are displayed by blue color. By presenting red, green and blue channels in histogram, the distinction between benign and malignant tumor is clear. In the SWE image of the benign tumor, red and green histograms are left-biased, and blue

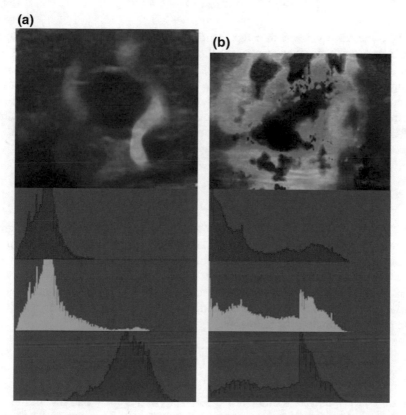

Fig. 3 Shear-wave elastography (SWE) images of **a** benign and **b** malignant tumors and their corresponding red, green, and blue channel histograms

is center-weighted. In contrast, the malignant tumor image is well-distributed in red, green and blue histograms. Histogram distributions of RGB channels were quantified in the experiment as classification features.

In the quantification process, the 24-bit depth color image was decomposed into 8-bit red, green, and blue channels image. Mean, variance, skewness, and kurtosis are calculated according to the follow formula to represent the histogram distribution.

$$\text{Mean}_c = \frac{1}{N} \sum_{i=1}^{N} P_{ci} \tag{15}$$

$$\text{Variance}_c = \frac{1}{N} \sum_{i=1}^{N} (P_{ci} - Mean_c)^2 \tag{16}$$

$$\text{Skewness}_c = \frac{1}{N} \sum_{i=1}^{N} \sum (P_{ci} - Mean_c)^3 \tag{17}$$

$$\text{Kurtosis}_c = \frac{1}{N} \sum_{i=1}^{N} (P_{ci} - Mean_c)^4 \tag{18}$$

P_{ci} is the pixel value with c representing the color channel of red, green, and blue. Mean is calculated by averaging all pixel values or the summation of all pixel values divided by total number of pixels. It represents the center location of the histogram distribution. Variance measures the spread from the mean. Skewness indicates the level of symmetry in distribution. Kurtosis is opposite of skewness. It is a measure of 'tailedness' in the distribution. There are 12 single channel features (3 RGB channels × 4—mean, variance, skewness, and kurtosis): *Rmean, Gmean, Bmean, Rvar, Gvar, Bvar, Rskew, Gskew, Bskew, Rkur, Gkur,* and *Bkur.*

3.2.2 Multi-channel Features

The measurement of elasticity is continuously presented in the order of blue, green, yellow, and red, indicating soft to hard tissue. To better separate hard from soft tissue, vector quantization [32] was performed by compartmentalizing continuous color expression into discrete color of pure red, green, blue, and yellow. R, G, and B channel represent each pixel color in the SWE image. The conceptual distance from each pixel to either blue, green, red, or yellow was calculated by Euclidean distance. The formula is as following:

$$ED_{PMi} = \sqrt{(P_R - M_{iR})^2 + (P_G - M_{iG})^2 + (P_B - M_{iB})^2} \tag{19}$$

where ED_{PMi} is the vector difference between a pixel color P and one of the main colors M_i = (blue, green, yellow, red) in the R, G, and B channels. The nearest color was selected to replace the old pixel color. When the pixel numbers of each four-color clusters were divided by the total number of pixels in the ROI, a new set of features are formed: *Bdensity, Gdensity, Ydensity,* and *Rdensity.* The average of elasticity was calculated based on color-weighted elasticity calibration with the following formula:

$$ColorAvg = B_{Num} \times 36 + G_{Num} \times 72 + Y_{Num} \times 108 + R_{Num} \times 144 / B_{Num} + G_{Num} + Y_{Num} + R_{Num}$$

(20)

where *Num* is the number of color cluster after vector quantification. The coefficients in numerators are the corresponding elasticity measurement of each color.

In addition to elasticity value, spatial information was also taken into consideration to minimize the noise around skin. In some cases, color close to skin resembling peri-tumor area where there was no pathology change of interest for malignancy diagnosis. Spatial correlation was in cooperated into elasticity color image by the application of an intensity decreasing function such as the following formula:

$$SpatialAvg = \frac{\sum_{P} P_{ij}(kPa) \times \left((HMid + WMid) - \left(\|P_i - WMid\| + \|P_j - HMid\|\right)\right)}{\sum_{P} \left((HMid + WMid) - \left(\|P_i - WMid\| + \|P_j - HMid\|\right)\right)}$$

(21)

where $P_{ij}(kPa)$ is the elasticity value in kPa unit of a pixel in coordinate i and j; *HMid* and *WMid* are the midway of the vertical and horizontal location of the ROI, respectively; P_i is the pixel coordinate i (horizontal); and P_j is the pixel coordinate j (vertical)

3.3 Performance Evaluation

In order to develop a model for tumor classification, SWE features were combined by binary logistic regression with backward stepwise elimination. The representative features set were chosen with the minimum error rate. Leave-one-out cross validation was performed by selected features where each time one case is left out for testing while the remaining are training set. All cases were tested by accordingly.

The cases in this study are composed of 2 (2%) tumors in BI-RADS 2 (benign), 17 (19%) in BI-RADS 3 (probably benign), 52 (59%) in BI-RADS 4 (suspicious abnormality), and 17 (19%) in BI-RADS 5 (highly suggestive of malignancy). The performance of the proposed CAD system based on SWE features for tumor classification on each BI-RADS categories was also investigated. CAD system is designed as a helper for radiologist. In order to investigate if quantified elasticity features have added value in diagnosing breast cancer, it was combined with BI-RADS assessment from radiologist. The overall performance on diagnosing malignant tumor with or without SWE features was explored.

ROC curve was drawn to have a closer look on trade-offs between sensitivity and specificity. Area under the ROC curve (Az) was compared. Chi-Square test was utilized to analyze the performance of two feature sets. Other tests were performed on SPSS software (version 16 for Windows; SPSS, Chicago, IL, USA).

3.4 Results and Discussion

All 18 proposed features and the biopsy-proven result were correlated in binary logistic regression to develop a prediction model for distinguishing malignant and benign tumor. Predicted probability = 0.5 was used as a cutoff point to diagnose a malignant tumor. The diagnostic performance of CAD system on different BI-RADS categories was also evaluated. The CAD system classified poorly in BI-RADS category 5 cases with only accuracy of 59% (10/17). In other BI-RADS categories, the achieved accuracies are 100% (2/2), 94% (16/17), and 83% (43/52) in BI-RADS category 2, 3, and 4, respectively. Due to the heterogeneities of malignant tumors, more correct diagnosis was established when BI-RADS category 5 cases were interpreted as malignant under the B-mode features assessed by radiologists. The overall performance of CAD system in combination with radiologist interpreted BI-RADS category 5 went up to accuracy of 88% from 81%. Az was also significantly improved.

Elasticity features extracted from SWE image was not sufficient on characterizing BI-RADS category 5 tumors. The tumor in this category is often found to exhibit characteristic of taller-than-wide, irregular shape, speculation, and hypoechogenicity [8]. These characteristics contain morphology and texture information, which can be extracted from B-mode image. By taking into the consideration of regarding BI-RADS category 5 tumors as malignant, the performance of the CAD system improved. Az improved from 0.77 to 0.89 (Fig. 4, p-value = 0.0048) with sensitivity improvement from 61 to 81%. The results are consistent with previous studies conducted by human review [30, 31].

The CAD system based on the proposed SWE features achieved an accuracy of 81%, sensitivity of 61%, and specificity of 91%. A high specificity indicates that SWE features on elasticity might be useful in avoiding unnecessary biopsy. To take a closer look on these features, the performance of CAD system on each BI-RADS category was calculated. A high performance of CAD system was achieved in BI-RADS category 3 group with accuracy of 94% (16/17), sensitivity of 100% (2/ 2), specificity of 93% (14/15), PPV of 62% (2/3), and NPV of 100% (14/14). BI-RADS category 3 is probably benign, but with <2% likelihood of malignancy [11]. It is where a more accurate diagnosis is in need. The result implies CAD based on SWE features might be an effective second reader to determine whether a biopsy should be pursued instead of a long follow up period of 6 months.

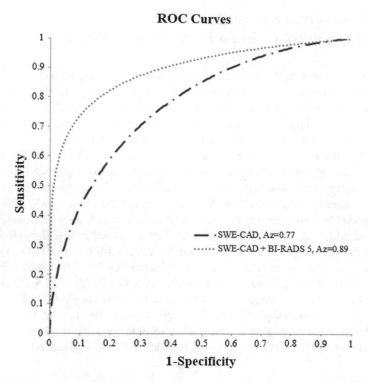

Fig. 4 The ROC curves illustrate that the Az was improved from 0.77 (SWE-CAD) to 0.89 (SWE-CAD + BI-RADS 5)

SpatialAvg was better than *ColorAvg*. The elimination of artifact caused by over compression of probe using intensity-decreasing function on the border of ROI indeed showed a better result. The example in Fig. 3 on the extraction of histograms on R, G, and B channels was for the purpose of showing case the feasibility of using those features on tumor classification. By using mean and standard deviation of pixel values from R, G, and B channels only resulted in an accuracy of 68%, much lower than the accuracy of 81% achieved by CAD system using all 18 SWE features.

Previous studies had suggested the inclusion of peri-tumor area [33] and the proposal of adaptive ROI for different tumors [34]. The SWE-based CAD system in this study with features extracted from whole and center ROI achieved an accuracy of 81 and 72%. Center ROI is only one-fourth the area of whole ROI. The area and location of ROI was pre-defined. The tumor and peri-tumor area could not have totally enveloped. As the result indicates, the accuracy is compromised when some of the tumor or peri-tumor areas are lost by the pre-selection of ROI. Hence, tumor segmentation from B-mode image will be performed in the future for the creation of more robust CAD system.

4   The Integration of Qualitative BI-RADS
and Quantitative Strain Features in Elastography

Recently, elastography features are extracted for the development of CAD system to classify breast tumors. The strain image of elastography was obtained through respiratory movement of patient. Such design minimizes the variation introduced by operator and possibly offers a more reproducible result than operator compression. The algorithm of the proposed CAD system is shown in Fig. 5.

Firstly, tumor contour was delineated in B-mode image by level-set segmentation. By overlapping strain image with the tumor contour segmented in B-mode image, tumor area was portrayed in elastogram. Secondly, fuzzy c-means (FCM) clustering was applied to the strain image for feature extraction. FCM re-categorize the 8-bit gray-scale image into a new image only containing black, gray, and white color. Strain features were then extracted to highlight strain area. Finally, the strain features were combined for the classification of tumor types.

B-mode and strain features are well established in many previous studies. The discrepancies of mass characteristics on elastography image and B-mode image were used for distinguishing malignant and benign lesions [35–37]. The ratio of tumor size in elastography and B mode image (strain-to-B-mode ratio) greater than 1.0 has high likelihood of malignancy. The stiffness contrast and normalized shear strain area are also elastography image features for differentiating malignancy

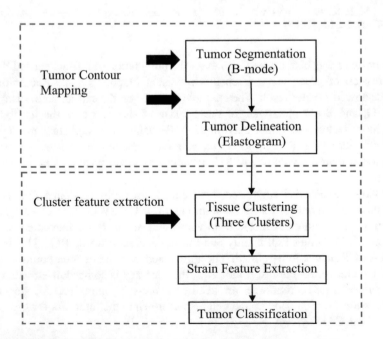

Fig. 5 The flowchart of the diagnostic procedure for elastography

[38–40]. Stiffness contrast is the mean strain ratio of background and within masses. Shear strain area is normalized with tumor size in B-mode.

4.1 Patients and Data Acquisition

The cases came from 90 patients who were examined by US model ACUSON S2000 (Siemens Medical Solutions, Mountain View, CA) with 9L4 linear-array transducer. Both B-mode and elastography images were acquired through the same transducer. The acquisition of elastography image on ACUSON S2000 is based on eSie Touch technique. The deformation of mass (strain) is induced by respiration movement of the patient with the transducer lightly place in contact with skin. Then, a gray-scale elastography image is displayed side-by-side with the B-mode image. Both images are 8-bit gray-scale image with pixel value ranges from 0 to 255.

There were 90 sets of core needle biopsy proven samples. 45 each were benign and malignant. Within the cases with benign lesions, there were 23 fibroadenomas, 14 fibrocystic change, and 8 intraductal papillomas. Malignant cases were composed of 37 invasive ductal carcinomas (IDC), 2 invasive lobular carcinomas (ILC), and 6 ductal carcinoma in situ (DCIS). The lesion sizes were 1.21 ± 0.73 and 1.37 ± 0.39 cm for benign and malignant cases. Patient age ranged from 18-80 years old (mean $= 44 \pm 12$ years old), and 39–83 years old (mean $= 54$ 12 years old).

4.2 Tumor Segmentation

In order to reduce operator-dependency on tumor contour delineation, a semi-automated method by level-set segmentation was applied to pre-processed B-mode image. The pre-processing filters and level-set segmentation were based on an effective method of contrast enhancement, and homogenous region separation used in previous study [41]. Firstly, sigmoid filter was applied to enhance image contrast and bring out tumor with weak edges. Secondly, the contrast-enhanced image was processed by gradient magnitude filter to generate a gradient image of which homogenous regions are better separated. The gradient magnitude filter accomplished such crucial step by analyzing the intensity variation in horizontal and vertical direction. Thirdly, contrast-enhancement by sigmoid filter is done on the gradient image. This step further segregates the range of gray-scale value of pixel to either small (black) or large (white) pixel value. The strengthened contrast in these pre-processing steps suppressed small variations such as speckle noises and conserved tumor contour defined by strong intensity gap.

4.3 Quantitative Features

4.3.1 Strain Features

The elastography image is composed of 8-bit gray-scale pixels with value of 0–255 (Fig. 6b). Soft tissue is indicated by pixels close to 255 (light color), and hard tissue close to 0 (dark color). FCM clustering [41] was applied to re-categorize pixel values into 0, 128, and 255 representing black, gray, and white color (Fig. 6c). The clusters with the following three pixel values were defined because this

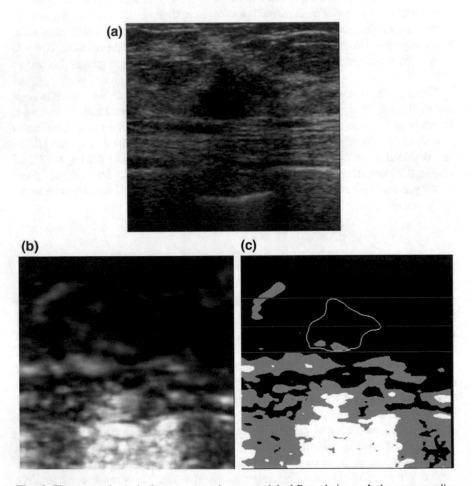

Fig. 6 The automatic strain features extraction **a** an original B-mode image **b** the corresponding elastography image **c** fuzzy c-means (FCM) clustering image with white, gray and black and the identification of maximum diameter on tumor contour in B-mode image, FCM clustering image. Red line indicates maximum diameter on tumor region in strain image. Blue lines highlight the size of strain area

combination resulted in a close resemblance of the original gray-scale distribution. From FCM clustered image and original elastography image, a set of strain features were derived.

Firstly, the two strain features extracted by using the delineated tumor region on original elastography image.

$$StrainMean = \left(\sum_{E(i,j) \in T} E(GrayScale) \right) / TN \qquad (22)$$

$$StrainVAR = \frac{StrainMean}{\left(\sum_{E(i,j) \in T} (E(GrayScale) - StrainMean)^2 \right) / TN} \qquad (23)$$

StrainMean [42] is the average of original elastography gray-scale values $E(i, j)$ where the sum of gray-scale values in tumor contour (T) divided by the number of pixels (TN). Conceptually, this variable represents the general stiffness of the tissue within tumor area.

StrainVAR [42] measures the deviation-fold of gray-scale values $E(i, j)$ where the sum of *StrainMean*-subtracted gray-scale values of tumor contour (T) in the power of 2 divided by the number of pixels (TN) is in the denominator term. The division of *StrainMean* by this term expresses strain heterogeneity in tumor area. The higher the variation of gray-scale within tumor contour, the smaller the value of *Strain-VAR*. This is an important term for malignancy prediction because it encompasses the change of elasticity when there is angiogenesis and necrosis, which are the histology proof of aggressiveness [43]. The concept of *StrainVAR* is similar to elastography signal-to-noise ratio (SNRe). It indicates the quality of strain estimation in elastography by relating measured data with parameters of ultrasound system [44].

Secondly, the difference of tumor area in B-mode and hard (black) area in FCM-clustered elastography was calculated and used as features. Stiffness on the surrounding area of tumor might be caused by desmoplastic reaction of stroma with abundant collagens accumulation. Radiologists commonly used the tumor size difference between B-mode and strain image for tumor diagnosis [28, 35, 45]. A 5-point elasticity scoring system based on comparison of B-mode image and elastography visually was also developed [46]. Nonetheless, all of these study relied on the visual inspection of human. Great interobserver variability is demonstrated with such set-up [28]. More training and experience could certainly close the gap of inconsistent diagnosis between observers. Furthermore, this visual-inspected quality could be quantified. The automated measurement of size difference between B-mode and FCM-clustered strain image was based on maximum length expressed by the following formula:

$$LengthRatio = \frac{length(j_{max}, B_{FCM})}{length(j_{max}, T_{B\,mode})}, j_{max} = \arg\max \, length(j, T_{B\,mode}) \qquad (24)$$

By reading through each j row in delineated tumor of B-mode image (T_{Bmode}), j_{max} is the row of maximum tumor length. By referring to the j_{max} row number acquired from B-mode image, *Strainlength* is the corresponding length in j_{max} row by calculating the number pixels in black area in FCM-clustered elastography image. The red line in Fig. 6c illustrates *Strainlength*.

Extending in 2-dimensional region of FCM-clustered strain image along the upper and lower bound defined by B-mode tumor contour. *GlobalDarkLevel* and *GlobalStrainLevel* are derived. *GlobalDarkLevel* is the total number of black pixel in FCM-clustered elastography image enclosed by the upper and lower bound of tumor contour. *GlobalStrainLevel* is the summation of all gray-scale pixel values in the same region.

$$GlobalDarkLevel = \sum B_{FCM}(i,j), j \geq \arg\min\ row(T_{B\,mode}), j \leq \arg\max\ row(T_{B\,mode})$$
(25)

$$GlobalStrainLevel = \sum E(i,j), j \geq \arg\min\ row(T_{B\,mode}), j \leq \arg\max\ row(T_{B\,mode})$$
(26)

4.3.2 Fuzzy c-means (FCM) Clustering

FCM is a useful technique in pattern recognition [41]. Here, the goal is to convert an 8-bit gray-scale elastography image into an image represented by only black, gray, and white. Altogether, there are N numbers of pixel in the image. By scanning through each pixel in the original image and pre-defined cluster, the below formula is minimized to categorize 8-bit gray-scale into cluster of 3 in this study. Then, the pixels in these clusters are represented in color of black, gray, and white. The classification is done by minimizing the following function:

$$J = \sum_{i=1}^{N} \sum_{j=1}^{C} u_{ij}^{m} \|x_i - c_j\|^2$$
(27)

x_i is the pixel value. c_j is the centroid of cluster j. m is an under-defined variable. u_{ij} is the membership of pixel value difference between x_i and c_j where it characterizes how close the pixel value x_i is to centroid pixel value of cluster c_j.

FCM algorithm is conducted by the initiation of membership matrix $U^{(0)}$ where the summation of membership u_{ij} in c number of clusters equal to 1 [47, 48]. The membership u_{ij} or pixel values difference between x_i and c_i centroid of cluster j can be conceptualized as the probability of x_i pixel values fall into the region of c_i centroid of cluster j.

$$\sum_{j=1}^{c} u_{ij} = 1, \forall j = 1 \ldots c \tag{28}$$

In each iteration, centroid values c_j of each cluster are calculated by the following formula.

$$c_j = \frac{\sum_{i=1}^{N} u_{ij}^{m} \cdot x_i}{\sum_{i=1}^{N} u_{ij}^{m}} \tag{29}$$

The u_{ij} membership of each pixel x_i with members of each cluster (in this case, only 3) is calculated by comparison to the difference in pixel value x_i to each pixel value of possible c_k cluster. It is referring to the following formula where k cannot be equal to j.

$$u_{ij} = \frac{1}{\sum_{k=1}^{c} (\frac{\|x_i - c_j\|}{\|x_i - c_k\|})^{\frac{2}{m-1}}} \tag{30}$$

The iteration keeps going until the centroids of each cluster could result in the smallest possible sum of difference between pixel values of x_i to c_j. Otherwise, new centroids are calculated for the next iterations. The memberships iteratively update while the influences of noise and outliers are reduced. The elastography image is consisted of wide range of gray-scale. The update of centroids and memberships in each iteration leads towards a more accurate classification.

This method provides flexibility to different elastography image setting. Unlike k-means clustering, FCM clustering does not cluster the value of each pixel into membership of 1 cluster only. Instead, FCM clustering focuses on strength of association between each pixel to a particular cluster. It indicates the strength of associations between an element and the all clusters by all memberships separately. The comparison of FCM and k-means clustering was further studied in prior literature [49, 50].

4.3.3 B-mode Features

The characteristics in B-mode images are inseparable part of most ultrasound examination in clinical setting. The ACR BI-RADS of ultrasound descriptors includes shape, orientation, margin, lesion boundary, echo pattern, and posterior acoustic features. These characteristics were used in the development of breast CAD system. The results were promising in distinguishing malignant and benign lesions [12, 17, 18].

Malignant tumor is described as uncontrolled growth pattern with irregular shape. A benign tumor is described as round and smooth. Tumor shape is the most commonly used feature to distinguish malignant from benign tumor. In previous studies, geometric properties such as irregularity and ellipse shape were extracted from tumor contour for differentiation of malignant and benign tumor [12, 16]. Best-fit eclipse of a tumor contour is used to estimate tumor size and position. Roundness metric is another feature related to best-fit eclipse. It is defined by circumference ratio between tumor contour and best-fit eclipse. Furthermore, the ratio of major and minor axes of the best-fit ellipse differentiates round from ellipse shape tumor [17, 18]. Normalized radial length (NRL) is based on Euclidean distance from the center of the mass to the lesion margin. It is normalized to the maximum radial length of lesion [51]. Estimation of tumor contour compactness level is obtained by the ratio of contour perimeter and area. Echogenic texture was quantified using gray level co-occurrence matrices (GLCM) as previously discussed in Sect. 2.4 of this chapter [23].

4.4 Statistical Analysis

The performance of each strain and B-mode feature was evaluated for distinguishing benign and malignant lesions. Kolmogorov-Smirnov test was utilized to determine the distribution of each feature was either normal or non-normal. Student's t-test was used on normal features and Mann-Whitney U-test for non-normal features. p-values <0.05 was regarded as statistical significance. Prediction model was constructed by using the feature set of strain, B-mode, and the combination of both. The tumor classification of feature sets were evaluated by using binary logistic regression with backward stepwise elimination. The analysis is initiated in whole set of features. One at a time, a feature with the minimum predictive residual error sum of squares is removed. The features with the lowest error rate in the set was selected and placed in the classifier for diagnosis. Leave-one-out cross-validation was used to validate the performance of selected features where each time one case is left out for testing while the remaining are training set. All cases were tested accordingly. Corresponding to 90 cases used in this experiment, there were 90 iterations executed. The final results were obtained by the average of these 90 iterations.

Prediction is compared with biopsy-proven result for each case. Tumors with predicted probability >0.5 were classified as malignant by the prediction model. Accuracy, sensitivity, specificity, positive predictive value (PPV), and negative predictive value (NPV) were calculated. Chi-Square test was utilized to compare the performance of two feature sets. ROC curve was drawn to have a closer look on trade-offs between sensitivity and specificity. Area under the ROC curve (Az) was compared. Chi-Square test was utilized to analyze the performance of two feature sets in SPSS software (version 16 for Windows; SPSS, Chicago, IL, USA).

Bivariate chi-square test was utilized to compare area under the ROC curve (Az) in ROCKIT software (Metz, University of Chicago, Chicago, IL, USA).

4.5 Results and Discussion

The 6 proposed strain features were *StrainLength*, *LengthRatio*, *GlobalDarkLevel*, *GlobalStrainLevel*, *StrainMean* and *StrainVAR*. Their performances on tumor classification were investigated individually. *GlobalStrainLevel* was the only feature not statistically significance. All 15 B-mode features were statistically significance. These features are tumor area, minor axis length, tumor compactness level, NRL features, and spiculation numbers on tumor contour, GLCM textures, intensity difference around tumor boundary, tumor-to-surrounding tissue, and tumor-to-posterior area.

The prediction model built by strain feature set out-performed B-mode feature set. Azs of ROC were 0.84 and 0.70 (*p*-value = 0.0443). Strain features achieved an accuracy of 80% (72/90), a sensitivity of 80% (36/45), and a specificity of 80% (36/45). When strain feature set is combined with B-mode feature set, Az improved to 0.93. The improvement of combined feature set is statistical significance compared to only using individual strain (*p*-value = 0.0176) or B-mode feature set (*p*-value = 0.0000).

FCM clustering was previously proposed to re-categorize elastography image into simple strain image for stiffness estimation [41]. Here, the extraction of strain features was based on this method. In addition, strain feature set from FCM-clustered image was combined with B-mode features. A better Az was achieved (Az = 0.93). The complementary effect of strain and B-mode feature is indicated. This result is consistent with previous study which achieved Az = 0.95 with combination of strain and B-mode features [52].

The spiculation number of tumor contour is usually higher in malignant tumor. However, the result showed otherwise. Previous studies support malignant tumor as round shape [16] and some invasive cancer with size >1 cm is round [20]. The spiculation number of a round malignant tumor contour might be close to 0. Furthermore, an ellipse-like benign tumor may have spiculation number of 2. This is still an area of controversy. More studies need to be done to examine the correlation of spiculation number and tumor type.

The heterogeneity within or around malignant tumor in strain image limits the usefulness of some strain feature such as *StrainLength*. The non-uniformity of pixels even after FCM clustering caused the underestimation of *StrainLength* and the misclassification. The use of *StrainVAR* offers a complementary effect to the diagnosis of malignancy with *StrainLength*. *StrainVAR* determines strain heterogeneity of tumor. It is defined by the ratio of *StrainMean* and sum of *strainMean*-subtracted gray-scale values of tumor contour (*T*) in the power of 2 divided by the number of pixels (*TN*). Smaller value of *StrainVAR* resulted from more variation of pixels in tumor area.

5 Conclusion

There is still a huge gap between a well-trained radiologist and a CAD system in terms of diagnosis capability. In order for a CAD system to be helpful, the result has to be accurate and precise. As it is shown in this chapter, the performances of CADs can be improved with the implementation of new algorithms. Maybe there is no one algorithm that can solve all diagnostic problems. The key is to keep questioning what more could be done to improve. Most of the time, there are already answers by referring to the precious clinical experience of radiologist. Interpreting the clinical experience as well as possible would be the challenge of a CAD based on image processing and artificial intelligence. The progress of medicine will be carried forward. More CADs are expected to be developed.

References

1. Siegel, R.L., Miller, K.D., Jemal, A.: Cancer statistics, 2015. CA Cancer J. Clin. **65**, 5–29 (2015)
2. Hoerger, T.J., Ekwueme, D.U., Miller, J.W., Uzunangelov, V., Hall, I.J., Segel, J., Royalty, J., Gardner, J.G., Smith, J.L., Li, C.: Estimated effects of the national breast and cervical cancer early detection program on breast cancer mortality. Am. J. Prev. Med. **40**, 397–404 (2010)
3. Smart, C.R., Byrne, C., Smith, R.A., Garfinkel, L., Letton, A.H., Dodd, G.D., Beahrs, O.H.: Twenty-year follow-up of the breast cancers diagnosed during the breast cancer detection demonstration project. CA Cancer J. Clin. **47**, 134–149 (1997)
4. Tabár, L., Vitak, B., Chen, H.-H.T., Yen, M.-F., Duffy, S.W., Smith, R.A.: Beyond randomized controlled trials. Cancer **91**, 1724–1731 (2001)
5. Jiang, M., Zhang, S., Li, H., Metaxas, D.N.: Computer-aided diagnosis of mammographic masses using scalable image retrieval. IEEE Trans. Biomed. Eng. **62**, 783–792 (2015)
6. Berg, W.A., Gilbreath, P.L.: Multicentric and multifocal cancer: whole-breast US in preoperative evaluation. Radiology **214**, 59–66 (2000)
7. Kelly, K.M., Dean, J., Comulada, W.S., Lee, S.J.: Breast cancer detection using automated whole breast ultrasound and mammography in radiographically dense breasts. Eur. Radiol. **20**, 734–742 (2010)
8. Stavros, A.T., Thickman, D., Rapp, C.L., Dennis, M.A., Parker, S.H., Sisney, G.A.: Solid breast nodules: use of sonography to distinguish between benign and malignant lesions. Radiology **196**, 123–134 (1995)
9. Weigel, S., Biesheuvel, C., Berkemeyer, S., Kugel, H., Heindel, W.: Digital mammography screening: how many breast cancers are additionally detected by bilateral ultrasound examination during assessment? Eur. Radiol. **23**, 684–691 (2013)
10. Mendelson, E., Böhm-Vélez, M., Berg, W., Merritt, C., Rubin, E.: ACR BI-RADS Ultrasound, ACR BI-RADS Atlas, Breast Imaging Reporting and Data System. American College of Radiology, Reston, VA (2013)
11. Leung, J.W.T., Sickles, E.A.: The probably benign assessment. Radiol. Clin. **45**, 773–789 (2007)
12. Drukker, K., Giger, M.L., Metz, C.E.: Robustness of computerized lesion detection and classification scheme across different breast US platforms. Radiology **237**, 834–840 (2005)
13. Lo, C.M., Moon, W.K., Huang, C.S., Chen, J.H., Yang, M.C., Chang, R.F.: Intensity-invariant texture analysis for classification of BI-RADS category 3 breast masses. Ultrasound Med. Biol. **41**, 2039–2048 (2015)

14. Lo, C.M., Chang, Y.C., Yang, Y.W., Huang, C.S., Chang, R.F.: Quantitative breast mass classification based on the integration of B-mode features and strain features in elastography. Comput. Biol. Med. **64**, 91–100 (2015)

15. Lo, C.M., Lai, Y.C., Chou, Y.H., Chang, R.F.: Quantitative breast lesion classification based on multichannel distributions in shear-wave imaging. Comput. Methods Programs Biomed. **122**, 354–361 (2015)

16. Moon, W.K., Lo, C.-M., Chang, J.M., Huang, C.-S., Chen, J.-H., Chang, R.-F.: Quantitative ultrasound analysis for classification of BI-RADS category 3 breast masses. J. Digit. Imaging **26**, 1091–1098 (2013)

17. Moon, W.K., Lo, C.-M., Chang, J.M., Huang, C.-S., Chen, J.-H., Chang, R.-F.: Computer-aided classification of breast masses using speckle features of automated breast ultrasound images. Med. Phys. **39**, 6465–6473 (2012)

18. Moon, W.K., Lo, C.-M., Huang, C.-S., Chen, J.-H., Chang, R.-F.: Computer-aided diagnosis based on speckle patterns in ultrasound images. Ultrasound Med. Biol. **38**, 1251–1261 (2012)

19. Berg, W.A., Blume, J.D., Cormack, J.B., et al.: Combined screening with ultrasound and mammography versus mammography alone in women at elevated risk of breast cancer. JAMA **299**, 2151–2163 (2008)

20. Chung-Ming, L., Rong-Tai, C., Yeun-Chung, C., Ya-Wen, Y., Ming-Jen, H., Chiun-Sheng, H., Ruey-Feng, C.: Multi-dimensional tumor detection in automated whole breast ultrasound using topographic watershed. IEEE Trans Med. Imaging **33**, 1503–1511 (2014)

21. Masotti, M., Lanconelli, N., Campanini, R.: Computer-aided mass detection in mammography: false positive reduction via gray-scale invariant ranklet texture features. Med. Phys. **36**, 311–316 (2009)

22. Min-Chun, Y., Woo Kyung, M., Wang, Y.C.F., Min Sun, B., Chiun-Sheng, H., Jeon-Hor, C., Ruey-Feng, C.: Robust texture analysis using multi-resolution gray-scale invariant features for breast sonographic tumor diagnosis. IEEE Trans. Med. Imaging **32**, 2262–2273 (2013)

23. Haralick, R.M., Shanmugam, K., Dinstein, I.H.: Textural features for image classification. IEEE Trans. Syst. Man Cybern. **SMC-3**, 610–621 (1973)

24. Kim, K.G., Cho, S.W., Min, S.J., Kim, J.H., Min, B.G., Bae, K.T.: Computerized scheme for assessing ultrasonographic features of breast masses. Acad. Radiol. **12**, 58–66 (2005)

25. Costantini, M., Belli, P., Lombardi, R., Franceschini, G., Mulè, A., Bonomo, L.: Characterization of solid breast masses: use of the sonographic breast imaging reporting and data system Lexicon. J. Ultrasound Med. **25**, 649–659 (2006)

26. Barr, R.G., Zhang, Z., Cormack, J.B., Mendelson, E.B., Berg, W.A.: Probably benign lesions at screening breast US in a population with elevated risk: prevalence and rate of malignancy in the ACRIN 6666 trial. Radiology **269**, 701–712 (2013)

27. Cho, N., Moon, W.K., Chang, J.M., Yi, A., Koo, H.R., Park, J.S., Park, I.A.: Sonoelastographic lesion stiffness: preoperative predictor of the presence of an invasive focus in nonpalpable DCIS diagnosed at US-guided needle biopsy. Eur. Radiol. **21**, 1618–1627 (2011)

28. Burnside, E.S., Hall, T.J., Sommer, A.M., Hesley, G.K., Sisney, G.A., Svensson, W.E.: Differentiating benign from malignant solid breast masses with US strain imaging. Radiology **245**, 401–410 (2007)

29. Bercoff, J., Tanter, M., Fink, M.: Supersonic shear imaging: a new technique for soft tissue elasticity mapping. IEEE Trans. Ultrason. Ferroelectr. Freq. Control **51**, 396–409 (2004)

30. Evans, A., Whelehan, P., Thomson, K., Brauer, K., Jordan, L., Purdie, C., McLean, D., Baker, L., Vinnicombe, S., Thompson, A.: Differentiating benign from malignant solid breast masses: value of shear wave elastography according to lesion stiffness combined with greyscale ultrasound according to BI-RADS classification. Br. J. Cancer **107**, 224–229 (2012)

31. Berg, W.A., Cosgrove, D.O., Doré, C.J., Schäfer, F.K.W., Svensson, W.E., Hooley, R.J., Ohlinger, R., Mendelson, E.B., Balu-Maestro, C., Locatelli, M., Tourasse, C., Cavanaugh, B. C., Juhan, V., Stavros, A.T., Tardivon, A., Gay, J., Henry, J.-P., Cohen-Bacrie, C.: Shear-wave elastography improves the specificity of breast US: the BE1 multinational study of 939 masses. Radiology **262**, 435–449 (2012)

32. Huang, P.-C., Li, P.-C.: Vector quantization of RF channel data for ultrasound imaging. Ultrason. Imaging **35**, 3–16 (2013)
33. Chang, J.M., Moon, W.K., Cho, N., Yi, A., Koo, H.R., Han, W., Noh, D.Y., Moon, H.G., Kim, S.J.: Clinical application of shear wave elastography (SWE) in the diagnosis of benign and malignant breast diseases. Breast Cancer Res. Treat. **129**, 89–97 (2011)
34. Evans, A., Whelehan, P., Thomson, K., McLean, D., Brauer, K., Purdie, C., Jordan, L., Baker, L., Thompson, A.: Quantitative shear wave ultrasound elastography: initial experience in solid breast masses. Breast Cancer Res. **12**, R104 (2010)
35. Jung, H.J., Hahn, S.Y., Choi, H.Y., Park, S.H., Park, H.K.: Breast sonographic elastography using an advanced breast tissue-specific imaging preset: initial clinical results. J. Ultrasound Med. **31**, 273–280 (2012)
36. Stachs, A., Hartmann, S., Stubert, J., Dieterich, M., Martin, A., Kundt, G., Reimer, T., Gerber, B.: Differentiating between malignant and benign breast masses: factors limiting sonoelastographic strain ratio. Ultraschall Med. **34**, 131–136 (2013)
37. Garra, B.S., Cespedes, E.I., Ophir, J., Spratt, S.R., Zuurbier, R.A., Magnant, C.M., Pennanen, M.F.: Elastography of breast lesions: initial clinical results. Radiology **202**, 79–86 (1997)
38. Xu, H., Rao, M., Varghese, T., Sommer, A., Baker, S., Hall, T.J., Sisney, G.A., Burnside, E. S.: Axial-shear strain imaging for differentiating benign and malignant breast masses. Ultrasound Med. Biol. **36**, 1813–1824 (2010)
39. Xu, H., Varghese, T., Jiang, J., Zagzebski, J.A.: In vivo classification of breast masses using features derived from axial-strain and axial-shear images. Ultrason. Imaging **34**, 222–236 (2012)
40. Thittai, A.K., Yamal, J.M., Mobbs, L.M., Kraemer-Chant, C.M., Chekuri, S., Garra, B.S., Ophir, J.: Axial-shear strain elastography for breast lesion classification: further results from in vivo data. Ultrasound Med. Biol. **37**, 189–197 (2011)
41. Moon, W.K., Chang, S.C., Huang, C.S., Chang, R.F.: Breast tumor classification using fuzzy clustering for breast elastography. Ultrasound Med. Biol. **37**, 700–708 (2011)
42. Lo, C.-M., Chen, Y.-P., Chang, Y.-C., Lo, C., Huang, C.-S., Chang, R.-F.: Computer-aided strain evaluation for acoustic radiation force impulse imaging of breast masses. Ultrason. Imaging **36**, 151–166 (2014)
43. Davnall, F., Yip, C.S., Ljungqvist, G., Selmi, M., Ng, F., Sanghera, B., Ganeshan, B., Miles, K.A., Cook, G.J., Goh, V.: Assessment of tumor heterogeneity: an emerging imaging tool for clinical practice? Insights Imaging **3**, 573–589 (2012)
44. Kallel, F., Ophir, J.: A least-squares strain estimator for elastography. Ultrason. Imaging **19**, 195–208 (1997)
45. Leong, L.C., Sim, L.S., Lee, Y.S., Ng, F.C., Wan, C.M., Fook-Chong, S.M., Jara-Lazaro, A. R., Tan, P.H.: A prospective study to compare the diagnostic performance of breast elastography versus conventional breast ultrasound. Clin. Radiol. **65**, 887–894 (2010)
46. Itoh, A., Ueno, E., Tohno, E., Kamma, H., Takahashi, H., Shiina, T., Yamakawa, M., Matsumura, T.: Breast disease: clinical application of US elastography for diagnosis. Radiology **239**, 341–350 (2006)
47. Bezdek, J.C., Ehrlich, R., Full, W.: FCM: the fuzzy c-means clustering algorithm. Comput. Geosci. **10**, 191–203 (1984)
48. Chuai-Aree, S., Lursinsap, C., Sophasathit, P., Siripant, S.: Fuzzy c-mean: a statistical feature classification of text and image segmentation method. Int. J. Uncertain. Fuzziness Knowl. Syst. **09**, 661–671 (2001)
49. Kannan, S.R.: A new segmentation system for brain MR images based on fuzzy techniques. Appl. Soft Comput. **8**, 1599–1606 (2008)
50. Sombutkaew, R., Kumsang, Y., Chitsobuk, O.: 14th International Conference on Presented at the Control, Automation and Systems (ICCAS) (2014) (unpublished)
51. Nie, K., Chen, J.H., Yu, H.J., Chu, Y., Nalcioglu, O., Su, M.Y.: Quantitative analysis of lesion morphology and texture features for diagnostic prediction in breast MRI. Acad Radiol **15**, 1513–1525 (2008)

52. Alhabshi, S.M., Rahmat, K., Abdul Halim, N., Aziz, S., Radhika, S., Gan, G.C., Vijayananthan, A., Westerhout, C.J., Mohd-Shah, M.N., Jaszle, S., Harlina Mohd Latar, N., Muhammad, R.: Semi-quantitative and qualitative assessment of breast ultrasound elastography in differentiating between malignant and benign lesions. Ultrasound Med. Biol. **39**, 568–578 (2013)

Categorization of Lung Tumors into Benign/Malignant, Solid/GGO, and Typical Benign/Others

Yasushi Hirano

Abstract In this chapter, various categorization methods for lung tumors in chest X-ray CT images are described. These categorization methods include not only a method for benign/malignant classification, but also methods for solid/Ground-glass opacity (GGO) classification and typical benign/others classification. Furthermore, extraction methods for lung tumors and lung blood vessels are also are described as the fundamental techniques for the structural analysis leading up to these categorization methods.

1 Extraction

1.1 Lung Tumors

1.1.1 Overview

Extraction of lung tumor regions plays an important role in classification of lung tumors. Extracted tumor regions can be used for analysis of their behavior such as texture and shape of the tumors themselves and peripheral anatomical structure of the tumors. The method introduced here is a threshold-based interactive method for extraction of lung tumors from chest X-ray CT images. Although many methods of extracting tumor regions have been proposed, most of these methods are based on simple thresholding or shape modeling [1, 2]. These methods have potential risks to miss-extract marginal structures of the tumors.

The proposed method consists of the following two stages: the rough extraction of central tumor regions and adding detailed marginal structures of the tumors to the central tumor regions. These two kinds of regions are extracted by using the threshold-based and distance transformation-based methods. And it is assumed that the rough locations of centers of the tumors are indicated manually. If the tumor

Y. Hirano (✉)
Yamaguchi University, Yamaguchi, Japan
e-mail: yhirano@yamaguchi-u.ac.jp

© Springer International Publishing AG 2018
K. Suzuki and Y. Chen (eds.), *Artificial Intelligence in Decision Support Systems for Diagnosis in Medical Imaging*, Intelligent Systems Reference Library 140, https://doi.org/10.1007/978-3-319-68843-5_8

regions are incompletely extracted, the users can interactively add parts of the tumor regions to the incomplete tumor regions. Additionally, all operations can be performed only using mouse operations. The authors applied this method to 78 clinical CT images, and showed its effectiveness [3].

1.1.2 Proposed Method

The outline of the proposed method is shown below, and the flow chart is shown in Fig. 1. Note that the voxel values of the foreground (figure) voxels are 1, those of the background voxels are 0, and the set of gray-valued voxels which belongs to a figure is called as a gray-tone connected component in the explanation.

[**Step 1**] Thresholding of CT numbers for CT image. The voxels with higher values than the threshold become foreground, and those with lower values are background. Additionally, the foreground regions outside of lung region are deleted. The remaining regions are called "vessel regions", but note that these regions contain vessel regions, bronchial wall regions, and tumor regions.

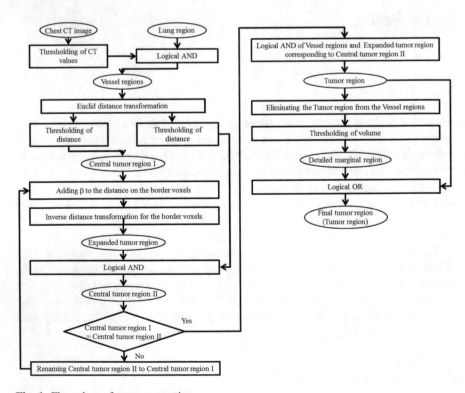

Fig. 1 Flow chart of tumor extraction

[**Step 2**] Performing the Euclidean distance transformation to the vessel region. The distance value on the voxel P_{sp} that is specified as the center of the tumor is D_{sp}.

[**Step 3**] Thresholding of distance values for vessel regions. The threshold is T_{dist} $(= D_{sp} - \alpha)$, where α is a constant. The voxel values which are lower than T_{dist} are changed to 0.

[**Step 4**] Foreground voxels which have longer distance than D_{sp} from P_{sp} are changed background voxels. The obtained gray-tone connected component is called as the central tumor region I. The maximum distance value in the central tumor region is D_{max}.

[**Step 5**] Performing the inverse distance transformation for the border voxels of the central tumor region I after adding β to the distance value on the border voxels. β is a constant. The obtained region is called as the expanded tumor region.

[**Step 6**] A set of voxels which have larger than $D_{max} - \alpha$ as the distance values in the product set of the vessel region and the expanded tumor region is named the central tumor region II.

[**Step 7**] If the central tumor region I coincides with the central tumor region II, go to [Step 8]. Otherwise, rename the central tumor region II to the central tumor region I, and go to [Step 5].

[**Step 8**] Performing logical AND of the expanded tumor region and the vessel region. Further, eliminate regions which do not contain P_{sp}. The obtained region is called the tumor region.

[**Step 9**] Eliminating the tumor region from the vessel regions.

[**Step 10**] Eliminating sets of voxels which are larger than T_v in volume. The obtained regions are named the detailed marginal region.

[**Step 11**] Performing logical OR of the tumor region and the detailed marginal region. The obtained region is the tumor region.

Figure 2 shows the illustrations of a part of the above procedure. In this example, because the central tumor region II in Step 6 (second) and Step 6 (third) coincide with each other, the iterative procedure for determination of central tumor region is terminated at Step 6 (third). Then Step 8 will be executed after the conditional branching in Step 7. Note that the central tumor region II in Step 6 is the same region as the central tumor region I in Step 6 in the previous iteration.

If the obtained tumor region is not enough, the users can complement the tumor region by specifying the rough center of the deficient region, performing the above procedure, and merging the original tumor region and newly obtained region.

The proposed method was applied to 78 chest CT images which contained one tumor for each. The experimental results are shown in Table 1, and the examples of the extracted results are shown in Fig. 3.

1.1.3 Experiment and Result

It is shown that the numbers of over extraction and poor cases are larger in solid type than in other types (Table 1). It is thought that over extraction was caused by

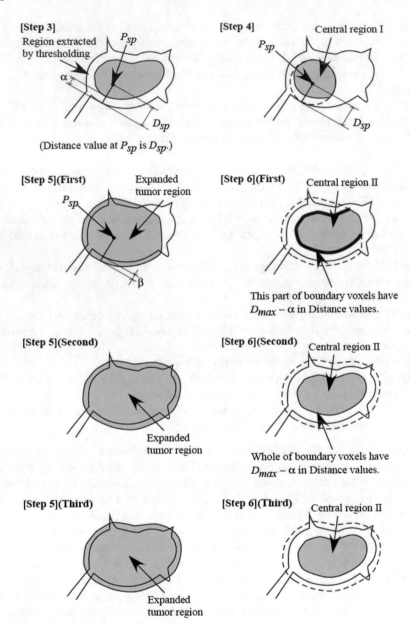

Fig. 2 Illustration of the procedure [3, 4]

convergence of vessels. This phenomenon is often observed in the cases of malignant tumors, and vessels around tumors become larger and connecting with tumors. These vessels were failed to recognize as parts of tumors. In the case of poor extracted cases, the tumors have cavities or they are separated more than one part.

Table 1 Evaluation of the experimental result for a single specified voxel

	Good	Overextraction	Poor
Solid	33	7	6
Mixed	6	0	5
GGO	13	1	2
Unknown	3	1	1
Total	55	9	14

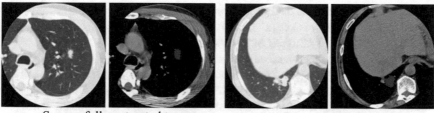

Successfully extracted tumor   Poor extracted tumor

Fig. 3 Examples of experimental results [4] (Red regions indicate extracted tumor regions). Successfully extracted tumor Poor extracted tumor

The additional voxels were manually specified by the user as the center of the missing tumors for the poorly extracted cases. As the result of that, for 12 cases of those cases, tumor regions were correctly extracted. Tumors in the other 2 cases were not able to be extracted because of their low CT numbers or widespread lesion.

By using the proposed method, lung tumors in chest X-ray CT images can properly be extracted with convenient operations.

1.2 Lung Blood Vessels

1.2.1 Overview

Lung vessel regions can be utilized to analyze the characteristics of lung tumors and the structure in lung regions. For instance, many adenocarcinomas present with the specific phenomenon. This phenomenon means the convergence of lung arteries and bronchi toward to adenocarcinomas, and quantification of the convergence gives us a hint for classification of lung tumors into malignant and benign tumors [5]. For another example, lung regions can be separated into five lung lobes by structural analysis of lung blood vessels [6]. For these application, peripheral thin vessels are more useful than thick vessels, because thin vessels tend to be stronger affected by the convergence, and they are located near the boundaries of lung lobes.

In this section, a method to extract lung vessel region based on curvatures. In three-dimensional space, the measure of bentness is presented by 2 curvatures. These curvatures are the maximum normal curvature and the minimum normal curvature of the surface of the object, where the 2 normal sections for each normal curvature are perpendicular to each other. Further, the Gauss curvature and the mean curvature are calculated from the maximum and the minimum normal curvatures. Every local surface can be categorized into one of 8 types using the Gauss and the mean curvatures. Note that characteristics of the curvatures mentioned above are true for surfaces of objects in three-dimensional space, in other words, three-dimensional binary space (images). The three-dimensional gray image can be treated as the four-dimensional binary space by transforming gray level into gray axis as well as the spatial axes (x, y, z). In this four-dimensional space, there exist 3 normal curvatures and 42 types of local surfaces [7].

The method introduced here categorizes voxels in three-dimensional gray images into one of the 42 types based on 3 normal curvatures. Furthermore, specifying a single voxel that belongs to lung vessel region and calculating the type of curvatures on the specified voxel, the lung vessel region is extracted using the region-growing method of the type of the local surface [8].

1.2.2 Proposed Method

First, the CT image is represented as the set of local curved hyper surfaces by performing the curve fitting method on each voxel in the CT image. In this section, we use three-dimensional second-order polynomials as curved hyper surface to be fit. As is well known, the first and second order derivations on the point of interest (POI) are required to calculate normal curvatures, and they can be easily obtained from three-dimensional second-order polynomials. Next, 3 normal curvatures are calculated on each voxel in the input CT image, and each voxel is categorized into one of the 42 type based on curvatures [7]. Finally, the region growing method is performed to extract a specific region. In this section, a combination of type based on curvatures is used as the condition of the region growing method instead of CT numbers in the standard region growing method. It is assumed that the starting point is specified manually. If a voxel belonging to lung vessels is specified as the starting point, a lung vessel region might be extracted. And if a voxel belonging to other organ is specified, the organ region might be extracted.

1.2.3 Experiment and Result

The method introduced above is applied to a chest CT image. The conditions for the region growing are the following. These conditions are decided by analyzing the distribution of types of curvatures in lung vessel regions.

[Conditions for region growing]

The type based on the curvatures is any one of the following types:

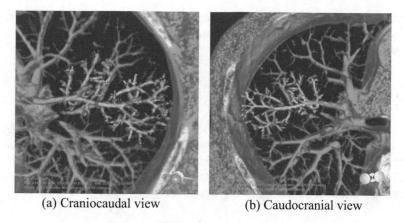

(a) Craniocaudal view   (b) Caudocranial view

Fig. 4 Extracted region rendered by volume rendering algorithm (Yellow regions) [7]

- Type 2 $k_1 > k_2 > k_3 = 0, |k_1| > |k_2| > |k_3| = 0$ and $k_1 + k_2 + k_3 > 0$ or
- Type 16 $k_1 > k_2 = 0 > k_3, |k_1| > |k_3| > |k_2| = 0$, and $k_1 + k_2 + k_3 > 0$,

where k_1, k_2, and k_3 are the normal curvatures, and $k_1 \geq k_2 \geq k_3$. And $k_{1max} \geq k_1 \geq k_{1min}$, where k_{1max} and k_{1min} are constant values.

The experimental results are shown in Fig. 4. Yellow regions are the extracted regions. A single voxel at the root of the lung vessel was specified as the starting point. It is shown that lung vessel regions are selectively extracted. Further thin vessel regions peripherally located are also extracted with the same conditions for thick vessels in the same region growing process. These thin vessel regions might not be extracted simple region growing methods using CT numbers.

The Jaccard index between the ground truth and the extracted vessel regions was 0.93.

2   Classification

2.1   Benign/Malignant Classification

Classification of lung tumors into benign/malignant tumors by using computer is important in the sense of reducing medical doctors' labor, and diagnosing objectively and universally. This section shows two features to quantify the state of the distribution of lung vessels and bronchi in three-dimensional space for analysis of peripheral structures of tumors. As mentioned above, the phenomenon named convergence is frequently observed in the case of adenocarcinoma. Two features introduced here were developed to quantify the degree of convergence of lung vessels and bronchi, and improvement of the classification accuracy for adenocarcinoma lead higher classification accuracy for lung tumors. These features are based on the concentration index and the Voronoi tessellation as described below.

2.1.1 Concentration Index

The concentration index quantifies the degree of the concentration of line figures (i.e. center line of blood vessel) in three-dimensional space toward an arbitrary point in the same three-dimensional space [5, 9]. First, line figures are divided into small line segment called the line element. Then the concentration index on the point P is calculated as the following equation:

$$C(\mathrm{P}) = \frac{\sum_{\mathrm{R}} \frac{ds|\cos\alpha|}{r}}{\sum_{\mathrm{R}} \frac{ds}{r}},$$

where, ds, r, R and α are the lengths of the line elements, the distance between the point P and the line element, the neighborhood region to calculate local concentration, and the angle between each line element and the line $\overline{\mathrm{PQ}}$, respectively. Point Q is a voxel on which each line element exists. The concentration index takes continuous value between 0 and 1, and if no concentration of line figures is observed, the concentration index takes the value 0. Figure 5 shows the examples of the values of concentration index for artificial line figures. The concentration index was calculated on each voxel in the binary images containing line figures. As the results of calculating the concentration index in whole images, the gray images are obtained. These gray images are called the concentration index images. In Fig. 5, a higher concentration index is represented whither. The upper row of Fig. 5

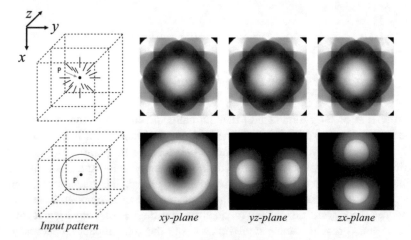

Input pattern   xy-plane   yz-plane   zx-plane

Fig. 5 Concentration index image for artificial line figures

shows the concentrating line figures toward to the center of the binary image, and cross sections of its concentration index image. The lower row shows the circular line figure (i.e. the line figure does not concentrate toward to the center of the binary image at all) and cross sections of the concentration index image.

In the concentration index image for the concentrating pattern, values of concentration index are higher in the center of the images, and very low in the surrounding region. For the circular pattern, the center of the concentration index image is very low. Thus it is thought that existence of concentration can be detected by the value of the concentration index.

Figure 6 shows the application results for the CT images. Figure 6a is the procedure to obtain line figures which represent the center lines of the lung blood vessel regions. Although images in Fig. 6a are presented in two-dimensionally, the images are processed in three-dimensionally. Lung blood vessel regions are extracted from chest CT images, and they are linearized by the thinning method [10]. By calculating the concentration index using these linearized vessel regions, the convergence of blood vessels are quantified. The left images in Fig. 6b-1 and b-2 are the slices of the original CT images, in which the centers of the tumors are located, and the right images in these images are the cross-sections of the concentration index images which are correspond to the slices of the CT images. The red circles indicate the locations of the tumors. In the concentration index images, whither voxels have higher concentration indexes. As shown in Fig. 6b-1 and b-2 the region corresponding to the tumor region in the case without convergence of

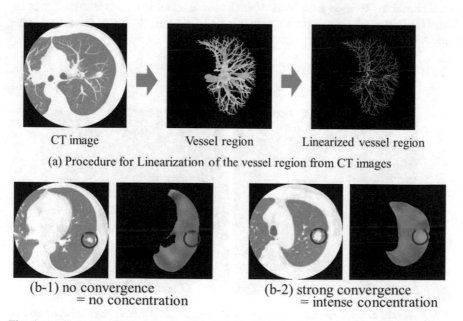

CT image   Vessel region   Linearized vessel region

(a) Procedure for Linearization of the vessel region from CT images

(b-1) no convergence   (b-2) strong convergence
      = no concentration   = intense concentration

Fig. 6 Application to CT images [9]. Red circles indicate the locations of tumors

blood vessels has very low values in the concentration index. On the other hand, for the case with strong convergence, that has high values.

2.1.2 Voronoi Tessellation-Base Feature

A feature which quantifies the difference of the density of line figures was developed [11]. This feature is based on the 3D extended Voronoi tessellation, and defined as the ratio of average volumes of Voronoi regions at the neighborhood of the specific point to the average volume of the Voronoi regions over the whole image. In the application to medical images, the former is the average volume of the Voronoi region surrounding tumors, and the latter is that in lung region. The feature is defined as the following equation:

$$M_r = \frac{M_{aver}}{M_{sp_r}},$$

where M_{aver} and M_{spr} are the average volumes of Voronoi regions in whole lung region, and the average volume of the Voronoi regions surrounding the tumor region (Fig. 7). If the line segments are densely distributed in the neighborhood of the tumor, the feature M_r takes large value, because the Voronoi regions tend to be small for densely distributed generators.

The linearized lung blood vessels (i.e. line figures) are divided into short line segments. In this experiment, the line segments obtained from vessels with 4–6 mm in diameter are used as generators of the Voronoi tessellation. As the result that the linearized lung blood vessels with smaller or larger vessels out of the above range are deleted, short line segments are remained.

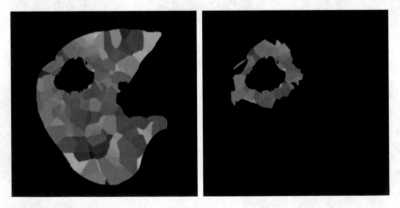

Fig. 7 Results of the Voronoi tessellation of whole lung region (left) and neighborhood of tumor (right) [11]. The black region inside the lung region corresponds to the tumor region

2.1.3 Classification Result

The benign/malignant classification was performed using the nearest-neighbor decision rule. The leave-one-out cross-validation method was employed for performance evaluation. When four features (the concentration index, the complexity in the shape of the tumor region, the average of CT numbers in the peripheral of the tumor region, and the volume of the peripheral of the tumor region [12]) were employed, the correct classification ratio was 85.9%. When three features (the feature M_r, the entropy of CT numbers in the tumor region, and the variance of CT numbers in the peripheral of the tumor region) were used, the correct classification ratio was 82.1%.

2.2 Solid/GGO Classification

2.2.1 Overview

Classification into Solid and GGO tumors is important for accurate benign/malignant discrimination, because the different decision rules are applied for Solid and GGO tumors to discriminate between benign and malignant tumors. In the field of the computer-aided diagnosis, it is thought that the accuracy of benign/malignant discrimination will be improved, if the different decision rules can be applied. This section introduces a method to classify tumors into solid tumors and GGO.

2.2.2 Proposed Method

First, the tumors are extracted by using the method mentioned above [3]. Then, they are classified nearest-neighbor classifier in the feature space consisting of the average value and the variance of CT number in the tumor [12].

2.2.3 Experiment and Result

53 cases were used in this experiment. The detail of the cases is shown in Table 2. GGO cases tend to be malignant in the cases used in this experiment.

Table 2 Detail of the cases used in this experiment

	Malignant	Benign	Total
Solid	25	18	43
GGO	9	1	10
Total	34	19	53

204 Y. Hirano

Table 3 Classification result

Medical doctor	Computer	
	Solid	GGO
Solid	0.93 (40/43)	0.07 (3/43)
GGO	0.20 (2/10)	0.80 (8/10)

Table 4 Result of discrimination between benign and malignant tumor

		Correct classification rate	Sensitivity	Specificity
After solid/GGO classification	Solid	0.90	0.90	0.86
	GGO	0.93	1.00	0.67
Without solid/GGO classification		0.88	0.76	0.84

Classification result is shown in Table 3. The numbers which are enclosed in parentheses are number of cases classified by computer and the number of the true types. For example, (8/10) at the bottom right of Table 3 means that 8 true GGO tumors are correctly classified as GGO tumors, and the total number of true GGO tumors is 10. The leave-one-out method was used in the performance evaluation. The correct classification rate ($= (TP + TN)/$(number of all cases)) is 0.91 ($= (40 + 8)/53$). Although solid tumors are classified with high accuracy, accuracy of the result for GGO is not enough. The reason of this result is caused by the fact that the vessels with high CT number have almost the same CT numbers as solid tumors, but GGO have lower CT numbers than vessels. Therefore GGO is misclassified because of vessels in GGO tumors.

Table 4 shows the result of discrimination between benign and malignant tumor. It is shown that higher performance can be obtained due to solid/GGO classification except for the specificity in GGO.

2.3 Typical Benign/Others Classification

2.3.1 Overview

Progression of CT scanners, small tumors have been found aside from the target tumors. Because most of these small tumors are benign but some of these are malignant, it is required to perform invasive study or a long-term follow-up to decide their malignancy even if they are benign. Therefore a method to classify these small tumors with a single volume of CT image is important. On the other hand, some of skillful radiologists can discriminate these tumors into typical benign tumors and others without invasive study or a long-term follow-up because of their

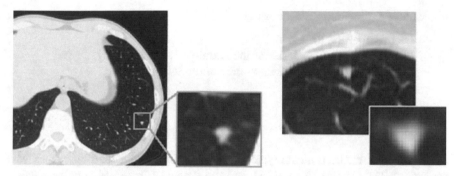

Fig. 8 Examples of typical benign tumors [13]

accumulated medical findings. Note that the "others" does not contain "typical benign tumors" but contain non-typical benign tumors or malignant tumors. So that means "typical benign tumors" are tumors that can be determined as benign by skillful radiologists with their common sense, and most of these typical benign tumors consist of granuloma or lymphoid hyperplasia. They arise in a single secondary lobule, rarely change their size or density according to time course.

In this section, a method to discriminate typical benign tumors is introduced. Figure 8 shows examples of typical benign tumors [13].

2.3.2 Proposed Method

The features used in this classification are based on the findings of medical doctors. The findings utilized in diagnosis are as follows:

- Diameter is less than 10 mm.
- Distance between tumor and chest wall is between 5 and 10 mm.
- Border of tumor is linear, or perimeter of tumor is polygonal.
- Density inside tumor is almost uniform.
- Linear structure is sometime observed between tumor and chest wall.

These medical findings are quantified by the methods in the papers [14, 15]. The following features are used in the experiments.

- Features in two-dimensional space

  - Complexity of the boundaries of the nodule
  - Uniformity of CT numbers in the nodule
    Distance between the nodule and the pleura
  - Existence of linear structures between the nodule and the pleura

- Features in three-dimensional space

  - Diameter of the nodule
  - Planarity of the boundaries of the nodule
  - Connection of blood vessels to the corners of the nodule.

2.3.3 Experiment and Results

An experiment to discriminate typical benign nodules from the other types was performed. The classifier is an SVM, and the kernel of the SVM is polynomial.

The number of the CT images is 78 which contain 43 typical benign tumors and 35 other type of tumors. All tumors are solid type and their diameters in three-dimensional space are smaller than 10 mm.

The accuracy, precision and recall are defined as the following equations:

$$\text{accuracy} = (\text{TP} + \text{TN})/(\text{TP} + \text{TN} + \text{FP} + \text{FN})$$
$$\text{precision} = \text{TP}/(\text{TP} + \text{FP})$$
$$\text{recall} = \text{TP}/(\text{TP} + \text{FN})$$

The accuracy of the classification was 100% using the resubstitution method and 74.4% using the leave-one-out method. In the result using the leave-one-out method, the precision is 73.5% and the recall is 83.7%. It takes about 2 min to calculate features after the user designated the tumors in interest by mouse operation with observing the CT image and about 1 min for classify.

3 Discussion

Because the changes of CT numbers mean the changes of kinds of tissues (cells), extraction of lung tumors should be basically done by thresholding of CT numbers. The method for extracting lung tumors introduced in this chapter is based on this concept, and the almost all lung tumors were successfully extracted including detailed peripheral regions. On the other hand, vessel regions connecting to lung tumors are excluded. Needless to say, although other methods such as the shape model-based methods could be exclude connecting vessel regions, these methods might spoil the detailed peripheral information of tumors. For this reason, the tumor regions using the method introduced in this chapter can be used for various kinds of tumor classifications such as those introduced in the latter half of this chapter. In the experiment, two lung tumors could not be successfully extracted. These lung tumors have very low CT numbers, or widely diffuse. The adaptive parameter (e.g. thresholds of CT numbers and distance) setting is required for improvement of the accuracy.

In the extracting method of lung vessel regions, the lung vessel regions are segmented based on combinations of curvatures calculated on each voxel. It is efficient to use the curvature-based method to extract regions which have particular kinds of distributions of gray levels. For instance, the vessel regions used in the experiment have only two major combinations of curvatures, and these combinations rarely exist in other region in the lung region. Parallel use of the curvature information and the region growing method could extract vessel regions accurately.

The author introduced three classification methods for lung tumors. Benign/ malignant classification and solid/GGO classification show that the correct classification rate of benign/malignant classification is improved after solid/GGO classification according to clinical manner. The correct classification rates in benign/ malignant classification of solid and GGO are 0.90 and 0.93, respectively. These values are higher than that without solid/GGO classification, and it is thought that it is high enough for clinical use. Furthermore, it is confirmed that criterion to discriminate benign tumors from malignant tumors for solid tumors might be different from that for GGO tumors. The third classification method presented in this chapter is developed to pick up benign tumors which can be easily diagnosed as benign by skillful radiologists. The features used in this classification are based on medical findings. Although the performance is not enough at this point in time, it will be improved by adding other features based on other medical findings.

4 Conclusion

In this chapter, three classification methods of lung tumors were introduced, that is, benign/malignant, Solid/GGO, and typical benign/others classifications. Methods for extracting lung tumor regions and lung vessel regions for characterizing the tumors themselves and the surrounding structure of the tumors were also introduced. The features used in the tumor classification were designed in order to match with the diagnostic manner of medical doctors. Both the extraction methods for lung tumor regions and lung vessel regions were designed as interactive methods in order to expand the target regions with simple operations if the automatically extracted regions were insufficient. These two methods extracted target regions for each method accurately, and it was confirmed that they were adapted to uses of classifications of lung tumors.

References

1. Kim, D.-Y., Kim, J.-H., Noh, S.-M., Park, J.-W.: Pulmonary nodule detection using chest Ct images. Acta Radiol. **44**(3), 252–257 (2003)
2. Way, T.W., Sahiner, B., Chan, H.-P., Hadjiiski, L., Cascade, P.N., Chughtai, A., Bogot, N., Kazerooni, E.: Computer-aided diagnosis of pulmonary nodules on CT scans: improvement of

classification performance with nodule surface features. Med. Phys. **36**, 3086 (2009). https://doi.org/10.1118/1.3140589

3. Hirano, Y., Hasegawa, J., Toriwaki, J., Ohmatsu, H., Eguchi, K.: Extraction of tumor regions keeping boundary shape information from chest X-ray CT images and benign/malignant discrimination. In: Proceedings of Computer Assisted Radiology and Surgery (CARS) 2001, pp. 617–622 (2001)

4. Hirano, Y., Hasegawa, J., Toriwaki, J., Ohmatsu, H., Eguchi, K.: Interactive method to extract tumor regions from chest X-ray CT images and its application to benign/malignant discrimination. J. Inst. Electron. Inf. Commun. Eng. **J87-D-II**(1), 237–247 (2004) (in Japanese)

5. Hirano, Y., Mekada, Y., Hasegawa, J., Toriwaki, J.: Quantification of the spatial distribution of line segments with applications to CAD of chest X-ray CT images. In: Asano, T., Klette, R., Ronse, C. (eds.) Geometry, Morphology, and Computational Imaging (LNCS2616), pp. 22–38 (2003)

6. Ukil, S., Reinhardt, J.: Anatomy-guided lung lobe segmentation in x-ray ct images. IEEE Trans. Med. Imaging **28**, 202–214 (2009)

7. Hirano, Y., Shimizu, A., Hasegawa, J., Toriwaki, J.: A tracking algorithm for extracting ridge lines in three dimensional gray images using curvature of four-dimensional hyper surface. Syst. Comput. Jpn. **32**(12), 25–37 (2001)

8. Hirano, Y., Kunimitsu, K., Hasegawa, J., Toriwaki, J.: A region growing method using hyper surface curvature and its application to extraction of blood vessel region from chest X-ray CT images. J. Comput.-Aided Diagn. Med. Images **7**(3), 19–28 (2003). (in Japanese)

9. Hirano, Y., Mekada, Y., Hasegawa, J., Toriwaki, J.: Three dimensional concentration index as a feature of line pattern distribution in three dimensional space. FORMA **13**(3), 233–245 (1998)

10. Saito, T., Toriwaki, J.: A sequential thinning algorithm for three dimensional digital pictures using the euclidean distance transformation. In: Proceedings of 9th Scandinavian Conf. on Image Analysis, pp. 507–516 (1995)

11. Hirano, Y., Hasegawa, J., Toriwaki, J., Ohmatsu, H., Eguchi, K.: Quantification of shrinkage of lung lobe from chest CT images using the 3D extended voronoi division and its application to the benign/malignant discrimination of tumor shadows. In: Proceedings of the 16th International Conference on Pattern Recognition (ICPR 2002), pp. I-751–I-754 (2002)

12. Hirano, Y., Hasegawa, J., Toriwaki, J., Ohmatsu, H., Eguchi, K.: Classification of tumor shadows into the air-containing type or the solid type from chest X-ray CT images and its application to discrimination between benign tumors and malignant tumors). J. Jpn. Soc. CT Screening (Supplement) **8**(3), 201–204 (2001)

13. Hirano, Y., Seki, N., Eguchi, K.: Plug-in modules on PLUTO for identifying inflammatory nodules from lung nodules in chest X-ray CT images. In: Proceedings of International Workshop on Advanced Image Technology (IWAIT) 2009, Paper No. 0073 (2009)

14. Miyashita, K., Hirano, Y., Mekada, Y., Murase, H., Hasegawa, J., Toriwaki, J., Seki, N., Eguchi, K., Matsumoto, T., Omatsu, H., Mogami, H., Nakata, M.: Method for identifying inflammatory nodules from lung nodules extracted from chest X-ray CT images for computer-aided diagnosis. Med. Imag. Tech. **23**(3), 161–171 (2005). (in Japanese)

15. Morita, Y., Hirano, Y., Kitasaka, T., Mori, K., Suenaga, Y., Toriwaki, J., Seki, N., Eguchi, K.: Development of feature for recognizing inflammatory nodules from chest CT images using nodule shape and connecting point of blood vessel. IEICE Technical Report, MI2004–100, pp. 109–114 (2005). (in Japanese)

Fuzzy Object Growth Model for Neonatal Brain MR Understanding

Saadia Binte Alam, Syoji Kobashi and Jayaram K Udupa

Abstract This chapter summaries a brain region segmentation method for newborn using magnetic resonance (MR) images. The method deploys fuzzy object growth model (FOGM) which is an extension of fuzzy object model. It is a 4-dimensional model which gives a prior knowledge of brain shape and position at any growing time. First we calculate 4th dimension of FOGM, called growth index in this chapter. Because the growth index will be different from person to person even in the same age group, the method estimates the growth index from cerebral shape using Manifold learning. Using the growth index, FOGM is constructed from the training dataset. To recognize the brain region in evaluating subject, it first estimates the growth index. Then, the brain region is segmented using fuzzy connected image segmentation with the FOGM matched by the growth index. To evaluate the method, this study segments the parenchymal region of 16 subjects (revised age; 0–2 years old) using synthesized FOGM.

1 Introduction

Neonatal cerebral disorders deteriorate the quality of life (QoL) for patients and also their families as these disorders cause developmental delay, and/or reduce cerebral function. For example, most epilepsy patients show a brain formation disorder. To

S. B. Alam · S. Kobashi (✉)
Graduate School of Engineering, University of Hyogo, Kobe, Japan
e-mail: kobashi@eng.u-hyogo.ac.jp

S. B. Alam
e-mail: saadiabinte@gmail.com

S. B. Alam
International University of Business Agriculture and Technology, Dhaka, Bangladesh

J. K. Udupa
Department of Radiology, University of Pennsylvania, Philadelphia, PA, USA
e-mail: jay@mail.med.upenn.edu

© Springer International Publishing AG 2018
K. Suzuki and Y. Chen (eds.), *Artificial Intelligence in Decision Support Systems for Diagnosis in Medical Imaging*, Intelligent Systems Reference Library 140,
https://doi.org/10.1007/978-3-319-68843-5_9

monitor the long-term progress of cerebral disorders, magnetic resonance imaging (MRI) is useful because of its noninvasiveness [1, 2]. However, diagnosis from newborn brain MR image is very difficult and takes more time, because it requires high skill to interpret newborn brain MR image, and it is often subjective as well. Computer-aided diagnosis (CAD) systems can bring in image quantification and analytics to increase diagnostic efficiency and accuracy. CAD systems for adult brain have been proposed [3], however, they usually cannot operate on neonatal brains as neonatal brains change rapidly due to natural growth. Therefore, CAD systems for neonatal brains are needed.

To develop a CAD system for neonatal brains, we need brain shape templates corresponding to each time point. One of the methods of analyzing a developing brain is via a growth model. Ref. [4] proposed a method for generating a growth model using subjects' age, because the growth rate of newborn children varies among subjects even for the same age. Ref. [5] has proposed a method of generating a growth model by employing manifold learning (ML) on newborn brain images. The method normalizes brain images and applies ML using the amount of change observed during normalization. However, it is difficult to apply the method to various subjects because the technique of normalization does not work well for newborn brains. Thus, alternative strategies which do not use normalization are desirable.

In our work, we define an entity called *brain growth index* using ML. We bring several concepts together to build what we call a 4-dimensional fuzzy object growth model (FOGM)—fuzzy connectedness [6] and image segmentation [7, 8], fuzzy object model (FOM) [9], and brain growth index. FOM [10] is an object model which encodes prior knowledge of brain position and shape in the form of a fuzzy set. FOM is generated from training data composed of subjects' MR images. To synthesize consistent FOMs, the subjects' group should be controlled. Since newborn brain shape changes rapidly due to natural growth, we deal with subjects by their revised age. The method improves the segmentation accuracy by using FOM as we previously demonstrated. However, the accuracy of FOM-based method will suffer when an inappropriate FOM is utilized for a subject whose brain growth age is out of the age group. In order to improve the applicability of the FOM based method, we describe a method of synthesizing growable FOMs.

This work proposes the concept of FOGM by extending FOM to take into account growth. FOGM is defined as a growth index weighted FOM [11–13]. To evaluate this model, we segment brain regions and compare among different strategies—using FOGM, revised age weighted FOM, and single FOM.

2 Proposed Method

2.1 Growth Index

A key marker of a subject's growth is age. However, it is difficult to estimate the progress of brain development using only age because the deformation of the neonatal cerebrum due to natural growth varies considerably from subject to subject. Deformation due to brain growth is known to be continuous. Our idea is that when the growth indexes of two subjects are similar, their brain shape should be similar. Therefore, growth index can be defined based on similarity of brain shape. To implement this idea, ML can be employed on the MR image derived brain shape to estimate growth index.

This section introduces the concept of growth index and presents a method for its estimation from training image data. The proposed ML method calculates distances among all combinations of training data sets in a high dimensional space, and resolves eigenvalue of the graph Laplacian to project the training data to a low dimensional space. ML is basically a method of dimensionality reduction [14]. The Laplacian eigenmaps approach, a sort of ML technique, makes a neighbor graph in a high dimensional space, and then calculates a Laplacian of the neighbor graph to project it into a low dimensional space.

Consider k points, $a_1, ..., a_k$, in a high dimensional space, and corresponding points, $v_1, ..., v_k$, in a low dimensional space. The Laplacian eigenmap approach employs 3 steps to find the correspondence of points between the high and low-dimensional spaces.

Step 1. Calculate the weight (or distance) between all combinations of subjects in the high-dimensional space, and obtain a weight matrix W between two subjects, i and j, defined by

$$W_{i,j} = \exp\left(-\frac{a_i - a_{j2}^2}{t}\right) \qquad (1)$$

where t is a normalization parameter.

Step 2. Calculate a diagonal matrix $D_{i,j} = \sum_{j=1}^{k} W_{i,j}$ and a graph Laplacian

$$L = D - W.$$

Step 3. Solve a generalized eigenvalue problem formulated by Eq. (2), and obtain non-zero eigenvalues λ. The eigenvector $v_{low} = [v_1, ..., v_k]^T$ corresponding to the lowest eigenvalue λ_{low} shows corresponding points in the low-dimensional space.

$$Lv = \lambda Dv \qquad (2)$$

According to the above steps, at first, the following 11 brain anatomical land-marks are detected manually: the inferior extremity of genu corporis callosi, the inferior extremity of splenium corporis callosi, interpeduncular cistern, the right and the left cross points of the superior frontal sulcus and the precentral sulcus, the right and the left anterior extremity points of temporal lobe, the right and the left anterior extremity points of frontal lobe, and the right and the left posterior extremity points of occipital lobe. These landmarks are shown in Fig. 1. The proposed method then

(a)

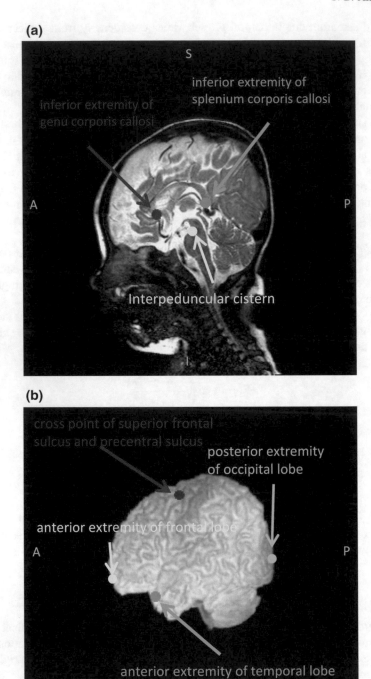

Fig. 1 Feature points used in manifold learning

calculates Euclidean distances between all 55 pairs of these selected landmarks. The calculated distances are used as a characteristic vector of subject i, $\boldsymbol{a}_i = [a_1(i), a_2(i), \ldots, a_{55}(i),]^T$. Using the characteristic vectors, $\boldsymbol{a}_1, \boldsymbol{a}_2, \ldots, \boldsymbol{a}_k$, all subjects in the training dataset are represented in a high-dimensional space. The method calculates neighborhood relations among these vectors using Eq. (1), and then solves a generalized eigenvalue problem to project the high dimensional data into a 1-dimensional space.

The eigenvalues in the 1-dimensional space are normalized to a value between 0 and 1 by liner conversion. The normalized values $v_1, \ldots, v_k$ are defined as growth indexes of subjects in the training dataset. The maximum and minimum growth index were set to 1 and 0, respectively.

Now, let us examine the problem of estimation of growth index for a new data set. The generalized eigenvalue problem given by Eq. (2) can be transformed to Eq. (3) below by multiplying $\boldsymbol{D}^{-1}$ on both sides.

$$\boldsymbol{D}^{-1}\boldsymbol{L}\boldsymbol{v} = \lambda\boldsymbol{v} \tag{3}$$

If the number of subjects in the training dataset is N, $\boldsymbol{X} = \boldsymbol{D}^{-1}\boldsymbol{L}$ is a $N \times N$ square matrix, and Eq. (3) can be transformed to

$$v_e = \frac{\sum_{i=1}^{N} X_{ei} \times v_i}{(\lambda - 1)}, \quad i \neq e \tag{4}$$

where v_i and λ have been obtained by applying the ML process on the training data sets. The value of $\boldsymbol{W}$ can also be calculated by Eq. (1) using the characteristic vector of the evaluating subject and the vectors of training data, once the anatomical landmarks are detected manually. Therefore, both $\boldsymbol{D}$ and $\boldsymbol{L}$ can be calculated using $\boldsymbol{W}$, and then the growth index of the evaluating subject can be estimated.

2.2 Construction of Fuzzy Object Growth Model

A brain segmentation method using FOMs was proposed in [9]. FOM is generated from training data sets composed of subjects' MR images. To build consistent FOMs, the subjects' group should be properly controlled and represented at the model building stage as well as at the time of using the model on a given subject. Because the newborn brain shape deforms quickly by natural growth, the subjects need to be controlled by the revised age.

The proposed method synthesizes FOGM using training datasets which are composed of MR images acquired from different subjects with various growth indexes. The flowchart of the proposed method is shown in Fig. 2. FOGM is an

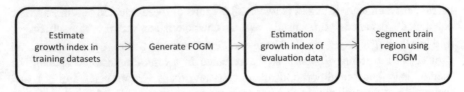

Fig. 2 Flowchart of proposed method

extension of FOM, where each voxel has a fuzzy degree between 0 and 1. Fuzzy degree means a degree of belonging to a target region (*i.e.*, brain region). The value of fuzzy degree 1 means that the position is completely inside the target region, and the value of fuzzy degree 0 means the position is completely outside the target region.

Each voxel in FOGM has a set of distances from the target contour for each training subject, and FOGM has a table of growth indexes of the training subjects. The method consists of 4 steps. FOGM is generated only once from the training subject image data sets, and the model can be used subsequently to analyze evaluating subjects.

[Algorithm] FOGM generation

[Step 1]   For each training subject, experts delineate the brain region in MR images manually or using interactive tools.

[Step 2]   Calibrate the pose/position of each brain region to a coordinate system because there is variability among subjects. The coordinate system used is illustrated in Fig. 3. The inferior extremity of genu corporis callosi is the origin. A line which connects the origin to the inferior extremity of splenium corporis callosi is the anterior-posterior (AP) axis, and the line of fissure longitudinalis cerebri denotes the superior-inferior (SI) axis. The landmarks detected manually are shown in Fig. 1.

Fig. 3 Coordinate system for calibration of brain pose/position. A: anterior; P: posterior; S: superior; I: inferior; L: left; and R: right

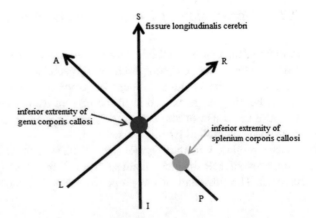

(a)

4	3	4
3	0	3
4	3	4

(b)

8	7	8
7	6	7
8	7	8

Fig. 4 3-D chamfer distance mask. **a** is used in the current slice. **b** is used in the previous and the next slice

$$D(p) = \{d_1(p), d_2(p), \ldots, d_N(p)\}.$$

[Step 3] For each voxel in all training data, calculate the 3D chamfer distance (Fig. 4) to the delineated brain surface. Each voxel in the reference coordinate system has a set of distances whose number is the same as the number of training data, N. At a voxel p, the distances are represented by

[Step 4] Estimate growth indexes using methods described above and denote them by $V = \{v_1, v_2, \ldots, v_N\}$

[End]

After generating FOGM, the method synthesizes FOM at a certain growth index when analyzing evaluation subjects. Consider a FOM generation for a growth index value v_t ($0 \leq v_t \leq 1$). We define a fuzzy membership degree for every voxel, p, as follows by utilizing the index values.

First, we calculate weighted average and variance of distances at voxel p by Eqs. (5), (6) and (7)

$$m(p) = \frac{\sum_{i=1}^{N} w_i \times d_i(p)}{\sum_{i=1}^{N} w_i} \tag{5}$$

$$\sigma^2(p) = \frac{\sum_{i=1}^{N} w_i(d_i(p) - m(p))^2}{\sum_{i=1}^{N} w_i} \tag{6}$$

$$w_i = e^{-\frac{(v_i - v_T)^2}{K}} \tag{7}$$

Here K is fuzzification parameter and has positive value. The shape of Eq. (7) is illustrated in Fig. 5. When K is smaller, FOM is generated over a wider range of growth index. As K becomes larger, this range becomes smaller. The relationship between K and half-width at half-maximum (*HWHM*) of Gaussian function is

$$K = HWHM/\sqrt{2 \ln 2} \tag{8}$$

Fig. 5 Weighting function for calculate average and variance. This function has Gaussian distribution shape

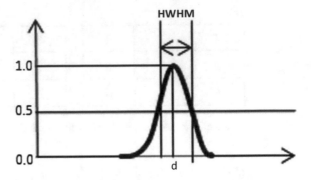

Fig. 6 Fuzzy membership function

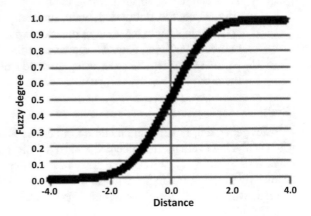

The fuzzy degree $\mu(p)$ at voxel p can then be calculated using weighted average $m(p)$ and variance $\sigma^2(p)$ by Eq. (9).

$$\mu(p) = \begin{cases} 0 & \text{if} \quad m(p) \leq -\frac{1}{2}\sigma^2 \\ \frac{1}{2}sin\left(\frac{m(p)}{\sigma^2}\pi\right) + \frac{1}{2} & \text{if} \quad -\frac{1}{2}\sigma^2 < m(p) < \frac{1}{2}\sigma^2 \\ 1 & \text{if} \quad m(p) \geq \frac{1}{2}\sigma^2 \end{cases} \tag{9}$$

When a voxel of interest is on the cerebral surface, the value of fuzzy degree is 0.5. If the voxel falls outside from the cerebral surface, the fuzzy degree will be smaller. And, when the voxel comes inside the brain, the fuzzy degree will be bigger. That is illustrated in Fig. 6. The gradient is determined by the variance of distance. When the variance becomes larger, the gradient becomes smooth. In contrast, when the variance becomes smaller, the gradient becomes steep.

2.3 Fuzzy Connected Image Segmentation with Fuzzy Object Growth Model

Proposed method estimates growth index of target subject and generates FOGM and 4-dimensional normalize brain which is created using voxel value as $d(p)$ by Eqs. (5) and (6). Thus, two fuzzy degrees, $\mu_s(p)$ and $\mu_I(p)$ are obtained for voxel p. These show fuzzy degrees belonging to the brain region with respect to shape and intensity at the position, respectively. Using the fuzzy degrees, the fuzzy degree $\mu(p)$ of belonging to the cerebral parenchyma is estimated by

$$\mu(p) = \alpha(p)\mu_1(p)$$

$$\alpha(p) = \begin{cases} 1 & \text{if } \mu_s(p) > th_s \\ \frac{\mu_s(p)}{th_s} & otherwise \end{cases} \tag{10}$$

where th_S is a parameter between 0 and 1.

Secondly, the proposed method extracts seed voxels by thresholding fuzzy degree belonging to the cerebral parenchyma, $\mu(p)$. To assemble with FOM, fuzzy affinity is defined between voxel c and voxel d as

$$\mu_k(c,d) = \alpha(d)\sqrt{\mu_\psi(c,d)\mu_\phi(c,d)} \tag{11}$$

where $\mu_\Psi(c,d)$ is homogeneity affinity defined in Ref. [11]. $\mu_\Phi(c,d)$ is object affinity, and is defined by;

$$\mu_\phi(c,d) = min(\mu_0(c), \mu_0(d)) \tag{12}$$

$\mu_0(p)$ is an object feature estimated by using both of seed objects and fuzzy object models, and is defined by,

$$\mu_0(p) = max(\mu_{seed}(I(p)), \mu(p)), \tag{13}$$

where $\mu_{seed}(x)$ is a fuzzy membership function defined by a Gaussian function whose mean and variance are those of seed voxels. It expresses how MR signal x is similar to the MR signal of seed voxels. Applying *growth index* estimation method, affinity to the cerebral parenchyma is estimated based on two aspects, one from the given images, and the other from FOM. Fuzzy connectedness [7] can be calculated, which is the maximum fuzzy affinity among all possible paths from seed voxels to a voxel of interest. Finally, the brain region was segmented by thresholding fuzzy connectedness.

3   Image Data

This research recruited 16 newborn subjects, with informed consent from all their parents. The revised ages of the infants were lower than 2 years. The mean and standard deviation of the revised age was 122.13 ± 191.62 days. The revised age is defined as an age calculated by normal fetal weeks (40 weeks) for premature babies. According to diagnosis by radiologists, significant cerebral disorders were not found at the time of MR image acquisition.

T2-weighted MR images were acquired using 3.0T MR scanner (Intera, Philips Medical Systems) with a circularly polarized head coil used as both transmitter and receiver. The images were acquired with the following parameters: echo time (TE), 106–165 ms; repetition time (TR), 2000 ms; slice thickness, 1.5 mm; space between slices, 0.75 mm; field of view (FOV) and number of slices were also adjusted by the size of the target head size (120–200 mm), image matrix, 320×320 voxels; resolution, $0.75 \times 0.75 \times 0.75$ mm^3.

4   Experimental Results

First, the estimated growth index was compared with both the revised age and cerebral volume for evaluating the performance as shown in Fig. 7. The cerebral volume was calculated by segmenting the cerebral region manually. Correlation coefficients are 0.786 and 0.952, respectively, for revised age and cerebral volume, and these are significant ($p < 0.01$).

The method was evaluated by conducting a leave-one-out cross validation (LOOCV) test. ML was applied to all subjects except an evaluating subject. The growth index of the evaluating subject was then estimated. The truth values were growth indexes estimated by ML using all data. The corresponding experimental results are shown in Fig. 8. where mean absolute error (MAE) is 0.028. Accuracies declined a bit for subjects whose growth indexes are close to the maximum (1.0) or

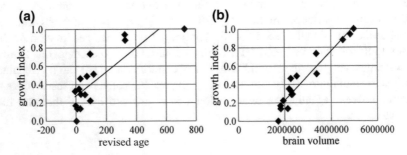

Fig. 7 Comparison of growth index. **a** compares the growth index with the revised age. The unit of revised age is day. **b** compares the growth index with the cerebral volume. The unit of brain volume is cc. The lines are regression lines

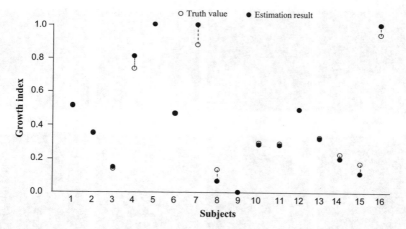

Fig. 8 Estimation result of growth index

the minimum (0.0). One of the reasons for this behavior is that it requires extrapolation for the subjects. The expected accuracy was improved by increasing the number of training subjects.

Secondly, the segmentation method using FOGM was also tested using the LOOCV test. The analysis parameter t of Eq. (1) was set to 4000, and th_S was set to 0.7. These were chosen experimentally. Figure 9 shows the segmented region using the proposed method for $HWHM = 0.1$.

The experimental results were evaluated by using the false-positive volume fraction (*FPVF*), false-negative-volume-fraction (*FNVF*), and Jaccard index (*JI*) defined below.

$$FPVF = \frac{FP}{FP + TN} \tag{14}$$

$$FNVF = \frac{FN}{TP + FN} \tag{15}$$

$$JI = \frac{TP}{FN + TP + FP} \tag{16}$$

Finally, to evaluate this result, the revised age weighted FOM and single FOM were constructed. The first type was generated by same flow of proposed method using revised age instead of growth index, and the latter type was synthesized by the average of subjects whose age was under a month. From the summarized result (Tables 1 and 2), it is obvious that the proposed method's *JI* is the best, whereas Table 2 depicts single FOM's *JI* is the best, and so it can be concluded that the

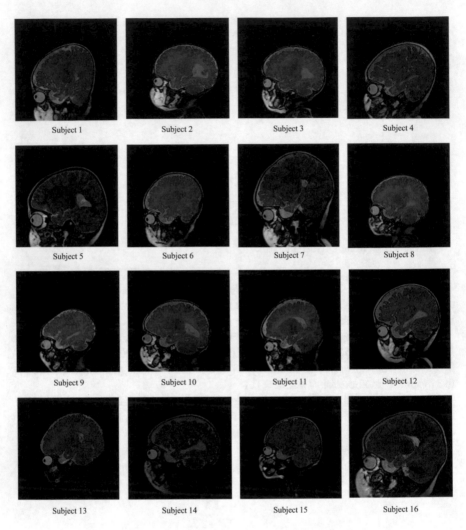

Fig. 9 Segmented brain region (red area) using the proposed method

Table 1 Segmentation result under one month

	Proposed method	Single FOM	Age based method
FPVF	0.018 ± 0.007	0.021 ± 0.007	0.023 ± 0.008
FNVF	0.022 ± 0.019	0.007 ± 0.006	0.009 ± 0.007
J.I.	0.758 ± 0.038	0.740 ± 0.035	0.719 ± 0.033

proposed method is better than age based method, however, worse than single FOM because the number of subjects included in the data whose age was over a month is not sufficient.

Table 2 Segmentation result over one month

	Proposed method	Single FOM	Age based method
FPVF	0.022 ± 0.009	0.027 ± 0.011	0.025 ± 0.011
FNVF	0.097 ± 0.064	0.040 ± 0.036	0.104 ± 0.114
J.I.	0.690 ± 0.072	0.706 ± 0.092	0.662 ± 0.094

5 Conclusion

This research discussed a method to calculate an index of natural growth. FOGM was synthesized using the growth index. Neonatal brain regions were automatically segmented by using FOGM and fuzzy connectedness. The segmentation accuracy of subjects whose age were under a month (average ± standard division) is 0.758 ± 0.037 and over one month is 0.690 ± 0.073.

To compare results, both revised age weighted FOM and single FOM were created. Revised age weighted FOM's accuracy over subjects aged under a month was 0.719 ± 0.033, and over a month is 0.662 ± 0.094. These results illustrate that *growth index* is more effective than revised age in generating object models. Further, single FOM's accuracy for under a month aged subjects is 0.741 ± 0.035, and for subjects over a month is 0.706 ± 0.092. FOGM is better than single FOM in case of subjects of age under a month. However, although FOGM provides poor performance over single FOM for current data, subjects aged over a month, but we cannot reach a final decision that FOGM is worse than that of single FOM because the number of subjects whose age is over a month is not sufficient in available database.

Acknowledgements Authors would like to express their sincere appreciation to Mr. Ryosuke Nakano, University of Hyogo, JAPAN, who implements the method. This work was supported in part by JSPS Grant-in-Aid for Scientific Research on Innovative Areas (Multidisciplinary Computational Anatomy) JSPS KAKENHI Grant Number 15H01126.

References

1. Braak, H., Braak, E.: Neuropathologic staging of alzheimer-related changes. Acta Neuropathol. **82**(4), 239–259 (1991)
2. Kitagaki, H., Mori, E., Yamaji, S., Ishii, K., Hirono, N., Kobashi, S., Hata, Y.: Frontotemporal dementia and alzheimer disease: evaluation of cortical atrophy with automated hemispheric surface display generated with MR images. Radiology **208**(2), 431–439 (1998)
3. Padilla, P., Lopez, M., Gorriz, J.M., Ramirez, J., Salas-Gonzalez, D., Alvarez, I.: NMF-SVM based CAD tool applied to functional brain images for the diagnosis of alzheimer's disease. IEEE Trans. Med. Imaging **31**(2), 207–216 (2012)
4. Davis, B.C., Fletcher, P.T., Bullitt, E., Joshi, S.: Population shape regression from random design data. Int. J. Comput. Vis. **2010**(2), 255–266 (2010)

5. Aljabar, P., Wolz, R., Srinivasan, L., Counsell, S., Boardman, J.P., Murgasova, M., Doria, V., Rutherford, M.A., Edwards, A.D., Hajnal, J.V., Rueckert, D.: Combining morphological information in a manifold learning framework: application to neonatal MRI. Lect. Notes Comput. Sci. Med. Image Comput. Comput. Assist. Interv. **6363**, 1–8 (2010)
6. Udupa, J.K., Samarasekera, S.: Fuzzy connectedness and object definition: theory, algorithms, and applications in image segmentation. Graph. Models Process. **58**(3), 246–261 (1996)
7. Prastawa, M., Gilmore, J.H., Lin, W., Gerig, G.: Automatic segmentation of MR images of the developing newborn brain. Med. Image Anal. **9**(5), 457–466 (2005)
8. Xue, H., Srinivasan, L., Jiang, S., Rutherford, M., Edwards, A.D., Rueckert, D., Hajnal, J.V.: Automatic segmentation and reconstruction of the cortex from neonatal MRI. Neuroimage **38** (3), 461–477 (2007)
9. Kobashi, S., Udupa, J.K.: Fuzzy object models for newborn brain MR image segmentation. In: Proceedings of SPIE Medical Imaging 2013, vol. 8672 (2013)
10. Udupa, J.K., Odhner, D., Falcao, A.X., Ciesielski, K.C., Miranda, P.A.V., Vaideeswaran, P., Mishra, S., Grevera, G.J., Saboury, B., Torigian, D.A.: Fuzzy object modeling. In: Proceedings of SPIE Medical Imaging 2011, vol. 7964, pp. 79640B-1–10 (2011)
11. Nakano, R., Kobashi, S., Kuramoto, K., Wakata, Y., Ando, K., Ishikura, R., Ishikawa, T., Hirota, S., Hata, Y.: Fuzzy object growth model for newborn brain using manifold learning. In: Proceedings of 2014 IEEE International Conference on Fuzzy Systems, pp. 1809–1816 (2014)
12. Kobashi, S., Nakano, R., Kuramoto, K., Wakata, Y., Ando, K., Ishikura, R., Ishikawa, T., Hirota, S., Hata, Y., Kamiura, N.: Neonatal brain segmentation using 4-D Fuzzy object model. In: Proceedings of International Conference on Informatics, Electronics & Vision (2014)
13. Belkin, M., Niyogi, P.: Laplacian eigenmaps for dimensionality reduction and data representation. Neural Comput. **15**(6), 1373–1396 (2003)
14. Remy, E., Thiel, E.: Computing 3D medial axis for chamfer distances. Lect. Notes Comput. Sci. **1953**, 418–430 (2000)

Part IV
Computer-Aided Prognosis

Computer-Aided Prognosis: Accurate Prediction of Patients with Neurologic and Psychiatric Diseases via Multi-modal MRI Analysis

Huiguang He, Hongwei Wen, Dai Dai and Jieqiong Wang

Abstract Multi-modal magnetic resonance imaging (MRI) is increasingly used in neuroscience research, as it allowed the non-invasive investigation of structure and function of the human brain in health and pathology. One of the most important applications of multi-modal MRI is the provision of vital diagnostic data for neurologic and psychiatric disorders. As traditional MRI researches using univariate analyses can only reveal disease-related structural and functional alterations at group level which limited the clinical application, and recent attention has turned toward integrating multi-modal neuroimaging and computer-aided prognosis (CAD) technology, especially machine learning, to assist clinical disease diagnose. Research in this area is growing exponentially, and therefore it is meaningful to review the current and future development of this emerging area. Hence, in this paper, based on our own studies and contributions, we review the recent advances in multi-modal MRI and CAD technologies, and their applications to assist the clinical diagnosis of three common neurologic and psychiatric disorders, namely, Alzheimer's disease, Attention deficit/hyperactivity disorder and Tourette syndrome. We extracted multi-modal features from structural, diffusion and resting-state functional MRI, then different feature selection methods and classifiers were applied. In addition, we applied different feature fusion schemes (e.g. multiple kernel learning) to combining multi-modal features for classification. Our experiments show that using feature fusion techniques to integrate multi-modal features can yield better classification results for diseases prediction, which may outline some future directions for multi-modal neuroimaging where researchers can design more advanced methods and models for neurologic and psychiatric research.

H. He (✉) · H. Wen · D. Dai · J. Wang
Research Center for Brain-Inspired Intelligence, Institute of Automation,
Chinese Academy of Sciences, Beijing 100190, China
e-mail: huiguang.he@ia.ac.cn

H. He · H. Wen · D. Dai · J. Wang
University of Chinese Academy of Sciences, Beijing, China

H. He
Center for Excellence in Brain Science and Intelligence Technology,
Chinese Academy of Sciences, Beijing, China

© Springer International Publishing AG 2018
K. Suzuki and Y. Chen (eds.), *Artificial Intelligence in Decision Support Systems for Diagnosis in Medical Imaging*, Intelligent Systems Reference Library 140,
https://doi.org/10.1007/978-3-319-68843-5_10

225

Keywords Alzheimer's disease · Tourette syndrome · Attention deficit/ hyperactivity disorder · Diffusion tensor imaging · Support vector machine Multiple kernel learning

1 Introduction

In the last twenty years, advanced magnetic resonance imaging (MRI) techniques have allowed the non-invasive investigation of the structure and function of the human brain in health and pathology [1]. These techniques have been applied to patients with neurological or psychiatric disorders in order to identify possible biomarkers which could be used for early diagnosis, treatment planning and monitoring of disease progression. Many previous studies have revealed structural and functional alterations in several neurological or psychiatric disorders including, amongst others, Alzheimer's disease [2, 3], obsessive-compulsive disorder [4, 5], Attention deficit/hyperactivity disorder [6, 7], Tourette syndrome [8, 9], schizophrenia [10, 11] and generalised anxiety disorder [12, 13]. Nonetheless, the results of these studies have had minimal clinical impact and despite much interest in the use of brain scans for diagnostic and prognostic purposes, neurologists and psychiatrists are still forced to rely on traditional and often ineffective diagnostic and prognostic tools. One of the reasons for the limited impact of the findings on clinical practice is that neuroimaging studies have typically reported differences between patients and controls at group level; in contrast, doctors working in a neurologic and psychiatric ward have to make clinical decisions about individuals. For neuroimaging to be useful in a clinical setting therefore, one must be able to make inferences at the level of the individual rather than the group [14]. As our main study worked on combining multi-modal MRI and computer-aided prognosis (CAD) technology to assist the clinical diagnosis of neurologic and psychiatric diseases, especially Alzhermer's disease, Attention deficit/hyperactivity disorder and Tourette syndrome, the Sects. 1.1–1.3 will give introduction to the research status of multi-modal MRI, CAD technology and neurologic and psychiatric diseases.

1.1 Multi-modal MRI

The native approach in this field of study was the investigation of a single MRI parameter at a time: (a) anatomical 3D T1-weighted images, which allows the employment of several neuroanatomical techniques able to describe and quantify macrostructural changes by using probabilistic (voxel-based morphometry analysis) or quantitative research tools (manual/automatic region-of-interest volumetry, cortical thickness measurements). (b) diffusion-weighted imaging (DWI)/diffusion tensor imaging (DTI). DWI and DTI provide specific quantitative measurement of micro-structural changes within white and gray matter compartments. In particular DTI provides quantitative parameters, such as the mean diffusivity that increases with microscopic barrier disruption and extracellular fluid accumulation and the fractional anisotropy that provides information on the microstructural integrity of highly oriented microstructures (i.e., myelin). (c) blood oxygenation-level-dependent (BOLD) images/resting-state fMRI. The common observation in functional MRI studies is that increasing in the BOLD MRI signal represents increasing of neural activity. Such a neurophysiological "activation" results from elevated oxygen saturation levels (and reduced paramagnetic deoxyhemoglobin contents) of capillary and venous blood. These positive signal changes are considered the basis for the functional organization of the brain.

In the last five years, multi-modal neuroimaging has become the most popular approach to study pathophysiology of diseased brain. In fact, the aim of this field of study is to quantify the single or combined weight of MRI parameters in describing neurodegenerative processes. In other words, the possibility to measure MR parameters sensitive to complementary tissue characteristics (e.g., volume atrophy, iron deposition, and microstructural damage) could have great potential for investigating pathological changes in several neurologic or psychiatric diseases. At this moment, important new findings have been reported although several issues remain open [15].

1.2 Computer Aided Diagnosis

In radiology, computer-aided diagnosis (CADx), also called computer-aided detection (CADe), are procedures in medicine that assist doctors in the interpretation of medical images. Imaging techniques in MRI, X-ray, and Ultrasound diagnostics yield a great deal of information, which the radiologist has to analyze and evaluate comprehensively in a short time. Although CAD has been used in clinical environments for over 40 years, CAD cannot and may not substitute the doctor, but rather plays a supporting role. The doctor (generally a radiologist) is always responsible for the final interpretation of a medical image.

CAD has become one of the major research subjects in medical imaging and diagnostic radiology. However, it has been said that it would be arduous to develop CAD using MRI, because the image quality of MR images including specific artifacts and image noise could vary with imaging sequences and patients [16]. In recent years, various kinds of CAD methods have been developed in the neuro-radiology using MRI [17, 18]. Radiologists expect that CAD can improve their diagnostic abilities based on synergistic effects between the computer's and radiologist's high abilities by using the information analysis including the medical images.

However, few studies have looked at the potential of combining multi-modal MRI and CAD to earliest phase diagnosis of neurologic and psychiatric diseases, especially Attention deficit/hyperactivity disorder and Tourette syndrome, which may be a key to discovering etiology, prevention or treatment. To date, machine learning techniques and pattern recognition techniques have been applied to a range of MRI modalities for CAD on various neurologic and psychiatric diseases. Unlike group-based comparison approaches, machine learning techniques and pattern recognition classification methods are able to detect the fine-grained spatial discriminative patterns, which are critical for individual-based disease diagnosis [19]. Our studies mainly focused on applying off-the-shelf tools in statistical machine learning to differentiate neurologic and psychiatric diseases, with the most popular small-sample machine learning techniques, support vector machines (SVMs) [20], one of the most successful application of statistical learning theory and frequently-used classifiers in neuroimaging community, and have the capability of dealing with high dimensional data and perform well on generalization.

What is more, as indicated by Fjell et al. [21], different biomarkers may carry complementary information. Therefore combining multi-modal features, instead of depending on one is a promising direction for improving classification accuracy. Intuitively, one can combine multiple results from different classifiers with voting technique, or ensemble method. Moreover, concatenating several features into one single vector and then training a classifier can also be a practical option. In addition, several popular feature fusion algorithms, such as boosting [22] and multi-kernel learning (MKL) [23], have been introduced in neuroimaging community. These approaches also achieved remarkable results on classification.

1.3 Neurologic and Psychiatric Diseases

There are more than 600 neurologic diseases. Patients with neurological disease require special management considerations. These include pretreatment planning, therapeutic techniques, and post treatment requirements. Neurologic conditions facing the dentist include abnormalities associated with the cranial nerves, facial sensory loss, facial paralysis, and conditions such as epilepsy, Parkinson disease, multiple sclerosis, stroke, and myasthenia gravis. In this article, we focus on three common neurologic and psychiatric diseases: Alzheimer's disease, Attention deficit/hyperactivity disorder, Tourette syndrome.

Alzheimer's Disease
Alzheimer's disease (AD) is a progressive neurodegenerative disease which is characterized by memory loss, poor judgment, language deterioration and so forth. As the major form of dementia, AD affected 26.6 million people worldwide in 2006 and was predicted to affect 1 in 85 people by 2050 [24]. Mild cognitive impairment (MCI), commonly defined as a subtle but measurable memory loss, is considered as the transition stage between normal aging and dementia; and patients with MCI have been reported more prone to progress to AD than healthy people [25, 26]. A number of studies have indicated that structural changes such as gray matter atrophy can be identified in MCI and AD patients [27–30], which, in structural

magnetic resonance imaging (MRI), might be reflected on brain volume atrophy [27, 28] or cortical thickness thinning [29, 30] of all or specific regions of the patient's brain. These studies demonstrate the feasibility of discovering clinical biomarkers or developing an automatic diagnosis system to distinguish AD or MCI patients from the healthy elder.

In our work on AD, we present a framework for establishing individual structural networks and attempt to use these networks to distinguish AD (and MCI) patients from the normal controls (NC) [31]. To obtain a connectivity matrix for each subject, we first calculate the distance of pairs of cortical regions using mean cortical thickness; then a kernel function is applied to the distance to obtain the connection weight. For feature selection, the hybrid method is used including: (i) a filter method for fast and rough dimensionality reduction and (ii) a wrapper method for further precise feature selection. Totally three types of filters and two wrappers are attempted to combined together to form six different hybrid feature selection methods and the results of them are compared. Classification is performed via a kernel-based SVM. We apply our method to 83 subjects from the OASIS AD database and report the highest cross validation accuracy of 90.4%, at least 10% higher than that using the raw cortical thickness as features.

Attention Deficit/Hyperactivity Disorder

Attention deficit/hyperactivity disorder (ADHD), one of the most commonly neurological disorder, always present from childhood, which manifests itself with symptoms such as hyperactivity, forgetfulness, poor impulse control, and distractibility. ADHD affects at least 5% of school-age children, causing them to be difficult to control their behaviors or focus their attentions. These symptoms may persist into adulthood and result in a lifelong impairment [32]. In spite of a large amount of research efforts, the community has not yet comprehensively understood the pathology of ADHD. Moreover, the current practice in the diagnosis of ADHD is mainly according to the levels of symptoms listed in DSM-IV [33], and the diagnosis is usually conducted by the parents or teachers, which is unfortunately subjective. In fact, it is very difficult to draw a line between the normal levels of the ADHD symptoms and the clinically significant levels that require interventions. Thus, further studies on objective diagnosis of ADHD are of great significance. Recently, structural MRI (sMRI) and functional MRI (fMRI) have been widely used in examining the brain of ADHD patients, and various abnormalities have been reported. Studies using sMRI showed a totally decreased cerebral volume of 3–5% [34, 35], and abnormalities in several specific brain regions such as lateral prefrontal cortex, cingulate cortex, striatum, cerebellum, and corpus coliseum [34–38]. As for fMRI studies, abnormal brain activations were found in task-related experiments on the dorsal anterior cingulate cortex (dACC), the ventrolateral prefrontal cortex (VLPFC), and the putamen [39–41]. Resting-state fMRI was also used in ADHD studies and abnormalities were found in ACC, prefrontal cortex, putamen, temporal cortex, and cerebellum [42–45]. In addition, ADHD-related decreases of functional connectivity (FC) between anterior cingulate and precuneus/ posterior cingulate cortex regions, as well as between precuneus and other default-mode network components, including ventromedial prefrontal cortex and portions of posterior cingulate cortex were also found in previous study [46].

In our work on ADHD, we conducted extensive experiments on the features which were extracted from sMRI or rs-fMRI, as well as the combination of multi-modal features. In the final results released by ADHD-200 consortium, we were ranked the 6th out of 21 participants under the contest scoring policy, and our method performed the best in terms of sensitivity and J-statistic [47]. In this paper, we list and compare the performances of all kinds of features we used to provide a comprehensive understanding of potential useful information related to ADHD diagnosis.

Tourette Syndrome

Tourette syndrome (TS) is a common genetic neurological disorder with onset in childhood, characterized by multiple physical (motor) tics and at least one vocal (phonic) tic [48]. These tics characteristically wax and wane, can be suppressed temporarily, and are preceded by a premonitory urge. Tourette's is defined as part of a spectrum of tic disorders. Affected individuals typically have repetitive, stereotyped movements or vocalizations, such as blinking, sniffing, facial movements, or tensing of the abdominal musculature. TS is frequently concomitant with obsessive-compulsive disorder (OCD), attention-deficit hyperactivity disorder (ADHD), and other social and behavioral disturbances [49]. The incidence of TS is much higher than previously estimated [50], accounting for about 1% of children between the age 5–17 years [51, 52]. About 0.6% of the children also show symptoms of distress and impairment caused by their tics [53]. To date, the neural basis of TS remains largely unknown. While tics constitute the major diagnostic symptom, TS is quite heterogeneous and has a long-term prognosis that is difficult to accurately estimate. Moreover, TS is typically diagnosed by observing symptoms and by evaluating the history of their onset. Thus far, only clinical measures, and not any brain morphological parameters, have been developed to diagnose TS [8], and the diagnosis is usually conducted by the parents, which is unfortunately subjective. Thus, further studies on objective diagnosis of TS are of great significance.

Our work on TS mainly involved in two DTI analysis methods: Tract-Based Spatial Statistics (TBSS) analysis and structural networks analysis using tractography. TBSS analysis of DTI data was recently developed as an automatic, hypothesis-free and precise method for the assessment of integrity of the WM [54]. Some previous studies have used TBSS to indicate that significant axial diffusivity (AD) and mean diffusivity (MD) increases were found in anterior thalamic radiation, right cingulum bundle projecting to the cingulate gurus and forceps minor in early TS children [8]. On the other hand, diffusion MRI tractography can reconstruct the major WM tracts faithful to the known WM anatomy, allowing mapping of the brain's structural connectivity in vivo [55]. Some previous studies has reported tic generation link to disturbed networks of brain areas involved in planning, controlling and execution of action, particularly structural disorders in the striatum and cortico–striato–thalamo–cortical circuits [56]. Some studies used the probabilistic tractography algorithms to quantify the structural integration of CSTC circuits, and showed widespread structural abnormalities in CSTC white matter pathways in TS patients [9]. However, these findings are mainly obtained based on group-level statistical comparison, and thus are of limited value for individual-based disease diagnosis.

In our work on TS, we applied SVM classification with TBSS to assess the efficacy of each DTI metric for classification and the locations of the voxels that were most useful for discriminating between groups [57]. We also make diagnostic predictions about individuals using deterministic tractography methods and graph theoretical modeling of brain connectivity. We aimed to select the topological characteristics of structural network which were most efficient for classification and establish the effective diagnosis models for early TS children [58].

2 Method

The overview of our proposed classification pipeline was illustrated as follows. From the preprocessed multi-modal MRI images, we first extracted the respective voxel or regional features. Based on these features, a hybrid feature selection method which combines filter-based and wrapper-based method was applied to select the important features from each modality. Based on the selected features, feature fusion algorithms were further implemented, for classification by using SVM.

2.1 Image Preprocessing and Original Feature Extraction

In order to obtain potential features related to neurologic and psychiatric diseases, we employ different image processing techniques to extract multimodal features. For sMRI, cortical thickness (CT) and gray matter probability (GMP) are extracted, For diffusion MRI, TBSS and structural connectivity are extracted, while regional homogeneity (ReHo) and functional connectivity (FC) are extracted from resting-state fMRI. We selected these multimodal features because they were effective neuroimaging metrics to reveal structural and functional alterations in related neurological or psychiatric diseases especially in AD, ADHD and TS [3, 6, 7, 9, 59]. The following is the summary of features that we have considered in our framework.

Structural MRI
All T1-weighted images in this study were corrected for intensity non-uniformity using N3 algorithm [60] and were brain extracted to exclude the non-brain tissues and reoriented with the origin set close to the anterior commissure (AC).

Cortical Thickness

Cortical surface is reconstructed by FreeSurfer (surfer.nmr.mgh.harvard.edu/) using the methods described in [61, 62], The registered images are first classified into gray matter (GM), white matter (WM) and cerebrospinal fluid (CSF) using an artificial neural network classifier [61]. Then the inner (GM/WM) and outer (pial) cortical surfaces are extracted automatically from the segmented images through the Constrained Laplacian-based Anatomic Segmentation with Proximities (CLASP) algorithm [62]. Cortical thickness is calculated as the Euclidean distance between the linked vertices on the two surfaces. To increase the signal-to-noise ratio, the cortical thickness data were smoothed using surface-based diffusion smoothing with 20 mm FWHM. Finally, the brain of each subject is segmented using Automated Anatomical Labeling (AAL) atlas [63] which divides the whole brain volume into 116 anatomical regions. The cortical parcellation is produced by finding the highest occurrence at each vertex on the cortical surface; 40 cortical regions are identified for each hemisphere. The mean cortical thickness of regions is estimated by averaging the cortical thickness values over all vertices in the corresponding region, and used for construction of cortical connectivity for each subject. Figure 1 shows the pipeline of image pre-processing and mean cortical thickness extraction.

Construction of Individual Cortical Networks

A network, or graph, is typically defined as $G = (V, E)$, where V is the set of vertices (or nodes) and E is the set of edges (or links). For this work, we assume that a node is a cortical region as defined by the AAL atlas and an edge is a certain similarity of the mean cortical thickness between a pair of nodes. Thus each individual network, or graph, shares the same set of 80 vertices. This facilitates performing comparisons using only the weight of edges, which is measured by the kernel below. The mean cortical thickness features of all subjects form a $n \times V$ feature matrix, where n is the number of subjects and V is the number of vertices. Let $T_k(i)$ denote the cortical thickness of the i-th ROI of the k-th subject; then the connection weight $\omega_k(i, j)$ is defined as,

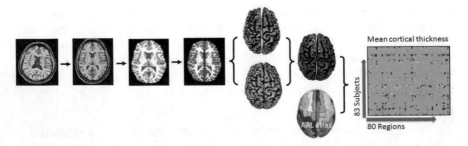

Fig. 1 The pipeline of pre-processing and mean cortical thickness extraction. Take AD samples for example (N = 83), both surfaces consist of 40,962 vertices and 81,920 polygons in each hemisphere

$$w_k(i,j) = k(d_k(i,j)) = \exp(-\frac{d_k(i,j)}{\sigma}) \tag{1}$$

where $k(\cdot)$ is a kernel function, and $d_k(i,j)$ is a function that measures the distance between the i-th and the j-th ROI. Specifically, the exponential kernel $k(d) = \exp(-d/\eta)$ is used here, which contains an input parameter η that determines how locally data is analyzed, and the distance function $d_k(i,j)$ is defined as the square of difference between the mean cortical thickness of any two regions,

$$d_k(i,j) = [T_k(i) - T_k(j)]^2 \tag{2}$$

Other kernel and distance functions could also be used to construct the networks. We choose the exponential kernel because it has several desirable properties, including non-negativity and monotonicity, and bounded range. The smaller the absolute difference of cortical thickness, the larger the connection weight between two regions. If two regions have the same value of cortical thickness, they have the strongest connection whose weight equals 1. The kernel width η partially determines the distribution of edge weight or the network density. In this study, we chose a set of different η to examine its influence on the final classification performance. These networks are pruned to reduce noise: edges with weight less than 0.01 are eliminated.

We attempt to make prediction of patients using the edge weight features of individual cortical networks. Each network has edges, and their weights are rearranged to form a long feature vector for each subject. Because of the high-dimensionality of the network features and small number of samples, namely, the curse of dimensionality, dimensionality reduction is considered to reduce the variance and improve the performance of classifiers. Because we are interested in interpretable results, we consider only canonical dimensionality reduction, a.k.a., feature selection (as opposed to feature extraction (or transformation), in which new dimensions are constructed as functions of the original dimensions such as principle component analysis).

Gray Matter Probability

All the structural images are preprocessed using voxcl-based morphometry (VBM) toolbox in Statistical Parametric Mapping software (SPM, www.fil.ion.ucl.ac.uk/spm). First the original anatomical images are segmented into gray matter (GM), white matter (WM), and cerebrospinal fluid images (CSF). Then the segmented images are registered to the Montreal Neurological Institute (MNI) template using 12-parameter affine transformation and non-linear deformation with a warp frequency cutoff at 25. A modulation process is also employed, which scales the final GM images by the amount of contraction required to warp the images to the template. The final result is GM volume maps for each subject, where the total amount of GM remains the same as in the original images. Finally, the normalized maps are smoothed using an 8-mm isotropic Gaussian kernel to improve signal-to-noise ratio and facilitate comparison across subjects. We use only GMP as the features.

Diffusion MRI

Following image acquisition, we used the FMRIB's Diffusion Toolbox (FDT2.0) within FSL v4.1 (http://www.fmrib.ox.ac.uk/fsl) for DTI processing. For each participant, 30 DTI volumes with 1000 s/mm^2 b-value were first affinely registered to the b0 volume for correction of eddy current distortion and simple head motion. Non-brain voxels were removed using Brain Extraction Tool (BET) of FSL; a fractional intensity threshold of 0.25 was selected, resulting in a brain-extracted 4D image and a binary brain mask for each subject. We then used the eddy-corrected 4D data and corresponding brain mask to fit the diffusion tensor model at each voxel by using the FDT. Eigenvalues of diffusion tensor matrix (λ_1, λ_2, λ_3) were obtained and maps of axial diffusivity (AD = λ_1), mean diffusivity (MD = (λ_1 + λ_2 + λ_3)/3), and fractional anisotropy (FA) were generated. Radial diffusivity (perpendicular eigenvalue, λ_{23} = (λ_2 + λ_3)/2) was calculated by averaging λ_2 and λ_3 maps.

Tract-Based Spatial Statistics

The Most-Representative-Subject TBSS (RS-TBSS) procedure [64] was then applied to the data which is recommended if the subjects are all young children. The FA images from each participant were co-registered to every other one using a nonlinear registration (FNIRT) provided by FSL, identify the "most representative" one, and use this as the target image. This target image is then affine-aligned into MNI152 standard space, and every image is transformed into 1 × 1 × 1 mm MNI152 space by combining the nonlinear transform to the target FA image with the affine transform from that target to MNI152 space. The resulting standard-space FA images of each participant were averaged to create a mean FA image, and then a skeleton image of WM tracts was created suppressing all non-maximum FA values in each voxel's local-perpendicular direction and subsequently comparing all remaining non-zero voxels with their nearest neighbors, thus searching for the center of fiber bundles. A threshold of 0.2 was selected to define the border distinguishing white from gray matter. Then, for each participant, we projected the local maximal FA intensity along the perpendicular direction of the WM tract to the mean FA skeleton to carry out the voxel wise statistics across subjects. The same projection method was applied to MD, AD, and RD images. For voxel-wise group comparisons between patients and normal control on the skeleton image, we used FSL's randomise tool. Essentially, randomise uses a permutation-based statistical inference that does not rely on a Gaussian distribution. Random Monte Carlo simulated samples of 10,000 permutations were used as null distribution. P < 0.05 were identified as significant and corrected for multiple comparisons with threshold-free cluster enhancement (TFCE) method [65] to avoid definition of an initial cluster-forming threshold or carrying out a large amount of data smoothing (Fig. 2 shows the pipeline). The *ICBM-DTI-81 white-matter labels* atlas, *JHU White-Matter Tractography* atlas and *Talairach Daemon Labels* atlas provided by FSL were used to identify the abnormal white matter tracts. Similarly, we also analyze MD, RD and AD TBSS results.

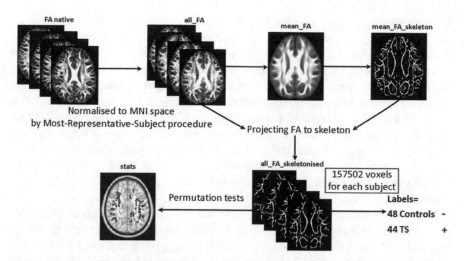

Fig. 2 Flow-chart of the RS-TBSS procedure. A WM skeleton is created in TBSS processing which is common to all subjects. Diffusion values are then extracted from every voxel in the WM skeleton. Data is then labelled as either Control or TS

Following TBSS analysis, a mask was created based on the WM skeleton that is common to all subjects and the skeletonised FA, AD, RD and MD images were analysed in Matlab. There were 157502 voxels in the WM skeleton and diffusion values for each DTI metric were extracted from each voxel in the WM skeleton. Classification between groups was undertaken using each DTI metric separately in order to determine the most efficient metric for classification.

Brain Structural Network

The whole brain fiber bundles linked different cortical regions form a huge complicated network. The most basic element network nodes and edges are defined as follows.

Network node definition: The entire brain is divided into multiple regions using the Automated Anatomical Labeling (AAL) atlas, where each region represents a network node [66]. Specifically, the individual FA image in native space was co-registered to its corresponding T1-weighted image using an affine transformation. The individual structural image was then non-linearly registered to the ICBM152 template. Based on the resultant transformations in these two steps, an inverse warping transformation from the standard space to the native DTI space can be obtained. AAL template in the standard space was then inversely warped back to individual native space by applying this inverse transformation [67].

Network edge definition: All the reconstructed fiber bundles in native space were taken into account for the composition of the network edge. We constructed networks using deterministic tractography. The whole brain fiber tracking was performed via the Fiber Assignment by Continuous Tracking (FACT) algorithm [68] by seeding from the center of each voxel, with the FA threshold of 0.2 and tracking turning angular threshold of 45°. For every pair of brain nodes/regions defined above, fibers with two end-points located in their respective masks were considered to link the two nodes. After defining the network edges, both the weighted and binary network analyses were performed. For the weighted networks, we defined the number, mean FA and averaged length of the connected fibers between two regions as the weights of the network edges. For the binary networks, we considered the existence/absence of fiber bundles in which the network edges were defined as 1 if the fiber number between the two regions was larger than the threshold (T = 3 in our case) and as 0 otherwise. As a result, for each participant, there were four different kinds of networks, namely fiber number (FN)-weighted, FA-weighted, fiber length (FL)-weighted and binary network, each of which was represented by a symmetric 90 * 90 matrix.

For each weighted or binary network, we computed three nodal (regional) characteristics of the structural networks, the nodal degree $D_{nodal}(i)$, nodal efficiency $E_{nodal}(i)$ [67] and nodal betweenness centrality $B_{nodal}(i)$ as the features. Classification between groups was undertaken using each characteristic of structural network separately in order to determine the most efficient characteristic for classification.

$$D_{\text{nodal}}(i) = \sum_{i \neq j \in G} w_{ij} \tag{3}$$

$$E_{\text{nodal}}(i) = \frac{1}{N-1} \sum_{i \neq j \in G} \frac{1}{L_{ij}} \tag{4}$$

$$B_{nodal}(i) = \sum_{s \neq i \neq t \in G} \sigma_{st}(i) \tag{5}$$

where w_{ij} is the edge weight between node i and node j in G, L_{ij} is the shortest path length between node i and node j in G, $\sigma_{st}(i)$ is the number of shortest paths from node s to node t passing through node i. $D_{nodal}(i)$ is the sum of edge w_{ij} linking to node i. $E_{nodal}(i)$ measures the average shortest path length between a given node i and all of the other nodes in the network. $B_{nodal}(i)$ measures the number of shortest paths that pass through a node.

Resting-State fMRI

Some image preprocessing steps should be conducted before features of rs-fMRI are extracted. The first 10 volumes of each functional time series are discarded for participant adaptation to the scanning. Then the image data are temporally realigned to remove time delay between different slices, and spatially realigned to remove head motions. If the head motions of a session are over the threshold of 2 mm [69], this session of the subject will be abandoned and other sessions are used. We further spatially normalize the realigned images to the MNI template. Considering the sMRI images of subjects are offered, T1 image unified segmentation [70] is applied to normalize the realigned images. Then the normalized images are resampled to voxels of $3 \times 3 \times 3$ mm^3. At last, linear drift detrend and temporal band-pass filtering ($0.01 < f < 0.08$ Hz) [71, 72] are performed to reduce low-frequency drift and high-frequency noise using the rs-fMRI data analysis toolkit [73] (REST V1.6, www.restfmri.net/).

Regional Homogeneity

Regional homogeneity was originally proposed by Zang et al. [74]. It uses Kendall's coefficient of concordance (KCC) to measure the regional synchrony for the given voxel and its $K - 1$ nearest neighbors, and is calculated as

$$W = \frac{\sum_i R_i^2 - n \cdot \overline{R}^2}{\frac{1}{12} K^2 (n^3 - n)} \tag{6}$$

where W is the KCC of the given voxel, ranging from 0 to 1; $K = 27$ is the number of neighborhood voxels and n is the number of time points; R_i is the sum of K voxels on the i-th time point; $\overline{R}$ is the mean of the R_i's. ReHo is calculated on each voxel of the whole brain to form a ReHo map using REST toolkit. A smoothing process is conducted on the ReHo map to reduce noise.

Functional Connectivity

Functional connectivity is measured as the correlation coefficient of time courses of any two voxels or ROIs. In this study, we mainly use ROI-based functional connectivity due to the low computational complexity. We utilize the CC400 atlas (which is conducted in Athena pipeline of ADHD preprocessed data, neurobureau. projects.nitrc.org/ADHD200/Introduction.html) to extract time courses of 351 ROIs. Then ROI-based functional connectivity is calculated for each subject as

$$FC(i,j) = \frac{\sum (X_i - \overline{X_i})(X_j - \overline{X_j})}{\sqrt{\sum (X_i - \overline{X_i}) \sum (X_j - \overline{X_j})}} \tag{7}$$

where X_i is the time courses of the i-th ROI and FC(i, j) presents the connection weight between the i-th and the j-th ROI. The calculated functional connectivity is pruned using an absolute threshold of 0.05 in order to reduce noise.

2.2 Feature Selection

The dimensionality of original brain features is usually much higher than the number of samples, which cannot be directly used to train classifier considering overfitting problem and computational complexity. Thus, dimensionality reduction is required to reduce the variance and improve the performance of the classifier. Feature selection is one of commonly used dimensionality reduction methods, as opposed to feature extraction (or transformation) such as PCA, in which new low-dimensional embedding is produced using the original features. Feature selection algorithms can be grossly subdivided into two categories: filter methods and wrapper methods [75]. A filter method such as t-test directly evaluates feature subsets through their information content while a wrapper method iteratively optimizes the performance of a specific classification algorithm. Thus filter methods tend to be more computationally efficient; they also tend to be less effective than wrapper methods for a specific classification problem. Hence, a hybrid approach is intuitively desirable to improve the accuracy of feature selection at relatively low computational cost. In our study, we try different combinations of filters and wrappers and compare their impacts on classification performance.

Filter Methods

Filter methods are used to filter the features on the original feature dimensions to eliminate features with small discriminative power. We consider four filter methods: (1) a two-sample t-test, (2) Pearson's correlation with classification labels, (3) the ratios of between-group sum of squares to within-group sum of squares (BSS/WSS), and (4) ReliefF algorithm.

Two-Sample t-test

First, a two-sample t-test is used to test whether there exists a statistically significant difference between the means of two data samples. For a two-tailed test, the null hypothesis is that the mean value of two groups are equal. The t-test yields a p value-the probability of mistakenly rejecting the null hypothesis-for this hypothesis testing. We assume the data are normally distributed and apply two-sample t-test on each feature dimension to retain the features which have a p-value smaller than some threshold.

Pearson's Correlation

Second, Pearson's correlation coefficient between a feature dimension and clinical labels may reveal the discriminative power of the feature; the larger the absolute Pearson correlation coefficient is, the more relevant a feature is to classification. Let f_{ij} denote the i-th feature of the j-th subject, and y_i denote the label of the j-th subject; Pearson's correlation coefficient of the i-th feature dimension is defined as follows,

$$r_i = \frac{\sum_j (f_{ij} - \bar{f}_i)(y_i - \bar{y})}{\sqrt{\sum_j (f_{ij} - \bar{f}_i)^2} \sqrt{\sum_j (y_i - \bar{y})^2}} \tag{8}$$

where $\bar{f}_i$ is the mean value of the i-th feature dimension across subjects and $\bar{y}$ is the mean value of labels. Pearson's correlation coefficient of each feature dimension are ranked and features with larger r_i are retained.

BSS/WSS

Third, the within-group sum of squares (WSS) measures the within-class scatter while the between-group sum (BSS) of squares measures the variation between the group means. A discriminative feature should have a larger BSS and a smaller WSS, or a larger ratio of BSS to WSS. Also we assume that f_{ij} is the value of the i-th feature of the j-th sample and c is the group label $(+1$ or $-1)$; the ratio (BSS/WSS) of the i-th feature is defined as,

$$ratio_j = \frac{BSS_j}{WSS_j} = \frac{\sum\limits_{i=1}^{n} \sum\limits_{r=1}^{2} I(y_i = r)(\overline{f_{rj}} - \overline{f._j})^2}{\sum\limits_{i=1}^{n} \sum\limits_{r=1}^{2} I(y_i = r)(f_{ij} - \overline{f_{rj}})^2} \tag{9}$$

where $\overline{f_{rj}}$ is the mean value of the j-th feature across subjects in group r and $\overline{f_j}$ is the mean value of the j-th feature across all n subjects; the index function I $(y_i = r)$ equals 1 if the i-th subject belongs to group r and equals 0 otherwise.

ReliefF

The feature selection algorithm "ReliefF" [76] was used to extract the most salient voxels. The basic idea of ReliefF is to draw instances at random, compute their nearest neighbors, and adjust a feature weighting vector to give more weight to features that discriminate the instance from neighbors of different classes. Given a set of training sample data $X = \{x_1, x_2, ..., x_n\}$, $x_i = \{x_{i1}, x_{i2}, ..., x_{iN}\}^T$, x_{iN} is the Nth feature value of the ith sample, λ is a $N \times 1$ matrix, representing the weight of each feature. ReliefF searches for R nearest neighbors from the same class called nearest hits h_j, $j = 1, 2, ..., R$, and also R nearest neighbors from each of the different classes, called nearest misses m_{ij}, $j = 1, 2, ..., R$, $1 \neq$ class(x_i). Assuming that diff_hit is a $N \times 1$ matrix, representing the difference between hj and xi on feature.

$$diff\_hit = \sum_{j=1}^{R} \frac{|x_i - h_j|}{max(X) - min(X)} \tag{10}$$

Assuming that diff_miss is a $N \times 1$ matrix, representing the difference between m_{lj} and x_i on feature.

$$diff\_miss = \sum_{1 \neq class(x_i)} \frac{P(l)}{1 - P(class(x_i))} \sum_{j=1}^{R} \frac{|x_i - m_{lj}|}{max(X) - min(X)} \tag{11}$$

where P(l) is the probability of class l, ReliefF then updates the weight λ based on the formulation.

$$\lambda = \lambda - \frac{diff\_hit}{R} + \frac{diff\_miss}{R} \tag{12}$$

The above four filter methods calculate the ranking scores independently for each feature; however they do not take into account the relationship (redundant or complementary) between features, in other words, they do not consider the features as a whole or do not optimize the feature subset for a specific classification problem; thus the selected features might not be the most optimal feature subset for the classification. In fact, features with weak discriminative power may contribute to the performance of classification if they are complementary to others, while those with strong power may affects the performance if redundant. To avoid this problem, we retain a little more features than in the common situation when using filter method, and then apply wrapper method (normally subset-based) for further feature selection.

Wrapper Methods

Compared to filter method which computes the ranking scores independently for each feature, the wrapper-based method takes into account the relationship between features.

SVM-RFE

One of the wrapper methods we use in this work is the well-known SVM-RFE [77]. It uses the selected feature subset to iteratively train a SVM. In each iteration, the weight w for each feature in the feature subset is calculated during the SVM training process (e.g., for linear SVM we can simply consider the weight of features as the w in $y = w * x + b$; however, the SVM-RFE algorithm a radial basis function kernel, which is a little complicated for estimation of the feature weight), and is considered as the score of the features. A portion of features with small score are eliminated in each iteration of SVM training until the classification accuracy is over a set value, or the number of remaining features is smaller than a set value. Note that SVM-RFE uses the accuracy of cross validation to estimate the goodness of feature subset, which may avoid overfitting problem as far as possible.

LLB

Another wrapper method is a local-learning-based feature selection method [78], whose algorithm can iteratively optimize the weight of feature to maximize a defined margin between the groups. In this algorithm, the distance of a sample to the nearest sample in the same group (nearest hit) and the distance to the nearest sample in the opposite group (nearest miss) are calculated; the margin of a sample is defined as the difference of the two distances. Because a weight is set to each feature, we should find the nearest hit and nearest miss in the weighted feature space, which cannot be estimated as in the original feature space according to the author. Thus the authors assume that every sample might be the nearest sample and the probability is estimated using the weight of feature. Then the margin is considered as the expectation of margins calculated using all possible nearest samples (For detail, see [78]). This method is especially suit to high dimensional data that contain lots of irrelevant features.

2.3 Classification Methods

Classification was then performed using SVM, which is a supervised classification tool that can automatically learn a classification hyperplane in a feature space by optimizing margin-based criteria. Let $x_i = \{x_i^1, ..., x_i^j, ..., x_i^m\}$ represent a feature vector of the i-th subject with m modalities and $y_i \in \{1, -1\}$ denote the corresponding class label. The primal optimization problem of the traditional SVM is given as:

$$
\begin{aligned}
&\min \frac{1}{2} \|w\|^2 + c \sum_{i=1}^{n} \xi_i \\
&s.t.\, y_i\left(w^T \cdot x_i + b\right) \geq 1 - \xi_i \\
&\xi_i \geq 0,\, i = 1, 2, \ldots, n
\end{aligned}
\tag{13}
$$

where ξ_i denotes non-negative slack variable which measures the degree of mis-classification of the data, c denotes the penalty parameter which controls the amount of constraint violations introduced by ξ_i, b denotes the bias term, w denotes the normal vector of hyperplane and $\cdot$ denotes the dot product.

We used an SVM with a radial basis function kernel to solve the classification problem. Let x1, x2 be the feature vectors, and RBF kernel is defined as

$$
K(x_1, x_2) = \exp\left(-\frac{\|x_1 - x_2\|^2}{2\sigma^2}\right)
\tag{14}
$$

where σ is the width of the kernel. The hyper-parameters of SVM such as the penalized coefficient C that adjusts the importance of the separation error in the creation of the separation surface, and the kernel width σ should be carefully tuned to obtain the optimal SVM model.

In our framework, a nested 10-fold cross-validation strategy was used to evaluate the classification performance. We apply an automatic searching method which uses grid search to tune parameters and CV to evaluate the goodness of them. Usually, this CV for parameter tuning is named inner CV because it is nested in another CV called outer CV. For outer CV, the data is randomly divided into 10 parts in which each class is represented in approximately the same proportions as in the full dataset. Each fold is held out in turn and the learning scheme trained on the remaining nine-tenths and the error rate is then calculated on the tenth fold. After all samples have been validated once, we calculate the average CV accuracy and consider it as the estimation of generalization [79].

This nested CV method can yield an unbiased assessment of the classification method and prevent overestimation. Figure 3 shows the flow chart of the evaluation method we used for nested CV.

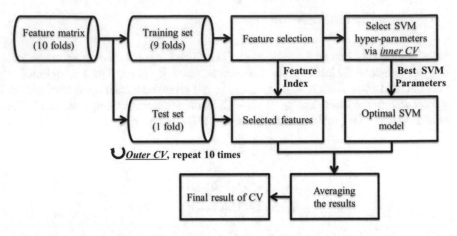

Fig. 3 Nested CV pipeline of our classification framework

2.4 Feature Fusion

In addition to using SVM as classifier, we also attempt to apply two methods to integrate multi-modal features.

Mixed One Single Vector

In our study on TS children using brain structural network, we combined several features into one single vector and then training a classifier can also be a practical option. Dyrba et al. [80] used the same method to combine DTI and MRI features for the automated AD detection. Specially, we merged the best feature subset of each network characteristic at peak performance level of classification. That means that the feature vector for each subject x_i was constructed by concatenating the nodal topological characteristics for each network: $x_i = [\text{node}_j^{(FN)}, ..., \text{node}_k^{(FN)}, ..., \text{node}_l^{(FA)}, ..., \text{node}_m^{(FA)}, ..., \text{node}_n^{(FL)}, ..., \text{node}_o^{(FL)}, \text{node}_p^{(Binary)}, ..., \text{node}_q^{(Binary)}]$. The same feature selection and classification procedure as the single type of feature was then applied to the combining features.

Multi-kernel Learning

In addition to using SVM as classifier, we also attempt to apply multi-kernel learning (MKL) to integrate multi-modal features. In MKL framework, each kind of feature can be presented using its own kernel matrix and the MLK algorithm can automatically search the optimal combination of these kernels to form a new kernel matrix, which could be better than any of single kernels. The output of MKL is defined as

$$y_i = \sum_k \beta_k \left(\sum_j \lambda_j^k y_j K_k \left(x_j^k, x_i^k \right) \right) + b \tag{15}$$

where k denotes the k-th kind of feature; y_i denotes the corresponding class label of i-th subject; K_k is the kernel matrix; β_k is the sub-kernel weight; λ_j^k is the Lagrange parameters; x_j^k is the support vector of training set; and x_i^k is the feature vector of the i-th test sample. Though MKL is theoretically better, it has more parameters to be tuned. Thus, the training process is much more time-consuming, and sub-optimal model tends to be obtained which might affect the effectiveness of MKL. In our experiments, MKL is implemented using Shogun (www.shogun-toolbox.org/).

2.5 Evaluation

For the analysis of results, accuracy, sensitivity, specificity, accuracy and the area under the curve for the receiver operated characteristic curve (AUC ROC) are shown. Accuracy is defined as (TP + TN)/(TP + TN + FN + FP), sensitivity is defined as TP/(TP + FN) and specificity is defined as TN/(FP + TN), where TP is the number of true positives (number of patients correctly classified), TN is the number of true negatives (number of NC correctly classified), FP is the number of false positives (number of NC classified as patients), and FN is the number of false negatives (number of patients classified as NC). Besides, the area under ROC curve (AUC) is an evaluation measure derived from receiver operating characteristic (ROC) curve. The ROC curve is a graph evaluation method, which illustrates the performance of a binary classifier as its decision threshold is varied. When the decision threshold of a classifier varies, sensitivity and specificity also change. ROC curve is created by plotting sensitivity and 1–specificity at different thresholds. A larger AUC commonly indicates a better classifier.

3 Result

3.1 Accurate Prediction of AD Patients

Classification Results Using Individual Cortical Networks
The LOOCV classification accuracy are showed in Fig. 4, in which we report the accuracy of classifying individual cortical networks (CTNet) that are constructed using kernel widths from 0.008 to 0.024. Each line represents the result using a different hybrid filter and wrapper feature selection combination. The filter we used includes two-sample t-Test (tTest), Pearson correlation with labels (Corr) and ratio of BSS to WSS (BSSWSS), while the wrapper includes local-learning-based feature selection (LLB) and SVM-RFE (RFE). Note that our methods automatically select features and classifier hyper-parameters within each fold of outer LOOCV; thus the selected features and hyper-parameters may change every time in each fold. This nested CV pipeline provides a good estimate of generalization error. Figure 4

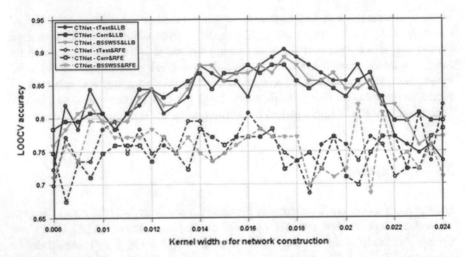

Fig. 4 The LOOCV accuracy of classification using six different hybrid feature selection. The best accuracy of 90.4% is achieved when using $\sigma = 0.0175$ for network construction and the combination of t-test and local-learning-based feature selection (CTNet–tTest&LLB)

shows that the performance of the predictive system is better and more stable when using LLB as the wrapper than RFE. The best LOOCV classification accuracy is 90.4% when using the kernel width $\sigma = 0.0175$ for network construction and the feature subset selected by the combination of t-test and local-learning-based feature selection methods. The best accuracy using six different hybrid feature selection methods and the corresponding are listed in Table 1.

Although the prediction accuracy is commonly used for the evaluation of classification system, it might be biased and not comprehensive when considering class prior and misclassification cost (operational conditions). Thus other methods are introduced for a more comprehensive evaluation. One evaluation method is to use true positive rate (TPR, or sensitivity) and false positive rate (FPR, or specificity). TPR and FPR can evaluate the prediction performance without considering operational conditions, in other words, for a classification problem, the prediction

Table 1 The best LOOCV accuracy of classification using six types of hybrid feature selection and the corresponding kernel width σ for network construction

	σ	Accuracy (%)	Sensitivity/ Specificity (%)	ROCCH	AUC
CTNet– tTest&LLB	0.0175	90.4	92.3/88.6	Yes	0.9610
	0.0180	89.2	92.3/86.3	No	0.9621
CTNet–Corr&LLB	0.0160	87.9	89.7/86.4	Yes	0.9528
	0.0170	87.9	89.7/86.4	Yes	0.9376
	0.0175	87.9	87.2/88.6	Yes	0.9429

(continued)

Table 1 (continued)

	σ	Accuracy (%)	Sensitivity/ Specificity (%)	ROCCH	AUC
CTNet– BSSWSS&LLB	0.0165	87.9	92.3/84.1	No	0.9522
	0.0175	89.2	92.3/86.4	Yes	0.9435
CTNet– tTest&RFE	0.0140	79.5	82.1/77.3	Yes	0.8537
	0.0160	80.7	79.5/81.2	Yes	0.8700
	0.0165	78.3	76.9/79.6	No	0.8700
	0.0240	81.9	74.3/88.6	Yes	0.8700
CTNet–Corr&RFE	0.0140	78.3	82.1/75.0	Yes	0.8462
	0.0165	77.1	76.9/77.2	No	0.8735
	0.0170	78.3	79.5/78.2	Yes	0.8526
	0.0235	77.1	69.2/84.1	Yes	0.8246
	0.0240	78.3	76.9/79.6	Yes	0.8473
CTNet– BSSWSS&RFE	0.0205	81.9	82.1/81.8	Yes	0.8922
	0.0215	80.7	76.9/84.1	Yes	0.8555

accuracy or expected error cost may change when class prior or misclassification cost varies, while TPR and FPR remain consistent. We can easily visualize and organize the performance of a set of discrete classifiers (predicting discrete labels such as +1 or −1) using TPR and FPR to plot the receiver operator characteristic (ROC) graph (note that ROC graph is different from ROC curve), in which each classifier is represented by a point (FPR, TPR). In ROC space, the (0, 1) point represents a perfect classifier (all samples are correctly predicted); thus the nearer a point to the (0, 1) point (more northwest), the better a classifier is. The convex hull of a set of classifiers in ROC graph consists of point (0, 0), (1, 1) and several "more northwest" points. A classifier is potentially optimal if and only if it lies on the convex hull regardless of operational conditions. Figure 5 shows the ROC graphs of classification using different hybrid feature selection schemes, in which each point represents classification using different kernel width for network construction. We aim to find the best kernel width in terms of ROC graph and list it in Table 1. On the other hand, ROC curve can be used for evaluation of ranking or continuous classifier, in which case each classifier is represented by a curve. This is because a classifier that export continuous value can be thresholded to make discrete binary prediction (such as SVMs commonly use a threshold of zero), and by varying the threshold a set of classifiers with different (FPR, TPR) can be produced so that a curve can be traced. A single measure of classification performance can be derived by calculating the area under ROC curve (AUC), e.g., a larger AUC indicate a better classifier. In Table 1, we also list the best AUC and the corresponding. For a review of ROC graph and ROC curve, see [37].

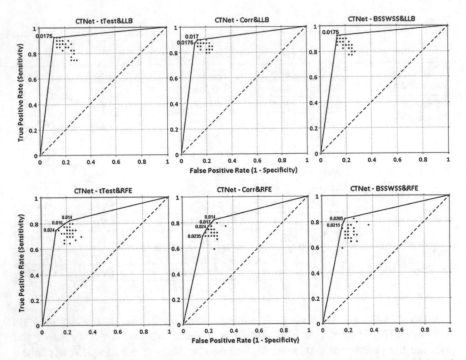

Fig. 5 The ROC graphs of classification using different hybrid feature selection, in which each point represents a classification using different kernel width for network construction. The convex hull of ROC graphs (ROCCH) is drawn and the corresponding is marked near the point on it. These points on convex hull present the potentially optimal classifiers in terms of ROC graph

Comparison with Classification Using the Raw Cortical Thickness

The proposed method for network construction actually projects the mean cortical thickness of AAL ROIs to much higher-dimensional network connectivity features (in this study from 80 to 3160), which may be the major cause of the curse of dimensionality. This compels us to reduce feature dimensionality in order to improve the performance of classifiers. Fortunately, modern sophisticated feature selection methods are powerful enough for large-scale dimensionality reduction, making it possible for learning more complex classifiers. To further demonstrate the effect of the proposed network method, we compare the prediction results of classification using individual cortical networks (CTNet) and raw mean cortical thickness (RawCT).

Because of the similar number of subjects versus raw cortical features (83 vs. 80), we can apply only wrapper methods instead of hybrid method for feature selection (because we use hybrid methods to reduce the computation time and avoid over-fitting of wappers caused by too much features), or even directly train the classifier using original features without feature selection. Therefore we implement the following three strategies before training a SVM using raw cortical thickness: (i) without feature selection (None); (ii) using local-learning-based feature selection

Table 2 The LOOCV accuracy of classifying raw cortical thickness

	Accuracy (%)	Sensitivity/Specificity (%)	AUC
RCT–None	75.9	74.3/77.3	0.8054
RCT–LLB	77.1	71.8/81.8	0.7931
RCT–RFE	79.5	76.9/81.8	0.8258

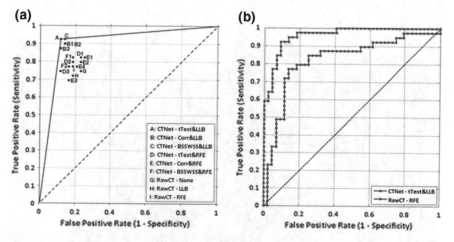

Fig. 6 a The ROC graph of the optimal classifiers (on convex hull in Fig) of 9 different methods. The convex hull of this ROC graph indicates that classification using for network construction and hybrid feature selection that combines t-test and local-learning-based f method is better than others regardless of operational conditions; **b** Comparison of ROC curves under the best condition using network features (CTNet–tTest&LLB) and raw cortical thickness features (RawCT–RFE)

(LLB); (iii) using SVM-RFE for feature selection (RFE). The LOOCV prediction accuracy and AUC of the three methods are summarized in Table 2. Obviously, the highest LOOCV classification accuracy using network edge features exceeds that using raw cortical thickness by more than 10%. The ROC graph in Fig. 6a visualizes the best classification results based on network features, as well as that based on raw cortical thickness. The convex hull consists of point (0, 0), A1 and (1, 1), indicating that the proposed network-based method using tTest&LLB feature selection (A1) is better than other methods regardless of operational conditions. In Fig. 6b, we compare the ROC curve under the best condition using network features and raw cortical thickness features.

Most Discriminative Features of Individual Networks

For network features, we find the features selected by local-learning-based method is more stable than SVM-RFE in the leave-one-out analysis, on which we will discuss in the next section. Here we only examine the most discriminative features under the best condition (CTNet–tTest&LLB, $\sigma = 0.0175$) which use 2-sample t-test and local-learning-based feature selection. The number of features selected by

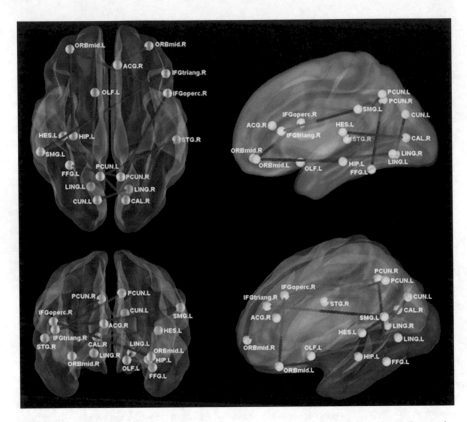

Fig. 7 A visualization of the 10 edges that have most discriminative power when using σ = 0.0175 for network construction and hybrid feature selection that combines t-test and local-learning-based method. The red (or blue) line indicates that the average weight of edges in normal group is larger (or smaller) than that in patient group

the tTest&LLB feature selection in leave-one-out (LOO) analysis ranges from 10 to 15; in total, 22 different edges were selected in at least one of the 83 folds of cross validation. We calculate the reproducibility ratio of each feature selected across LOO iterations to find which of them are almost consistent or chosen in most feature selections out of the 83 folds of cross validation, because these consistent features might encode the class-conditional signal. We find the selected edges connect several regions that are believed to be related with Alzheimer's disease, including hippocampus and parahipppocampus, anterior and middle cingulum, superior temporal gyrus, fusiform gyrus, precuneus, lingual gyrus, calcarine, supramarginal gyrus, and several regions in the frontal lobes such as orbitofrontal region. The most discriminative edges with high reproducibility ratio (>90%) are visualized in Fig. 7. The red (or blue) line connected to the related regions indicates that the weight of edge in AD (or MCI) is larger (or smaller) than that of normal controls.

3.2 Accurate Identification of ADHD Children

Classification Results Using Single Feature

The 10-fold CV classification results using single feature are listed in Table 3. We compare the CV results using cortical thickness (CT), gray matter probability (GMP), regional homogeneity (ReHo) or ROI-based functional connectivity (FC) as the feature to train the classifier. From the results we find classification using ReHo achieves the best CV accuracy. However, it does not work well in terms of J-statics and the area under ROC curve (AUC). This might be caused by the class imbalance, which we will discuss later. Classifiers using GMP and ROI-based FC both achieve good CV accuracy and AUC, as well as more balanced sensitivity and specificity. Figure 8a shows the ROC curve of the CV classification using different kinds of features.

We also test the classifier built using single feature on the test set of 169 samples (the labels for 26 samples from Brown University are not given) and the classification results are summarized in Table 4. Classifier using ROI-based FC as feature

Table 3 The CV classification results using single kind of feature and multimodal features

Feature	CV accuracy (2-class) (%)	Sensitivity/ Specificity (%)	J-statics	AUC	CV accuracy (3-class) (%)
CT	61.38	18.47/85.07	0.0353	0.5870	49.12
GMP	64.90	45.50/75.62	0.2112	0.6787	56.87
ReHo	65.87	22.52/89.80	0.1232	0.5982	56.15
FC	62.02	41.89/73.13	0.1502	0.6365	54.92
MKL	67.79	38.29/84.08	0.2237	0.7068	57.71

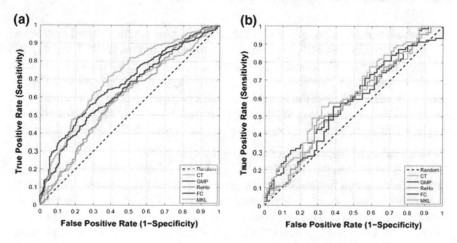

Fig. 8 **a** The ROC curve of CV classification on training set of 624 subjects; **b** The ROC curve of classification on test set of 169 subjects

Table 4 The classification results on test set using single kind of feature

Feature	Accuracy (2-class) (%)	Sensitivity/ Specificity (%)	J-statics	AUC	Accuracy (3-class) (%)
CT	55.62	22.67/81.91	0.0458	0.5212	44.1
GMP	56.80	34.67/74.47	0.0917	0.6065	52.6
ReHo	56.80	17.57/90.30	0.0788	0.5480	48.1
FC	59.17	44.00/71.28	0.1528	0.6187	53.2
MKL	61.54	41.33/77.66	0.1899	0.6288	54.1

achieves the best results in terms of all criteria. Although the classification results on test set are a little worse than the CV results on training set, the difference between them is not significant. This suggests that our CV classification framework could estimate the performances with little bias.

Classification Results Using MKL
In order to integrate the above four kinds of features, an MKL classifier is trained. To reduce computational complexity, we skip the feature selection step and directly use the same features selected in classifications using single feature, which might not be the optimal ones for MKL framework. However, the classification results on both training set and test set exceed the best ones of classification using only single feature. This might suggest that MKL that integrates multimodal features is potentially powerful, although it is more difficult to choose hyper-parameters and more time consuming. The classification results using MKL are listed in Tables 3 and 4, and the ROC curve can be found in Fig. 8.

3.3 Accurate Identification of TS Children

For each classification group and also for each DTI metric, nine reduced feature sets were created using ReliefF algorithm, containing 100 voxels, 250 voxels, 500 voxels, 750 voxels, 1000 voxels, 2000 voxels, 3000 voxels, 4000 voxels and 5000 voxels respectively. The choice of identifying these 9 feature sets is based on previous studies that have shown that this is an optimum range of data reduction for successful classification [81, 82]. However, compared to their method, our method employs feature selection on the training samples rather than the entire samples.

Quantification of Microstructural Changes with TBSS
Compared with healthy control children, TS children showed significantly ($p < 0.05$, corrected for multiple comparisons) reduced FA, increased RD and MD in multiple white matter skeleton clusters. We did not find any significant FA increase, RD and MD decreases compared with healthy children. Skeleton clusters showing no significantly changed AD at $p < 0.05$ (corrected for multiple comparisons). However, there was a trend towards higher AD values in TS children

relative to healthy control children (p < 0.05, not corrected for multiple comparisons).

SVM Classification of Control and TS

For the classification of control and TS children, the accuracy (88.04%), sensitivity (88.64%) and specificity (87.50%) were achieved in our method as peak performance of the SVM classifier was achieved using the AD metric with 2000 voxels feature set. For the FA metric, classification performance was slightly lower, with accuracy in the range of 68–86%. For RD and MD metrics, classification performance had the accuracy in the range of 65–85% (Fig. 9 shows all the measures). As peak performance was achieved the feature set of 2000 voxels, the ROC curve is shown for this feature set for all 4 DTI metrics (Fig. 10).

Regions Most Influential for Classification

Following classification, we subsequently created images depicting the location of some of clusters of voxels selected the ReliefF algorithm. For the control and TS children classification, we chose the AD feature set with the top 2000 voxels that produced the highest accuracy, sensitivity and specificity. Using *cluster* command provided by FSL, we present the largest 5 clusters (size ≥ 20) of voxels selected by ReliefF. The coordinates of the local maxima and cluster size are listed in Table 5.

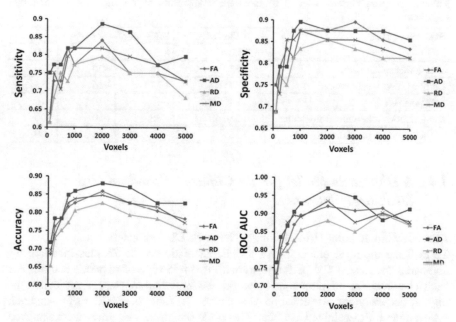

Fig. 9 Sensitivity, specificity, accuracy and the area under the curve for a receiver operating characteristic curve (ROC AUC) for control and TS children classification. Results are shown for the 9 feature sets. The voxels comprising these reduced feature sets were selected by the ReliefF algorithm

Fig. 10 Comparison of ROC
curve under the peak
performance of the SVM
classifier which occurs with
feature set of 2000 voxels.
True positives refer to TS
children that are correctly
classified as TS, and false
positives refer to healthy
children that are incorrectly
labelled as TS. The best
classification performance
was achieved using the AD
metric

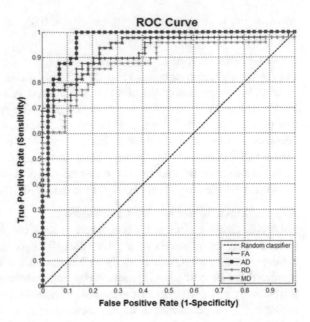

Table 5 Skeleton clusters selected by the ReliefF algorithm as the most salient for group classification

Skeleton clusters	Cluster	MNI coordinates (mm)		
	Size	x	y	z
Left corticospinal tract	83	−26	−20	29
Body of corpus callosum	34	−17	−16	35
Left putamen	24	−16	10	−15
Right inferior longitudinal fasciculus	21	48	−19	−20
Right cingulum (cingulate gyrus)	20	9	11	30

3.4 A Diagnosis Model for TS Children Based on Brain Structural Network

Classification Results Using a Single Network Characteristic

To evaluate the most efficient network characteristic on the TS classification, we
compared the nested CV performance with a single type of network feature. For
each characteristic of structural network, the best feature subset achieving the
highest accuracy for classification was shown in Table 6. For the FN-weighted,
FA-weighted, FL-weighted and binary network, the highest accuracy were achieved
respectively on the characteristic of FN-nodal degree (82.17%), FA-nodal efficiency
(78.04%), FL-nodal betweenness centrality (71.30%), Binary-nodal degree
(73.91%). The optimum parameters (C and γ) were estimate using grid search.

Table 6 The classification accuracy for each characteristic of structural network

Feature	Accuracy (%)	Sensitivity (%)	Specificity (%)	AUC (%)
FN-degree	82.17 ± 2.12	79.55 ± 5.57	84.58 ± 1.86	87.37 ± 2.67
FN-efficiency	71.74 ± 2.55	66.82 ± 3.45	76.25 ± 5.02	78.73 ± 0.81
FN-betweenness	73.48 ± 5.25	73.64 ± 2.59	73.33 ± 8.12	74.70 ± 3.78
FA-degree	74.57 ± 1.65	72.27 ± 4.37	76.67 ± 2.72	75.91 ± 1.13
FA-efficiency	78.04 ± 3.39	75.91 ± 1.24	80.00 ± 6.35	82.05 ± 1.86
FA-betweenness	65.00 ± 4.57	55.00 ± 7.43	74.17 ± 4.80	66.39 ± 5.02
FL-degree	62.39 ± 5.25	56.36 ± 5.88	67.92 ± 5.63	65.45 ± 3.94
FL-efficiency	66.96 ± 5.47	61.82 ± 5.88	71.67 ± 8.01	70.94 ± 5.52
FL-betweenness	71.30 ± 0.60	66.36 ± 2.49	75.83 ± 1.86	74.08 ± 0.98
Bi-degree	73.91 ± 1.09	69.09 ± 3.45	78.33 ± 1.86	76.85 ± 1.95
Bi-efficiency	71.96 ± 2.60	66.82 ± 4.43	76.67 ± 4.01	72.85 ± 2.77
Bi-betweenness	65.00 ± 4.44	60.45 ± 5.23	69.17 ± 7.42	65.33 ± 2.51
Multi-features	88.26 ± 1.79	82.73 ± 2.59	93.33 ± 1.74	94.77 ± 1.83

FN fiber numbers weighted network, *FA* mean FA values weighted network, *FL* averaged fiber length weighted network, *Bi* Binary network, *Degree/efficiency/betweenness* nodal degree/efficiency/betweenness centrality

Classification Based on Combining Features

In order to evaluate the benefits of integrating multiple network characteristic on the TS classification, we compared its performance with single network characteristic. The highest accuracy reaches 88.26% on the combing feature set. This suggests that integrating multi-features is a powerful classifier. The classification results using multi-features are also listed in Table 6, and the ROC curve can be found in Fig. 11. We can find that the ROC curve of multi-features classifier is better than single-feature based classifiers.

The Most Discriminative Network Node Regions

The current work also identifies the node regions which were most efficient characteristic for early TS classification. We summed the counts of each feature selected by our proposed method for each network characteristic. We summed the counts of each feature selected by our proposed method over the 5 rounds nested 10-fold CV. The top 19 selected features with the frequency more than 70% were provided in Table 7. We also used two-sample t-test to evaluate the variation trend of features in the selected node regions and whether each feature was significantly different in TS group compared to control group. The most discriminative node regions located mainly in bilateral angular gyrus and superior frontal gyrus, right amygdala, superior occipital gyrus and inferior frontal gyrus, left lenticular nucleus, puteman, parahippocampal gyrus, median cingulate and paracingulate gyri. It is worth noting that multiple features in the left lenticular nucleus, puteman, median cingulate and paracingulate gyri ranked within the top 19. It indicates that these regions may be highly related to TS pathology.

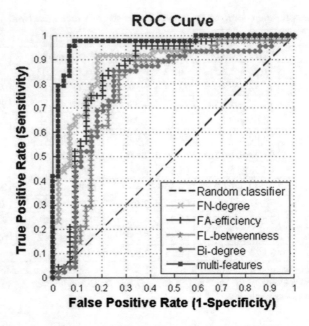

Fig. 11 The ROC curve of nested CV classification on 92 subjects. For the FN-weighted, FA-weighted, FL-weighted and binary network, only the single type of characteristic achieving the highest accuracy were shown

Table 7 The top 19 discriminative network features selected by the nested CV method as the most salient for group classification

Region	Feature	Num	Rate (%)	Trend	P	Abbreviation
Right amygdala	FL-efficiency	50	100	–	0.024	AMYG.R
Left lenticular nucleus, putamen	FL-efficiency	49	98	+	<0.001	PUT.L
Left angular gyrus	Bi-betweenness	49	98	–	0.003	ANG.L
Right rolandic operculum	FA-degree	48	96	+	0.024	ROL.R
Right superior frontal gyrus, dorsolateral	FA-betweenness	47	94	–	0.024	SFGdor.R
Left parahippocampal gyrus	FL-efficiency	47	94	+	0.037	PHG.L
Right angular gyrus	FL-efficiency	45	90	–	N.S.	ANG.R
Right inferior frontal gyrus, opercular part	FL-degree	43	86	+	0.019	IFGoperc.R
Right superior occipital gyrus	FL-degree	41	82	–	N.S.	SOG.R
Right inferior frontal gyrus, orbital part	Bi-degree	41	82	+	0.042	ORBinf.R

(continued)

Table 7 (continued)

Region	Feature	Num	Rate (%)	Trend	P	Abbreviation
Right middle temporal gyrus	FA-degree	40	80	+	N.S.	MTG.R
Left median cingulate and paracingulate gyri	Bi-efficiency	40	80	+	0.019	DCG.L
Right middle frontal gyrus	FA-betweenness	39	78	+	N.S.	MFG.R
Right precentral gyrus	FL-efficiency	39	78	−	0.109	PreCG.R
Left precuneus	Bi-efficiency	38	76	−	N.S.	PCUN.L
Left insula	FL-efficiency	37	74	−	N.S.	INS.L
Left lenticular nucleus, putamen	Bi-efficiency	37	74	+	0.027	PUT.L
Left median cingulate and paracingulate gyri	FN-efficiency	36	72	+	0.023	DCG.L
Right inferior occipital gyrus	Bi-efficiency	36	72	−	N.S.	IOG.R

Num the counts of each parameter selected by our proposed method over the 5 rounds nested 10-fold CV, *Rate* the frequency of being selected, equals Num/total times in 5 rounds nested 10-fold CV (50 times), +/− parameter is increased/decreased in TS group compared to control group, *P* p value of two sample t-test, *N.S.* parameter is not significantly different between groups

4 Discussion

4.1 Alzheimer's Disease

Network Representation Outperforms the Original Brain Measures
The proposed approach establishes individual cortical network for each subject through a kernel function using the mean cortical thickness of AAL regions. In fact, the raw cortical thickness features are transformed to high-dimensional network edge features, which makes complicated feature selection essential to the classification system due to the much larger number of features than samples. This results in more complex prediction system and demands more computation time to train it; nevertheless, it does work, as presented in the last section. We analyze the reasons why the proposed method works from three aspects. (i) The reliability and stability of the network patterns: we consider that the network features can seize the patterns of relationship between different ROIs, which are more reliable and stable than the original mean cortical thickness. This is because the human brain is so complex a non-linear system and has severe individual differences, in others words, the raw brain measures such as cortical thickness might not be easily modeled by a linear model with respect to age, gender, intracranial volume (ICV) and so forth. The individual differences might affect the accuracy of classification model, and moreover linear regression might not solve this problem well. An intuitive solution

is that we can find or produce patterns that are not, or hardly, affected by the individual differences. We consider that network features are just this kind of patterns, because networks focus on the relationships but not the cortical thickness values themselves and obviously the relationships are much more consistent across subjects than the values regarding individual differences. (ii) Sensitive to the disease: we think the network patterns are more sensitive to the changes caused by the diseases. Consider that a neuropathy may cause some organic changes such as gray matter atrophy or cortical thinning of a specific region. Such change might not be discovered by group analysis using raw cortical measures due to the individual differences, nonetheless it might be easily reflected in the variation of connection weight because the weight of edges connected to all other regions will be altered—those to regions with larger thickness will decrease and those to the regions with smaller thickness will increase. (iii) The perspective of kernel-based learning: for kernel-based learning, the original features are first projected to high-dimensional space (even infinite-dimensional space), in which data might be better organized or represented and prone to separate by linear model. The proposed method for network construction is sort of like this kernel trick. The kernel used for establishing network is actually a variant of RBF kernel. Although these two kinds of kernel tricks differ, they have the same intention: a better organization and representation of the data. Further investigation for the kernel trick used in network construction will be covered in future work.

Effect of Different Hybrid Feature Selection Methods

Hybrid feature selection combines filter and wrapper method: the filter method quickly removes most irrelevant features that have little discriminative power; while the wrapper method searches for the best feature subsets for classification. This consecutive feature selection method avoid the defects of both methods to some extent. Because the filter methods select features according to the content information but not the classification performance, although each of selected features has a better discriminative power when considering independently, they might be redundant to each other and not optimal for a specific classification problem. On the other hand, though the wrapper methods can optimize the feature subset for a specific problem, they are more computationally complicated and time-consuming; in addition, the overfitting problem is easily caused by high-dimensional data when using the wrapper. Thus, the thought of combining the both are quite intuitive. When examining the results of six combinations of feature selection, we find that the filter hardly influences the classification performance if adequate features are retained for the wrapper, in other words, it is the wrapper that determines the results of hybrid feature selection. However the filter is indispensable for accelerating the wrapper and reducing the probability of overfitting problem (because of the lower dimensional data). For the dataset in our experiment, local-learning-based feature selection (LLB) is much more stable and reliable than SVM-RFE, as shown in the results section. SVM-RFE iteratively eliminates feature to obtain a feature subset that has the best cross validation accuracy, which might be prone to cause the overfitting problem; while local-learning-based method aim to find the maximal margin in the deduced weight space. In addition, SVM-RFE is much slower than LLB because of the cross validation process. Thus, LLB is much more suitable for this AD dataset. In spite of this, we cannot say that LLB is better than SVM-RFE in all circumstances. In fact, we find in other studies that LLB can hardly output any feature if the dataset is not prone to be separated, in which condition, a forward or backward.

4.2 ADHD

Classification Using Multi-site Datasets
Because of the difficulty of collecting samples, datasets in imaging study are usually quite small in the neuroimaging community. One hundred samples are already quite large dataset and cost thousands of dollars and several months to collect. Thus, opening or exchanging neuroimaging data can produce much larger datasets, making the researches more reliable and convincing. This will benefit the whole community as the ADHD-200 datasets did. However, datasets from different sites usually vary in their scanning device or parameters, and the race of subjects may also be different. These factors might result in different baselines of extracted features. The impacts of multi-site datasets on each kind of feature are not similar, for instance, we also use scale-invariant feature transform (SIFT) to extract features for classification and we find that these features can even distinguish subjects from different sites, which means that they can hardly be used directly to predict ADHD patients because of the evidently distinct baseline. Several potential methods may alleviate this problem. The first is to regress the image by different factors before feature extraction. Nonetheless, this method might produce more uncertainty because the impacts of factors such as scanning parameters or races on the human brains are much more complicated than age or gender. Linear regression might not work for these factors. Another method is to normalize the features of subjects from different sites. Although this method may work well on other datasets, it is not suitable for ADHD-200 samples because datasets from some sites have only normal controls or few ADHD patients. We can use this method only when we abandon these datasets. The third method is to train classifier on each datasets from different sites. However, this method, in fact, does not take advantage of the large samples of multi-site datasets. Moreover, the ADHD-200 test set has some samples from new site which have to be predicted using samples from other sites. In short, how to use multi-site datasets is still a pending problem and worth future investigation. All the results we present in this paper do not use any of the aforementioned methods.

Impacts of Imbalanced Class on Classification
The ADHD-200 datasets have more TDC than ADHD patients (485 TDC vs. 281 ADHD). Such imbalanced datasets might cause bias of a classifier, making it more prone to classify samples to TDC. In fact, from the ADHD-200 competition results, we found that for most participants, the number of subjects that were

predicted as TDC was much more than the actual number of TDC in test set, which was one of the main cause of high specificity and low sensitivity in average (71.77% vs. 31.44%). (http://fcon_1000.projects.nitrc.org/indi/adhd200/results.html). A prediction system with an excessively imbalanced sensitivity and specificity is defective, which might at least suggest that the classifier is biased while training. We consider that we should pay more attention to other evaluation methods such as ROC graph rather than using only classification accuracy.

In this paper, we use the selected datasets containing 404 TDC and 222 ADHD patients, in which the ratio of the number of TDC to that of ADHD patients is 1.82. Without special handling of this imbalance, we obtain the specificity of 73.13% and the sensitivity of 41.89% (using FC as features). However, in the competition, we use much less TDC than in this paper—only 517 subjects with 303 TDC and 214 ADHD patients. The ratio of the number of TDC to that of ADHD patients is 1.42. The competition results show that we obtained the specificity of 66.4% and sensitivity of 52.3%—the highest sensitivity and highest J-statistics (specificity + sensitivity − 1) in the contest. The reason we reduce the TDC used in the competition is that we want to prevent the impacts of imbalanced datasets as far as possible. We do not know the priori of the test set. Thus, we assume it as 50%, that is, the probability of a sample being TDC or ADHD patient is equal in the test set. However, you can also assume the priori as the same of training set (as most participants did). In fact, the actual number of TDC is slightly more than that of ADHD patients (the ratio is only 1.21, much less than that in training set). Thus, we consider that imbalanced class of training set and almost balanced class of test set might be one of the main reasons that causes the mean specificity much more than the mean sensitivity. The results of this paper also demonstrate this trend, that is, when using more imbalanced datasets, we obtain a more imbalanced specificity and sensitivity, and the impacts of imbalanced datasets on classification are different for different kinds of features. However, we do not do any further experiments about this discovery so that it is yet a hypothesis.

4.3   TS

Classification Using TBSS

The current results show that it is possible to classify control and TS children with a high degree of accuracy using an automated procedure that combines TBSS with SVM. Our results achieved a highest accuracy of 88.04%, being able to classify group membership with 74% accuracy. It is worth noting that no significant AD change was found between the groups in our statistical results that are corrected for multiple comparisons, but the AD voxels feature sets selected by ReliefF achieved the most accurate classification using SVM. The reason for this lies in methodological differences between the two approaches. For TBSS, each voxel is assigned a t-value that is corrected for multiple comparisons, The level of correction for multiple comparisons is therefore extremely high due to the large number of total voxels to be considered. However, the SVM approach is underpinned by a different theoretical framework. Following the most salient voxels are selected by the ReliefF algorithm, the majority of voxels in the WM skeleton are discarded as irrelevant for subsequent SVM classification. Therefore, the SVM only considers the voxels identified by ReliefF in its calculation of a single parameter per subject, and does not run into the problem of multiple comparison biases.

The current work also identifies the regions selected by the ReliefF that are most influential for classification. The largest 5 clusters of voxels were located in left corticospinal tract and putamen, body of corpus callosum, right Inferior longitudinal fasciculus and cingulum (cingulate gyrus). Tics are the hallmark of TS, so the involvement of the corticospinal tract fits in well with clinical symptoms. Inferior longitudinal fasciculus and cingulum are long association fiber bundles. The modulation of tics by cortical activation depends on the long association fibre bundles within one hemisphere [83]. Our results conform to the previous study with TBSS which showed AD increase in these WM tracts [8]. The corpus callosum is the biggest commissural fibers and transfers information between the hemispheres. The corpus callosum is supposed to play an important role in modulation of tics by mediating the inhibiting influence by prefrontal cortices. The increased AD values in the body of corpus callosum in our data could be responsible for a diminished inhibitory influence. The increased AD in the putamen is discussed as a result of disrupted white matter projections to the globus pallidus and the microstructure change of globus pallidus led to some useful information cannot be passed to the cerebral cortex, causing the tics [84]. It also tallies with our result.

Classification Using Brain Structural Network
In this study, the current results show that it is possible to classify TS and healthy children with a high accuracy using an automated procedure that combines diffusion tractography, graph theoretical method and SVM. Our results achieved a highest accuracy of 88.26% better than the previous work which combined resting-state functional connectivity (RSFC) MRI and SVM for TS children classification and reached the accuracy of 74% [85].

Our study uses features extracted from multiple networks constructed from multiple parameters. The dimensionality of original features is much higher than the number of samples which cannot be directly used to train classifier. A wrapper feature selection method (SVM-RFE) is applied before training SVMs in order to prevent the overfitting problem and reduce the computational complexity. We also used a nested CV method to tune the hyper-parameters of classifiers and evaluate the performances of our method, which can yield unbiased estimation of classification method.

In addition to using a single kind of feature, our experiments show that combing multiple kinds of features can yield better classification results for early TS prediction. We used the same method to integrate features as a previous study [80] which combined several features into one single vector and then training a classifier. Wee et al. [86] also demonstrated that utilizing networks constructed from multiple DWI-derived parameters enhances classification performance.

The current work also identifies the discriminative node regions for classification which mainly located in the amygdala, basal ganglia (lenticular nucleus, putamen) and frontal cortico-cortical circuits. Our result showed the significantly reduced nodal efficiency in amygdala ranked as the most discriminative feature while the connectivity of the amygdala, for which a role in the pathophysiology of TS has been established [87]. Our result also tallied with previous related research where altered connectivity values were found in previous studies in basal ganglia and frontal cortico-cortical circuits [56]. These results support the contention that our diagnosis model may be efficient to capture the complexity of some brain disorders, and hold promise for early TS diagnosis.

5 Conclusion

We have presented our framework for neurologic and psychiatric diseases prediction. Multi-modal features are extracted from the brain images and used for training classifiers. A hybrid feature selection method is applied before training SVMs in order to prevent the overfitting problem and reduce the computational complexity. We have used a nested CV method to train the classifiers and evaluated the performances of our methods, which can yield unbiased estimation of classification method. In addition to using a single feature, we also employ some feature fusion techniques to integrate multimodal features. Our experiments show that using feature fusion techniques to integrate multimodal features can yield better classification results for neurologic and psychiatric diseases prediction.

Acknowledgements This work was supported by National Natural Science Foundation of China (91520202, 61271151), and Youth Innovation Promotion Association CAS.

References

1. Friston, K.J.: Modalities, modes, and models in functional neuroimaging. Science **326**, 399–403 (2009)
2. Zakzanis, K.K., Graham, S.J., Campbell, Z.: A meta-analysis of structural and functional brain imaging in dementia of the Alzheimer's type: a neuroimaging profile. Neuropsychol. Rev. **13**, 1–18 (2003)
3. Binnewijzend, M.A., Schoonheim, M.M., Sanz-Arigita, E., Wink, A.M., van der Flier, W.M., Tolboom, N., Adriaanse, S.M., Damoiseaux, J.S., Scheltens, P., van Berckel, B.N., Barkhof, F.: Resting-state fMRI changes in Alzheimer's disease and mild cognitive impairment. Neurobiol. Aging **33**, 2018–2028 (2012)
4. Stein, D.J., Fontenelle, L.F., Reed, G.M.: Obsessive-compulsive and related disorders in ICD-11. Revista brasileira de psiquiatria **36**(Suppl 1), 1–2 (2014)
5. Zhong, Z., Zhao, T., Luo, J., Guo, Z., Guo, M., Li, P., Sun, J., He, Y., Li, Z.: Abnormal topological organization in white matter structural networks revealed by diffusion tensor

tractography in unmedicated patients with obsessive-compulsive disorder. Prog. Neuropsychopharmacol. Biol. Psychiatry **51**, 39–50 (2014)

6. Hong, S.B., Zalesky, A., Fornito, A., Park, S., Yang, Y.H., Park, M.H., Song, I.C., Sohn, C. H., Shin, M.S., Kim, B.N., Cho, S.C., Han, D.H., Cheong, J.H., Kim, J.W.: Connectomic disturbances in attention-deficit/hyperactivity disorder: a whole-brain tractography analysis. Biol. Psychiatry **76**, 656–663 (2014)

7. Hart, H., Radua, J., Nakao, T., Mataix-Cols, D., Rubia, K.: Meta-analysis of functional magnetic resonance imaging studies of inhibition and attention in attention-deficit/ hyperactivity disorder: exploring task-specific, stimulant medication, and age effects. JAMA Psychiatry **70**, 185–198 (2013)

8. Liu, Y., Miao, W., Wang, J., Gao, P., Yin, G., Zhang, L., Lv, C., Ji, Z., Yu, T., Sabel, B.A., He, H., Peng, Y.: Structural abnormalities in early Tourette syndrome children: a combined voxel-based morphometry and tract-based spatial statistics study. PLoS ONE **8**, e76105 (2013)

9. Worbe, Y., Marrakchi-Kacem, L., Lecomte, S., Valabregue, R., Poupon, F., Guevara, P., Tucholka, A., Mangin, J.F., Vidailhet, M., Lehericy, S., Hartmann, A., Poupon, C.: Altered structural connectivity of cortico-striato-pallido-thalamic networks in Gilles de la Tourette syndrome. Brain **138**, 472–482 (2015)

10. Ellison-Wright, I., Bullmore, E.: Anatomy of bipolar disorder and schizophrenia: a meta-analysis. Schizophr. Res. **117**, 1–12 (2010)

11. Shergill, S.S., Brammer, M.J., Williams, S.C., Murray, R.M., Mcguire, P.K.: Mapping auditory hallucinations in schizophrenia using functional magnetic resonance imaging. Arch. Gen. Psychiatry **57**, 1033–1038 (2000)

12. Etkin, A., Wager, T.D.: Functional neuroimaging of anxiety: a meta-analysis of emotional processing in PTSD, social anxiety disorder, and specific phobia. Am. J. Psychiatry **164**, 1476–1488 (2007)

13. Liao, M., Yang, F., Zhang, Y., He, Z., Su, L., Li, L.: White matter abnormalities in adolescents with generalized anxiety disorder: a diffusion tensor imaging study. BMC Psychiatry **14**, 41 (2014)

14. Orrù, G., Pettersson-Yeo, W., Marquand, A.F., Sartori, G., Mechelli, A.: Using support vector machine to identify imaging biomarkers of neurological and psychiatric disease: a critical review. Neurosci. Biobehav. Rev. **36**, 1140–1152 (2012)

15. Cerasa, A., Cherubini, A., Peran, P.: Multimodal MRI in neurodegenerative disorders. Neurol. Res. Int. **2012** (2012)

16. Arimura, H., Magome, T., Yamashita, Y., Yamamoto, D.: Computer-aided diagnosis systems for brain diseases in magnetic resonance images. Algorithms **2**, 925–952 (2009)

17. Dorrius, M.D., Weide, M.D., Ooijen, P., Pijnappel, R.M.: Computer-aided detection in breast MRI: a systematic review and meta-analysis. Int. J. Med. Radiol. **21**, 1600–1608 (2011)

18. Hidetaka, A., Takashi, Y., Seiji, K., Kazuhiro, T., Hiroshi, K., Futoshi, M., Hiroshi, H., Shuji, S., Fukai, T., Yoshiharu, H.: Automated method for identification of patients with Alzheimer's disease based on three-dimensional MR images. Acad. Radiol. **15**, 274–284 (2008)

19. Liu, F., Wee, C.Y., Chen, H., Shen, D.: Inter-modality relationship constrained multi-modality multi-task feature selection for Alzheimer's Disease and mild cognitive impairment identification. Neuroimage **84**, 466–475 (2014)

20. Cherkassky, V.: The nature of statistical learning theory IEEE Trans. Neural Netw./A Publication of the IEEE Neural Networks Council **8**, 1564 (1997)

21. Fjell, A.M., Walhovd, K.B., Fennema-Notestine, C., McEvoy, L.K., Hagler, D.J., Holland, D., Brewer, J.B., Dale, A.M., Alzheimer's Disease Neuroimaging, I.: CSF biomarkers in prediction of cerebral and clinical change in mild cognitive impairment and Alzheimer's disease. J. Neurosci. **30**, 2088–2101 (2010)

22. Gerardin, E., Chetelat, G., Chupin, M., Cuingnet, R., Desgranges, B., Kim, H.S., Niethammer, M., Dubois, B., Lehericy, S., Garnero, L., Eustache, F., Colliot, O., Alzheimer's Disease Neuroimaging, I.: Multidimensional classification of hippocampal shape features discriminates Alzheimer's disease and mild cognitive impairment from normal aging. Neuroimage 47, 1476–1486 (2009)

23. Lanckriet, G.R., De Bie, T., Cristianini, N., Jordan, M.I., Noble, W.S.: A statistical framework for genomic data fusion. Bioinformatics 20, 2626–2635 (2004)

24. Brookmeyer, R., Johnson, E., Ziegler-Graham, K., Arrighi, H.M.: Forecasting the global burden of Alzheimer's disease. Alzheimers Dement. J. Alzheimers Assoc. 3, 186–191 (2007)

25. Petersen, R.C., Doody, R., Kurz, A., Mohs, R.C., Morris, J.C., Rabins, P.V., Ritchie, K., Rossor, M., Thal, L., Winblad, B.: Current concepts in mild cognitive impairment. Arch. Neurol. 58, 1985–1992 (2001)

26. Grundman, M., Petersen, R.C., Ferris, S.H., Thomas, R.G., Aisen, P.S., Bennett, D.A., Foster Jr., N.L.,, J.C., Galasko, D.R., Doody, R.: Mild cognitive impairment can be distinguished from Alzheimer disease and normal aging for clinical trials. JAMA Neurol. 61, 59–66 (2004)

27. Jack Jr., C.R., Shiung, M.M., Weigand, S.D., O'Brien, P.C., Gunter, J.L., Boeve, B.F., Knopman, D.S., Smith, G.E., Ivnik, R.J., Tangalos, E.G., Petersen, R.C.: Brain atrophy rates predict subsequent clinical conversion in normal elderly and amnestic MCI. Neurology 65, 1227–1231 (2005)

28. Detoledo, M.L., Stoub, T.M., Wilson, R.S., Bennett, D.A., Leurgans, S., Wuu, J., Turner, D. A.: MRI-derived entorhinal volume is a good predictor of conversion from MCI to AD. Neurobiol. Aging 25, 1197–1203 (2004)

29. Thompson, P.M., Mega, M.S., Woods, R.P., Zoumalan, C.I., Lindshield, C.J., Blanton, R.E., Moussai, J., Holmes, C.J., Cummings, J.L., Toga, A.W.: Cortical change in Alzheimer's disease detected with a disease-specific population-based brain atlas. Cereb. Cortex 11, 1–16 (2001)

30. Du, A.T., Schuff, N., Kramer, J.H., Rosen, H.J., Gorno-Tempini, M.L., Rankin, K., Miller, B.L., Weiner, M.W.: Different regional patterns of cortical thinning in Alzheimer's disease and frontotemporal dementia. Brain 130, 1159–1166 (2007)

31. Dai, D., Wang, J., Hua, J., He, H.: Classification of ADHD children through multimodal magnetic resonance imaging. Front. Syst. Neurosci. 6, 63 (2012)

32. Biederman, J., Mick, E., Faraone, S.V.: Age-dependent decline of symptoms of attention deficit hyperactivity disorder: impact of remission definition and symptom type. Am. J. Psychiatry 157, 816–818 (2000)

33. Trull, T.J., Verges, A., Wood, P.K., Jahng, S., Sher, K.J.: The structure of diagnostic and statistical manual of mental disorders (4th edn., text revision) personality disorder symptoms in a large national sample. Pers. Disord. 3, 355–369 (2012)

34. Seidman, L.J., Valera, E.M., Makris, N.: Structural brain imaging of attention-deficit/ hyperactivity disorder. Biol. Psychiatry 57, 1263–1272 (2005)

35. Valera, E.M., Faraone, S.V., Murray, K.E., Seidman, L.J.: Meta-analysis of structural imaging findings in attention-deficit/hyperactivity disorder. Biol. Psychiatry 61, 1361–1369 (2007)

36. Semrud-Clikeman, M., Steingard, R.J., Filipek, P., Biederman, J., Bekken, K., Renshaw, P.F.: Using MRI to examine brain-behavior relationships in males with attention deficit disorder with hyperactivity. J. Am. Acad. Child Adolesc. Psychiatry 39, 477–484 (2000)

37. Overmeyer, S., Bullmore, E.T., Suckling, J., Simmons, A., Williams, S.C., Santosh, P.J., Taylor, E.: Distributed grey and white matter deficits in hyperkinetic disorder: MRI evidence for anatomical abnormality in an attentional network. Psychol. Med. 31, 1425–1435 (2001)

38. Kates, W.R., Frederikse, M., Mostofsky, S.H., Folley, B.S., Cooper, K., Mazur-Hopkins, P., Kofman, O., Singer, H.S., Denckla, M.B., Pearlson, G.D., Kaufmann, W.E.: MRI parcellation of the frontal lobe in boys with attention deficit hyperactivity disorder or Tourette syndrome. Psychiatry Res. 116, 63–81 (2002)

39. Bush, G., Frazier, J.A., Rauch, S.L., Seidman, L.J., Whalen, P.J., Jenike, M.A., Rosen, B.R., Biederman, J.: Anterior cingulate cortex dysfunction in attention-deficit/hyperactivity disorder revealed by fMRI and the Counting Stroop. Biol. Psychiatry 45, 1542–1552 (1999)

40. Teicher, M.H., Anderson, C.M., Polcari, A., Glod, C.A., Maas, L.C., Renshaw, P.F.: Functional deficits in basal ganglia of children with attention-deficit/hyperactivity disorder shown with functional magnetic resonance imaging relaxometry. Nat. Med. **6**, 470–473 (2000)

41. Durston, S., Tottenham, N.T., Thomas, K.M., Davidson, M.C., Eigsti, I.M., Yang, Y., Ulug, A.M., Casey, B.J.: Differential patterns of striatal activation in young children with and without ADHD. Biol. Psychiatry **53**, 871–878 (2003)

42. Cao, Q., Zang, Y., Sun, L., Sui, M., Long, X., Zou, Q., Wang, Y.: Abnormal neural activity in children with attention deficit hyperactivity disorder: a resting-state functional magnetic resonance imaging study. NeuroReport **17**, 1033–1036 (2006)

43. Tian, L., Jiang, T., Wang, Y., Zang, Y., He, Y., Liang, M., Sui, M., Cao, Q., Hu, S., Peng, M., Zhuo, Y.: Altered resting-state functional connectivity patterns of anterior cingulate cortex in adolescents with attention deficit hyperactivity disorder. Neurosci. Lett. **400**, 39–43 (2006)

44. Zang, Y.F., He, Y., Zhu, C.Z., Cao, Q.J., Sui, M.Q., Liang, M., Tian, L.X., Jiang, T.Z., Wang, Y.F.: Altered baseline brain activity in children with ADHD revealed by resting-state functional MRI. Brain Dev. **29**, 83–91 (2007)

45. Liu, D., Yan, C., Ren, J., Yao, L., Kiviniemi, V.J., Zang, Y.: Using coherence to measure regional homogeneity of resting-state fMRI signal. Front. Syst. Neurosci. **4**, 24 (2015)

46. Xavier Castellanos, F., Margulies, D.S., Clare, K., Uddin, L.Q., Manely, G., Andrew, K., David, S., Zarrar, S., Adriana, D.M., Bharat, B.: Cingulate-precuneus interactions: a new locus of dysfunction in adult attention-deficit/hyperactivity disorder. Biol. Psychiatry **63**, 332–337 (2008)

47. Dai, D., He, H., Vogelstein, J.T., Hou, Z.: Accurate prediction of AD patients using cortical thickness networks. Mach. Vis. Appl. **24**, 1445–1457 (2013)

48. Cooper, J.: Diagnostic and statistical manual of mental disorders (4th edn., text revision) (DSM-IV-TR). Br. J. Psychiatry **179**, 85–85 (2001)

49. Stokes, A., Bawden, H.N., Camfield, P.R., Backman, J.E., Dooley, J.M.: Peer problems in Tourettes disorder. Pediatrics **87**, 936–942 (1991)

50. Lucas, A.R., Beard, C.M., Rajput, A.H., Kurland, L.T.: Tourette syndrome in Rochester, Minnesota, 1968–1979. Adv. Neurol. **35**, 267–269 (1982)

51. Knight, T., Steeves, T., Day, L., Lowerison, M., Jette, N., Pringsheim, T.: Prevalence of tic disorders: a systematic review and meta-analysis. Pediatr. Neurol. **47**, 77–90 (2012)

52. Mason, A., Banerjee, S., Eapen, V., Zeitlin, H., Robertson, M.M.: The prevalence of Tourette syndrome in a mainstream school population. Dev. Med. Child Neurol. **40**, 292–296 (1998)

53. Stern, J.S., Burza SRobertson, M.M.: Gilles de la Tourette's syndrome and its impact in the UK. Postgrad. Med. J. **81**, 12–19 (2005)

54. Smith, S.M., Jenkinson, M., Johansen-Berg, H., Rueckert, D., Nichols, T.E., Mackay, C.E., Watkins, K.E., Ciccarelli, O., Cader, M.Z., Matthews, P.M., Behrens, T.E.: Tract-based spatial statistics: voxelwise analysis of multi-subject diffusion data. Neuroimage **31**, 1487–1505 (2006)

55. Basser, P.J., Pajevic, S., Pierpaoli, C., Duda, J., Aldroubi, A.: In vivo fiber tractography using DT-MRI data. Magn. Reson. Med. **44**, 625–632 (2000)

56. Cheng, B., Braass, H., Ganos, C., Treszl, A., Biermann-Ruben, K., Hummel, F.C., Muller-Vahl, K., Schnitzler, A., Gerloff, C., Munchau, A., Thomalla, G.: Altered intrahemispheric structural connectivity in Gilles de la Tourette syndrome. NeuroImage Clin. **4**, 174–181 (2014)

57. Wen, H., Liu, Y., Wang, J., Zhang, J., Peng, Y., He, H.: Using support vector machines with tract-based spatial statistics for automated classification of Tourette syndrome children. In: SPIE Medical Imaging, pp. 97852Q–97852Q-97859. International Society for Optics and Photonics (Year)

58. Wen, H., Liu, Y., Wang, J., Zhang, J., Peng, Y., He, H.: A diagnosis model for early Tourette syndrome children based on brain structural network characteristics. In: SPIE Medical Imaging, pp. 97852R–97852R-97859. International Society for Optics and Photonics (Year)

59. Wen, H., Liu, Y., Wang, J., Rekik, I., Zhang, J., Zhang, Y., Tian, H., Peng, Y., He, H.: Combining tract- and atlas-based analysis reveals microstructural abnormalities in early Tourette syndrome children. Hum. Brain Mapp. **37**, 1903–1919 (2016)
60. Sled, J.G., Zijdenbos, A.P., Evans, A.C.: A nonparametric method for automatic correction of intensity nonuniformity in MRI data. IEEE Trans. Med. Imaging **17**, 87–97 (1998)
61. Hastreiter, P., Rezksalama, C., Tomandl, B., Eberhardt, K.E.W., Ertl, T.: BFb: Medical Image Computing and Computer-Assisted Intervention—MICCAI'98. Springer, Berlin (1998)
62. June Sic, K., Vivek, S., Jun Ki, L., Jason, L., Yasser, A.D.B., David, M.D., Jong Min, L., Sun, I., Kim, Evans, A.C.: Automated 3-D extraction and evaluation of the inner and outer cortical surfaces using a Laplacian map and partial volume effect classification. Neuroimage **27**, 210–221 (2005)
63. Tzourio-Mazoyer, N., Landeau, B., Papathanassiou, D., Crivello, F., Etard, O., Delcroix, N., Mazoyer, B., Joliot, M.: Automated anatomical labeling of activations in SPM using a macroscopic anatomical parcellation of the MNI MRI single-subject brain. Neuroimage **15**, 273–289 (2002)
64. Shiva, K., Ryan, N.S., Malone, I.B., Marc, M., David, C., Ridgway, G.R., Hui, Z., Fox, N.C., Sebastien, O.: The importance of group-wise registration in tract based spatial statistics study of neurodegeneration: a simulation study in Alzheimer's disease. PLoS ONE **7**, e45996–e45996 (2012)
65. Smith, S.M., Nichols, T.E.: Threshold-free cluster enhancement: addressing problems of smoothing, threshold dependence and localisation in cluster inference. Neuroimage **44**, 83–98 (2009)
66. Bullmore, E., Sporns, O.: Complex brain networks: graph theoretical analysis of structural and functional systems. Nat. Rev. Neurosci. **10**, 186 (2009)
67. Liu, Y., Duan, Y.Y., He, Y., Wang, J., Xia, M.R., Yu, C.S., Dong, H.Q., Ye, J., Butzkueven, H., Li, K.C., Shu, N.: Altered topological organization of white matter structural networks in patients with neuromyelitis optica. Mult. Scler. J. **19**, 666–667 (2013)
68. Mori, S., Crain, B.J., Chacko, V.P., van Zijl, P.C.: Three-dimensional tracking of axonal projections in the brain by magnetic resonance imaging. Ann. Neurol. **45**, 265–269 (1999)
69. Power, J.D., Barnes, K.A., Snyder, A.Z., Schlaggar, B.L., Petersen, S.E.: Spurious but systematic correlations in functional connectivity MRI networks arise from subject motion. Neuroimage **59**, 2142–2154 (2012)
70. Ashburner, J., Friston, K.J.: Unified segmentation. Neuroimage **26**, 839–851 (2005)
71. Fox, M.D., Snyder, A.Z., Vincent, J.L., Corbetta, M., Essen, D.C.V., Raichle, M.E.: The human brain is intrinsically organized into dynamic, anticorrelated functional networks. Proc. Natl. Acad. Sci. USA **102**, 9673–9678 (2005)
72. Meng, L., Yuan, Z., Tianzi, J., Zhening, L., Lixia, T., Haihong, L., Yihui, H.: Widespread functional disconnectivity in schizophrenia with resting-state functional magnetic resonance imaging. Neuroreport **17**, 209–213 (2006)
73. Xiao-Wei, S., Zhang-Ye, D., Xiang-Yu, L., Su-Fang, L., Xi-Nian, Z., Chao-Zhe, Z., Yong, H., Chao-Gan, Y., Yu-Feng, Z.: REST: a toolkit for resting-state functional magnetic resonance imaging data processing. PLoS ONE **6**, e25031 (2011)
74. Zang, Y., Jiang, T., Lu, Y., He, Y., Tian, L.: Regional homogeneity approach to fMRI data analysis. Neuroimage **22**, 394–400 (2004)
75. Kohavi, R., John, G.H.: Wrappers for feature subset selection. Artif. Intell. **97**, 273–324 (1997)
76. Kononenko, I.: Estimating attributes: analysis and extensions of RELIEF. In: Proceedings of European Conference on Machine Learning, vol. 784, pp. 356–361 (1996)
77. Guyon, I., Weston, J., Barnhill, S., Vapnik, V.: Gene selection for cancer classification using support vector machines. Mach. Learn. **46**, 389–422 (2002)
78. Sun, Y., Todorovic, S., Goodison, S.: Local-learning-based feature selection for high-dimensional data analysis. IEEE Trans. Pattern Anal. Mach. Intell. **32**, 1610–1626 (2010)

79. Wilson, S.M., Ogar, J.M., Laluz, V., Growdon, M., Jang, J., Glenn, S., Miller, B.L., Weiner, M.W., Gorno-Tempini, M.L.: Automated MRI-based classification of primary progressive aphasia variants. Neuroimage **47**, 1558–1567 (2009)
80. Dyrba, M., Ewers, M., Wegrzyn, M., Kilimann, I., Plant, C., Oswald, A., Meindl, T., Pievani, M., Bokde, A.L.W., Fellgiebel, A.: Combining DTI and MRI for the Automated Detection of Alzheimer's Disease Using a Large European Multicenter Dataset. Springer, Berlin (2012)
81. Grana, M., Termenon, M., Savio, A., Gonzalez-Pinto, A., Echeveste, J., Perez, J.M., Besga, A.: Computer aided diagnosis system for Alzheimer disease using brain diffusion tensor imaging features selected by Pearson's correlation. Neurosci. Lett. **502**, 225–229 (2011)
82. O'Dwyer, L., Lamberton, F., Bokde, A.L.W., Ewers, M., Faluyi, Y.O., Tanner, C., Mazoyer, B., O'Neill, D., Bartley, M., Collins, D.R., Coughlan, T., Prvulovic, D., Hampel, H.: Using support vector machines with multiple indices of diffusion for automated classification of mild cognitive impairment. PLoS ONE **7** (2012)
83. Church, J.A., Fair, D.A., Dosenbach, N.U.F., Cohen, A.L., Miezin, F.M., Petersen, S.E., Schlaggar, B.L.: Control networks in paediatric Tourette syndrome show immature and anomalous patterns of functional connectivity. Brain **132**, 225–238 (2009)
84. Neuner, I., Kupriyanova, Y., Stocker, T., Huang, R.W., Posnansky, O., Schneider, F., Shah, N.J.: Microstructure assessment of grey matter nuclei in adult Tourette patients by diffusion tensor imaging. Neurosci. Lett. **487**, 22–26 (2011)
85. Greene, D.J., Church, J.A., Dosenbach, N.U.F., Nielsen, A.N., Adeyemo, B., Nardos, B., Petersen, S.E., Black, K.J., Schlaggar, B.L.: Multivariate pattern classification of pediatric Tourette syndrome using functional connectivity MRI. Dev. Sci. (2016)
86. Wee, C.Y., Yap, P.T., Li, W., Denny, K., Browndyke, J.N., Potter, G.G., Welsh-Bohmer, K.A., Wang, L., Shen, D.: Enriched white matter connectivity networks for accurate identification of MCI patients. Neuroimage **54**, 1812–1822 (2011)
87. Werner, C.J., Stocker, T., Kellermann, T., Wegener, H.P., Schneider, F., Shah, N.J., Neuner, I.: Altered amygdala functional connectivity in adult Tourette's syndrome. Eur. Arch. Psychiatry Clin. Neurosci. **260**(Suppl 2), S95–S99 (2010)

Radiomics in Medical Imaging— Detection, Extraction and Segmentation

Jie Tian, Di Dong, Zhenyu Liu, Yali Zang, Jingwei Wei,
Jiangdian Song, Wei Mu, Shuo Wang and Mu Zhou

Abstract Radiomics, as a newly emerging technology, converts medical images into high-dimensional data via high-throughput extraction of quantitative features, followed by subsequent data analysis for decision support. It identifies general diagnostic or prognostic phenotypes with target clinical need, providing an unprecedented opportunity to improve individualized treatment in cancer at low cost. In this chapter, we will introduce radiomics from its development to its clinical

J. Tian (✉) · D. Dong · Z. Liu · Y. Zang · J. Wei · W. Mu · S. Wang
Institute of Automation, Chinese Academy of Sciences,
No. 95 Zhongguancun East Road, Beijing 100190, China
e-mail: jie.tian@ia.ac.cn

D. Dong
e-mail: di.dong@ia.ac.cn

Z. Liu
e-mail: zhenyu.liu@ia.ac.cn

Y. Zang
e-mail: yali.zang@ia.ac.cn

J. Wei
e-mail: weijingwei1992@hotmail.com

W. Mu
e-mail: wei_mu2016@163.com

S. Wang
e-mail: wangshuo2014@ia.ac.cn

J. Song
Sino-Dutch Biomedical and Information Engineering School,
Northeastern University, NO. 3-11, Wenhua Road, Heping District,
Shenyang 110819, China
e-mail: dr.j.song@ieee.org

M. Zhou
Stanford Center for Biomedical Informatics Research (BMIR),
Department of Medicine, and Department of Biomedical Data Science,
Stanford University, 1265 Welch Rd, Stanford, CA 94305-5479, USA
e-mail: muzhou1@stanford.edu

© Springer International Publishing AG 2018
K. Suzuki and Y. Chen (eds.), *Artificial Intelligence in Decision Support Systems for Diagnosis in Medical Imaging*, Intelligent Systems Reference Library 140,
https://doi.org/10.1007/978-3-319-68843-5_11

applications. We divide the clinical applications into three sections based on three most common medical modality, including computed tomography (CT), magnetic resonance imaging (MRI) and positron emission tomography (PET), to give a comprehensive introduction of how radiomics works with the example of a typical cancer type. The workflow and detailed technology skills are well described in each section.

1 Introduction

1.1 Computer-Aided Diagnosis

During the past few decades, owing to the rapid development of medical imaging, computer-aided diagnosis (CAD) has been made possible in many clinical scenarios. It plays an increasingly important role in routine diagnosis and relieves the burden on the radiologist. The diagnosis efficiency has been improved by the move from a purely visual inspection to computer-aided quantitative evaluation [40, 41].

In radiology, the basic concept of CAD is to provide a computer output as a "second opinion" to assist radiologists when reading images [41]. Modern medical scanners usually produce images with numerous slices. It is very time-consuming for a radiologist to examine an image in detail, whereas it is possible for a CAD system to analyze the image quickly and produce a report about it. Some typical applications can be found in the classification of lung nodules [4, 45, 69] and the diagnosis of breast cancer [51, 79, 80].

CAD is fundamentally based on many other technologies such as image processing, pattern recognition, and machine learning [58, 90, 98]. Any improvement in these technologies will in turn take CAD one step further.

1.2 Radiomics

Recent years have witnessed the growth in the medical imaging field. The large number of medical images has brought new opportunities to researchers: (a) they can give more robust and reliable medical image analysis reports based on a large amount of images; and (b) they can develop more advanced methods that rely on a large amount of samples, such as data mining and machine learning, which can be introduced into the field of medical image analysis. The fast evolution of medical imaging has fostered a comprehensive analysis method for medical images called radiomics. Radiomics generally refers to the extraction and analysis of large amounts of advanced quantitative imaging features with high throughput from medical images obtained using computed tomography (CT), positron emission tomography (PET) or magnetic resonance imaging (MRI) [1, 2, 59, 88, 92]. In comparison with the traditional practice of treating medical images as pictures intended solely for visual inspection, the aim of radiomics' analysis is the transformation of medical images into minable data combined with other patient clinical information. Using sophisticated bioinformatics tools, researchers are able to develop models that may potentially improve diagnostic, prognostic, and predictive accuracy [59].

Radiomics' analysis is mainly performed on medical images such as CT images where tumors are clearly visible. Tumors may be significantly different in terms of their properties, e.g., their shape, size, and composition. These characteristics are visible in CT images and most of them can be extracted using their mathematical expression. The radiomics' process is similar to a conventional CAD process in that they both extract features from medical images and performance feature analysis to facilitate the decision making of radiologists. However, the difference is that CAD usually focuses on the detection and diagnosis of lesions, while radiomics tries to make the most of the images to provide more comprehensive information based on the mined features. For example, researchers recently found that radiomics' features were highly correlated with lung cancer prognosis. By mining numerous features, they discovered that a subset of lung tumors shared four characteristics related to intra-tumor heterogeneity, and these cancers grew and proliferated faster than others, leading to worse patient outcomes [1, 2].

Radiomics also provides a complementary method of gene analysis. The hypothesis behind this is that gene expression or mutation is reflected in the tumor phenotype [55]. In the traditional gene analysis process, tumor tissue is sampled from a certain location of the tumor. However, a gene mutation may occur in other parts of the tumor that are not sampled. Thus, a traditional gene analysis may have sampling errors [59]. Radiomics' features are extracted from the whole tumor image, which contains much more complete information compared to a specific area of the tumor. It is expected that radiomics will complement traditional gene analysis.

1.3 Radiomics Pipeline

Similar to CAD, radiomics contains several steps, including data acquisition, lesion identification, lesion segmentation, feature extraction, and knowledge discovery. In addition, the recently emerging deep learning technology will also be introduced in this section as a new promising parallel pipeline to the current radiomics' pipeline.

1.4 Data Acquisition

Sufficient data are the basis of a reliable conclusion, as is radiomics. Radiomics relies on a large medical image database to reveal the correlation between quantitative features and clinical data. The emphasis on a large dataset is also in accordance with the "big data" trend. The medical image analysis community is more desperate for large datasets than many other communities because medical images are mostly stored at institutes or hospitals, and the number of medical images depends on the size of the patient population. Another challenge in building a large dataset is that the diagnostic data collection is extremely time consuming. It often takes years to fill out the follow-up records. Thus, contributions from institutes and hospitals around the country or even around the world are required to create large medical image datasets with abundant diagnostic information. Recently, The Cancer Imaging Archive (TCIA) established a data sharing platform [29]. TCIA provides the public with available cancer-specific medical images and metadata. More and more medical images from different institutes and hospitals are contributed to the platform. Based on those datasets, researchers and engineers can develop new medical image analysis methods and tools to validate their hypotheses or assist radiologists in making decisions. One of the large datasets held by TCIA is the Lung Image Database Consortium and Image Database Resource Initiative (LIDC-IDRI) [7, 108]. This dataset contains raw CT images and radiologist annotations, including both nodule locations and nodule sematic features, which help in the development of nodule detection and segmentation methods [37, 38, 131, 154].

Because these medical images are from different institutes and hospitals, it is common for them to be reconstructed with different software and protocols. Researchers using these datasets need to consider these differences to avoid possible unexpected influences on the results. It is also possible to investigate the most suitable protocol for the analysis of a specific disease by comparing different protocols.

1.5 Lesion Segmentation

Lesion segmentation is a basic processing step in radiomics, because it transforms the original medical images into feature-extraction-ready data. Although segmentation methods have been investigated for a long time, it is still far from a fully automated application, especially in the field of medical image analysis. The challenges come from several aspects. First, there is no ground truth segmentation of lesions or tumors, and the manual segmentation of medical images is quite time consuming. Radiologists have to go through each slice to delineate the lesion, and a segmentation mask may contain dozens of slices if the lesion is large. It is also acknowledged that there is large inter-reader variability in the interpretation of in-plane nodule boundaries by different radiologists [7]. Second, lesions are not geometric objects, and large morphological variation exists, which is difficult to model. Third, lesion edges are not well-defined and are often blurred by the partial volume effect. Moreover, the reproducibility of segmentation methods is also very important. Because the following extraction is performed on segmented lesions, reproducible segmentation will ensure that the extracted features are stable and reliable for the lesion. Despite the challenges previously mentioned, researchers are still improving segmentation methods tailored to specific scenarios [67, 154].

1.6 Feature Extraction and Selection

Features extraction is a critical process that bridges the segmented lesions and clinical results. Features can be divided into two categories: semantic features and non-semantic features.

Semantic features are those perceived by radiologists and are usually qualitatively described. They lack efficient mathematical expression such as lesion speculation, subtlety, and margin.

Non-semantic features can be quantitatively described by a mathematical expression. Currently, the common method to produce numerous non-semantic features is to extract them from segmented lesions based on their mathematical expressions. First, the segmented lesions can be regarded as a mask and used to extract shape-relevant features such as the volume, surface area, and compactness. Second, the intensity of each voxel inside the volume can be utilized to construct a large number of features. These are first-order, second-order, and high-order features [59]. First-order features are mostly related to the distribution of the intensity within the volume, such as the minimum, maximum, and median, and the entropy of the intensity histogram. The second-order features are mostly related to the statistical interrelationships between voxels and their neighbors, such as texture features, which are usually representative of lesion heterogeneity. High-order features such as wavelets and fractal analyses are used to represent repetitive or non-repetitive patterns [59].

In general, hundreds of features can be produced by the feature extraction step. However, most of these features may be correlated, and thus redundant. Feature selection is applied to filter the generated features. In [13], the authors first selected features with high reproducibility and high concordance correlation coefficients between repeated tests. Then, they used hierarchical clustering to obtain representative features by removing features with high dependency. They also proposed a metric called "dynamic range," which indicated the inter-patient variability, to remove features with little variability. In [1, 2], the authors took similar steps and constructed a radiomics' signature from four types of features. The number of features after feature selection is usually less than 100, which is much less than the number of extracted features before feature selection.

1.7 Knowledge Discovery

Once features are extracted and filtered, they are ready for the knowledge discovery step. The goal in this step is finding the correlation between the radiomics' features and clinically related information. In many application scenarios, the discovery task can be formulated as a classification task; for example, images related to gene mutation are classified by dividing them into two categories: images with gene mutation and images without gene mutation. Models are trained to learn the difference between the images in these two categories. The discovery of features related to patient survival is also an application of data mining technology. In this step, advanced machine learning models and artificial intelligence approaches are welcome and are expected to play important roles in knowledge discovery.

1.8 Deep Learning Pipeline

Deep learning is a recent emerging technology that is attracting the interest of many researchers. Convolutional neural networks (CNNs) have been some of the most popular technologies in the field of image analysis in recent years. The first successful application of CNNs dates back to the late 1990s, when LeCun et al. designed a LeNet-5 network for digit recognition [95]. The second wave of CNNs occurred in 2012 when a deep CNN ranked first in the Imagenet Large Scale Visual Recognition Challenge (ILSVRC) [85]. Because of the development of dedicated hardware like the modern graphics processing unit (GPU), researchers can now design large networks for more complex tasks. Many of the applications in medical image analysis have the goal of improving the current CAD systems such as for lesion detection [165] and diagnosis [148]. Recently, Kumar et al. introduced the concept of "discovery radiomics" for lung cancer detection using CT imaging data [87]. The proposed radiomics sequencer is based on a deep CNN and is tailored to the characterization of the lung tumor phenotype. The produced radiomics' sequence includes abstract imaging-based features. The benefits of using CNN are two-fold: (a) since CNN has an end-to-end machine learning architecture, the input can be a raw image without segmentation [148]; (b) discriminative features are automatically learned during the training process. These benefits are desirable. As previously mentioned, segmentation is a challenging but unavoidable step in the current radiomics' pipeline. Unreliable segmentation will affect the feature analysis and may yield an incorrect report. In the feature extraction step, it is still unproven what features are relevant to a certain kind of disease or associated with cancer prognosis. Thus, numerous features are extracted prior to feature analysis, which is very time-consuming and inefficient, whereas deep learning can greatly speed up the knowledge discovery in the current radiomics' process.

Despite the inspiring advantages that deep learning brings, researchers may face another issue. Although deep learning outperformed state of the art methods, are the obtained deep features explainable and how are they correlated with the diagnostic data? In other words, the generated features seem to be a black box for both researchers and radiologists. Further investigations are needed to make the method more understandable.

In the field of natural image analysis, there is an environment that encourages the sharing of a trained network so that other researchers can directly use the trained model for their own purposes without long-term training, which saves other researchers a significant amount of time. In the field of medical image analysis, deep learning is still at an early stage, and there is an increasing number of researchers interested in the application of the technology. It is possible that a similar model-sharing atmosphere can be constructed through the efforts of both researchers and communities.

1.9 Clinical Results

Radiomics is a rapidly developing area. Over the past several years, many studies [1, 2, 34, 133, 135] have shown that image features are related to cancer prognosis, gene expression patterns and so on. In [1, 2], by mining 440 features, researchers found heterogeneity-related features, and tumor compactness/sphericity were correlated with patient survival. Heterogeneity in the primary tumors was associated with worse survival, whereas tumors with high compactness/sphericity often had better survival probabilities. As previously mentioned, medical imaging may also reflect gene-expression patterns. Researchers also found that the radiomics' signature was associated with gene-expression patterns and different biological gene sets [1, 2]. Another investigation by Ozkan et al. also showed that image features such as contrast, correlation, and inverse difference moment texture features were associated with the epidermal growth factor receptor (EGFR) mutation status in adenocarcinoma of the lung [133]. Radiomics also plays a role in distant metastasis (DM) prediction. Researchers extracted 635 radiomics' features from CT images, and thirty-five of them were found to be prognostic for DM and twelve for survival. Compared with tumor volume, which was only moderately prognostic, the radiomics' signature was more powerful in predicting DM [34].

An increasing number of researchers are giving attention to radiomics and its role in clinical scenarios [1, 2, 21, 32, 66, 97, 135]. The current results indicate that radiomics' features can be a complimentary tool to facilitate radiologists' decisions. In the following section, more detailed applications of radiomics will be presented.

2 Radiomics in CT Imaging

2.1 Background Knowledge

2.1.1 Radiomics and CT Images

Based on numerous clinical images combined with engineering methods and clinical diagnostic experience, the aim of radiomics is to create a scientific, quantitative, and large data-driven analysis model for tumor prognosis, and then apply it to clinically aided diagnosis. As a further step in personalized medicine using the prognostic features extracted from medical images, the radiomics solution may not only allow a more accurate measurement of tumor progression, but also the non-invasive molecular and genetic profiling of tumors [56]. It also has the advantage of being able to measure the therapy response relatively early in the course of treatment before anatomical changes have not occurred [27].

As an effective non-invasive approach to acquiring diagnostic images, the German scientist Roentgen discovered the X-ray in 1895, which opened the door to modern medical imaging [60]. In the 1970s, Cormack and Hounsfield succeeded in inventing CT, which became the first accurate reconstructive imaging method for internal structures of objects [130]. CT has become basic equipment in a modern radiology department, and has been widely used in the industrial non-destructive monitoring field, allowing humans to directly observe internal structures.

1. **Law of Lambert–Beers and Basic Physical Principle of CT**

When a beam of monochromatic X-rays passes through a homogeneous material, its energy is attenuated according to the law of Lambert–Beers,

$$I = I_0 e^{-u \cdot \Delta x} \tag{2.1}$$

where I_0 and I are the X-ray intensities of the incident and exiting beams, respectively; Δx is the thickness of the material through which the X-ray passes; and u is the linear attenuation coefficient of the material. Let $u(\vec{x})$ represent the distribution of the attenuation coefficient of a non-homogeneous material. Then, for a monochromatic X-ray, its intensity along a straight line L is described by the following formula:

$$I = I_0 e^{-\int u(\vec{x}) d\vec{x}} \tag{2.2}$$

When both sides of Eq. (2.2) are divided by I_0, taking the negative logarithm,

$$g = -\ln\left(\frac{I}{I_0}\right) = \int_L u(\vec{x}) d\vec{x} \tag{2.3}$$

In fact, the method used to acquire the CT image involves a calculation from the given line integral of an object (or projection), along with the solution of the attenuation coefficient distribution of the object. Namely, the process of reconstruction is from g to u. Since the first clinical CT, efficient systems and advanced reconstruction algorithms have been proposed, and much progress on the hardware components and software algorithms of the CT system has occurred.

2. Development of CT Equipment

As previously mentioned, the problem of CT image acquisition by the measured projection of a given object is used to evaluate the attenuation coefficient of the object. The measurement of the projection reflects the development of the CT scanner. According to the detector system, the measurement of the projection can be divided into a parallel beam, fan beam, and cone beam. According to the scanning trajectory, it can also be divided into a circular orbit and spiral orbit, in which the general orbit may be represented as a saddle shape, circle-linear, double circle, etc.

From the invention of CT until the end of the 1980s, CT involved a continuous scan of a single layer. After scanning a layer, the patient or object had to move to the next layer for repeated scanning. Here, this is called circular orbit scanning. The scan mode, which is transferred to stop and turn, increases the scan time. The scanning speed improved until the appearance of the slip ring, when spiral scanning became a new technology in CT. A variety of general tracks have since been proposed, including saddle-shaped, round-linear, and double circle. Utilizing a flexible scanning trajectory could reduce a patient's dose and ensure the best images quality. Combinations of a parallel beam, fan beam, and cone beam with various scanning tracks generally reflect the development of the CT scanner. In the late 1980s, the combination of the fan beam with a spiral orbit was considered to be a leap forward in the development of CT, as was the spiral orbit multi-row CT in the middle of the 1990s. Presently, a cone beam spiral CT is being used, and a general track cone beam CT is also being developed.

The use of a digital flat panel detector in recent years, such as in high-precision micro-CT for small animals, has played an important role in the development of molecular imaging [74]. Strictly speaking, because of the lack of specific contrast agents (molecular probes), CT cannot currently be used to directly obtain molecular images. However, because of its high spatial resolution, it can provide anatomical images of small animals. Furthermore, it can also be used to quantitatively measure bone density, and for bone tumor detection, lung cancer detection, and other fields of research.

As for radiomics, CT imaging is noninvasive, widely available, and frequently used to stage the tumor before treatment. Tumor heterogeneity can be assessed in a user-defined region of interest (ROI) on CT images by phenotype analysis, using the texture to quantify the spatial pattern or arrangement of pixel intensities, spatial features to measure the sphericity or asymmetry, and lesion intensity statistics to characterize the uniformity of the pixel distribution in the ROI [1, 2].

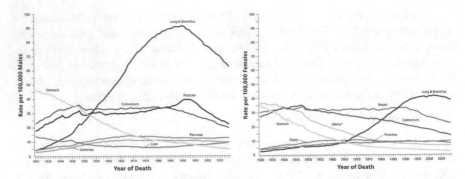

Fig. 1 Death rate trends among males (left) and females (right) for selected cancers, United States, 1930 to 2009. The rates are age adjusted to the 2000 US standard population. Because of changes in the International Classification of Diseases (ICD) coding, the numerator information has changed over time. The rates for cancers of the lung and bronchus, colorectum, and liver are affected by these changes (left). The rates for cancers of the uterus*, ovary, lung and bronchus, and colorectum are also affected by these changes (right) [150]. *Uterus includes uterine cervix and uterine corpus

In this chapter, we focus on the radiomics application of CT images. Lung cancer remains the number one cause of cancer-related mortality for men and women in the United States, as shown in Fig. 1, and its prevalence continues to increase worldwide [137]. Despite a potentially curative resection in early stage lung cancer, survival remains suboptimal, and recurrence rates are high [117]. In addition, some literature indicates that lung cancer causes the most cancer deaths in those 60 years of age and older [137].

Because non-small cell lung cancer (NSCLC) constitutes the vast majority of lung cancer cases, we will use NSCLC as the representative to discuss how to use the radiomics approach to analyze cancers via CT images. Figure 2 presents a clear structure of the human lung. The lungs are located in the chest on either side of the heart in the rib cage. The apex of the lung extends into the root of the neck, reaching just above the level of the sternal end of the first rib. The sac-enclosed lungs are divided into sections called lobes. The right lung has three lobes, while the left lung only has two. The lobes are further divided into bronchopulmonary segments and lobules. Both lungs have a central recession called the hilum at the root of the lung, where the blood vessels and airways pass into the lungs.

2.1.2 Heterogeneity of CT

Tumor heterogeneity refers to the divergence among different individuals with the same kind of malignant cancer or the diversity presented from genotype to phenotype among different tumor cells in one patient. This diversity occurring in different individuals may present as various genetic backgrounds such as the differences in the amount and quality of the chromosomes, cell pathological type,

Fig. 2 Lungs and nearby tissues

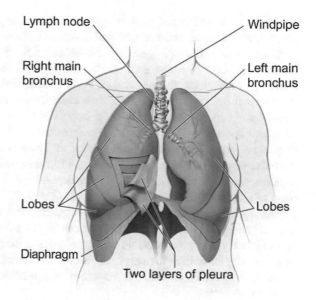

clinical stage, degree of differentiation, and evolution of the cells. Moreover, homogeneous tumors are significantly different at the molecular level: such as the gene expression profile or mutation spectrum. Tumors occurring in the same patient can present with different mutation spectra, biological characteristics, and other aspects, which reflect the high complexity and diversity of a malignant tumor in the evolution process. The heterogeneity of tumor cells in different parts of the same patient also includes intertumoral heterogeneity (different lesions, such as primary and metastatic tumors) and intratumor heterogeneity (different parts of the same lesion, as shown in Fig. 3). These are due to the presence of different subtypes of tumor cells within the tumor tissue. Therefore, different tumor cells show a diversity

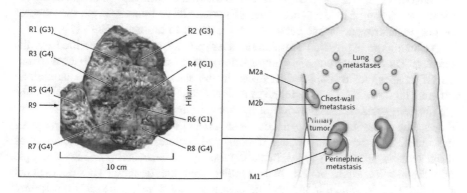

Fig. 3 Graph shows sites of core biopsies and regions harvested from nephrectomy and metastasectomy specimens. R denotes region and G indicates tumor grade [56]

of immune characteristics, growth speeds, invasion degrees, etc., resulting in different sensitivities to radiotherapy and anticancer drugs.

Changes in tumor cell genetics and epigenetics, the origin of tumor cells or tumor stem cells (cancer stem cells, CSC), and the selection of the tumor microenvironment are the major factors influencing intratumor heterogeneity and intertumoral heterogeneity. Tumor heterogeneity causes great difficulties for the treatment of cancer, and it has been an important scientific problem in the research on tumor genesis and development mechanisms. In recent years, with the rapid progress in genome sequencing and continuous breakthroughs in cancer research by the cross application of bioinformatics and big data science, the understanding of tumor heterogeneity has significantly accelerated and been given attention on the basis of individualized health "Precision Medicine". This mode tries to classify the disease according to traditional signs, symptoms, and molecular typing, with the goal of finding the most appropriate medication or treatment at the molecular level, and ultimately realizing accurate and personalized treatments for patients. Therefore, it is very important to analyze the biological characteristics and mechanism of tumor heterogeneity in order to transform the medical model into personalized treatment medicine.

Intratumor heterogeneity, as previously reported, may have important consequences for personalized medical approaches, which commonly rely on single tumor biopsy samples to portray tumor mutational landscapes. Intratumor heterogeneity could be described from the viewpoint of imaging and genetics. Genetic intratumor heterogeneity has shown treatment failure and drug resistance. The molecular heterogeneity of protein kinase C, which is expressed by individual enzyme characteristics, has some proteins that exhibit distinct patterns of tissue expression, indicating that different kinases may predict distinct functions in the processing and nodulation of a variety of physiological and pathological responses [122]. Research has shown that genetic intratumor heterogeneity was evident at the RNA-expression level, in expression signatures with good or poor prognoses detected in different regions of the same tumor. Reports related to the heterogeneity of monocytes indicated that with the improvement in our understanding of monocyte biology and the significance of these cells in inflammation, the issue of monocyte heterogeneity has become more relevant to human health [11].

As for image expression, intratumor heterogeneity could be quantified by different orders of magnitude. The tumor heterogeneity of the images showed (based on CT images, for example) differences in the same part of a tumor as seen in different layers of a CT image in the same layer, the tumor has different expressions for different parts. The expression of the same tumor showed diversity at different times. The quantitative analysis of these tumor characteristics is the basis of radiomics. The extraction of multidimensional features based on an analysis of characteristics grouped by types, including the texture, size, and shape is a hot topic in radiomics research. It has been verified that the quantitative measurement methods used to quantify tumor heterogeneity may play a role in the response assessment of cancers [181, 184, 185]. Intratumor heterogeneity parameters measured using the texture parameters of unenhanced and/or contrast material-enhanced

CT images between the baseline and initial post-therapy have been associated with overall survival in patients with colorectal cancer [121], metastatic renal cell cancer [62], esophageal cancer [53], and NSCLC [52, 54, 105]. More recently, another related study found that as the prognostic radiomics signature, reproducibility texture features were statistically significant in separating the samples into survival groups [13].

2.1.3 Decoding Tumor Phenotype

There is increasing number of proof that phenotypical characteristics with predictive ability can not only reduce clinical expenditures, but are also necessary for patients who need a timely follow-up treatment regimen. As previously mentioned, tumor heterogeneity refers to the divergence among different individuals with the same kind of malignant tumor or the diversity presented from genotype to phenotype among different tumor cells in one patient. The tumor phenotype is an increasingly important index for the evaluation of the degree of tumor malignancy. The correct decoding of the tumor phenotype not only assists in the prognosis of pathology, improving the personalized medical care for patients, but also achieves a further analysis of the genes. Extracting useful information from CT images and decoding it to obtain features that reveal the tumor heterogeneity and tumor progression is currently the main area of radiomics research.

As shown in Fig. 4, in order to obtain the complete heterogeneity information, different filters were used on a rectal tumor. This technique comprised an initial filtration step in which a Laplacian of Gaussian spatial band-pass filter was used to selectively extract features with different sizes and intensity variations. A series of derived images displaying features at different spatial scales from fine to coarse textures within a ROI drawn around the colorectal tumor were obtained using this filtration (Fig. 4). As can be seen in Fig. 4, an ROI was initially delineated around the tumor outline for the largest cross-sectional area. The ROI was further refined by the exclusion of areas of air using a thresholding procedure that removed any pixels with attenuation values below 250 HU from the analysis. Different features could be extracted from the ROI in the series of derived images.

A study reported that the dynamic imaging traits in noninvasive CT were systematically correlated with the global gene expression programs of primary human liver cancer [147]. First, the authors defined the traits from qualitative imaging features, and then defined coherent patterns of variation from gene expression profiles. They tried to prove that the imaging traits were likely to be correlated with the gene expression patterns in a complex manner, as shown in Fig. 5. Methods for relating the imaging to gene expression were used for and found that 78% of the global gene expression profiles could be reconstructed when using twenty-eight

(a)   **(c)**

(b)   **(d)**

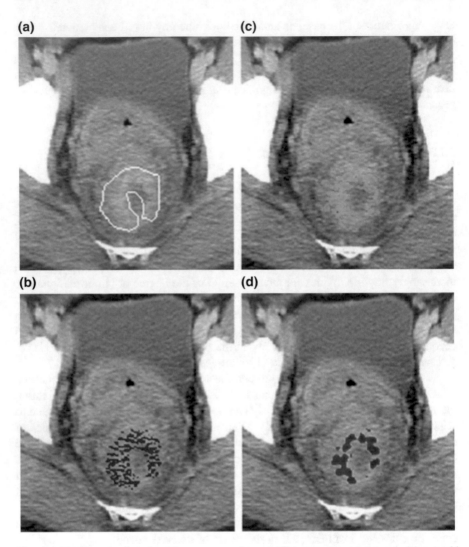

Fig. 4 a Fused anatomic and texture contrast-enhanced CT image of rectal tumor in 28-year-old woman. **b–d** Corresponding images in the same patient selectively display **b** fine, **c** medium, and **d** coarse textures and were obtained using filter values of 1.0 (2.72-mm width, 4 pixels), 1.5 (4.08-mm width, 6 pixels), and 2.5 (8.16-mm width, 12 pixels) [121]

imaging traits, which revealed the cell proliferation, liver synthetic function, and patient prognosis. It was concluded that the genomic activity of human liver cancers could be decoded by noninvasive imaging, thereby enabling noninvasive, serial and frequent molecular profiling for personalized medicine.

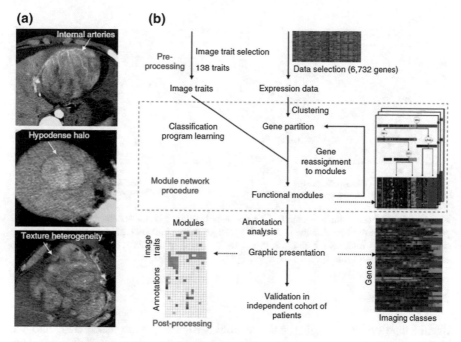

Fig. 5 Linking imaging traits and global gene expression. **a** Examples of imaging traits in HCC. **b** Strategy for constructing an association map between imaging traits and gene expression [147]

2.2 Radiomics Development of Lung Cancer

2.2.1 Pathology

Radiomics studies mainly explain the relationship between the pathology and imaging phenotype. As the basis of feature analysis, the accurate segmentation of tumors in CT images is the first step. Then, the prognostic information should be extracted from the ROI that has been segmented. Finally, appropriate automatic computed learning models are used to find the association between the pathology (such as the pathological staging, pathological type, and clinical stage) and phenotypical features. The research on lung cancer is especially prominent in this field. Song [153] found that the CT phenotypic features were significantly associated with the pathologic and clinical stage of NSCLC, as shown in Fig. 6. Another study indicated that the quantification of the entropy, uniformity, mean gray-level intensity, kurtosis, and standard deviation of the histogram could be used as prognostic biomarkers in patients with esophageal cancer who were treated with definitive chemotherapy and radiation therapy. Recently, a study found that a representative feature (the run-length gray-level nonuniformity) was statistically significant in separating the samples into survival groups [13].

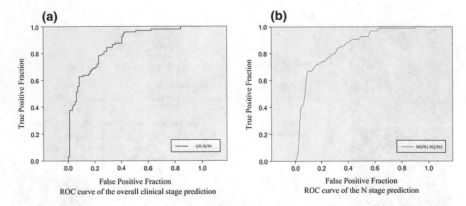

Fig. 6 Results from Song's research. The receiver operating characteristic curves of **a** is the prediction of overall clinical stage (stage I/II vs. stage III/IV) and **b** N stage (N0/N1 vs. N2/N3) when using the 25 features which are at top of the score list by support vector machine. The area under curves are 0.84 and 0.79, respectively [153]

2.2.2 Genomics

Segal proposed that imaging traits in noninvasive CT were associated with the global gene expression programs of primary human liver cancer in 2007, including research that indicated that the gene expression was significantly related to the tumor phenotype. The development of a description of the tumor phenotype has made the phenotypic characteristic an increasingly important factor for explaining the relationship between the disease progress and genes, as shown in Fig. 7.

The genomics concept involves the use of image information to analyze gene expression. The combination of genomics and radiomics is a further step toward personalized medicine at the pathology and gene level. Through the deep mining of image traits, and research on the relationship between image information and gene expression, the pathology and prognosis would be important research directions in personalized medicine.

2.3 Generic Radiomics Approach to Lung Cancer

As a quantitative analysis method based on images, radiomics needs to determine the ROI of the tumor in a CT image. Then, the phenotype characteristics are quantified in the ROI. Finally, a clinical aided diagnosis is obtained using a computed learning method. In this section, the application of radiomics to NSCLC will be introduced in the following steps: detection and segmentation of the ROI, feature extraction, quantification, and prognostic analysis of CT images, as described in Fig. 8.

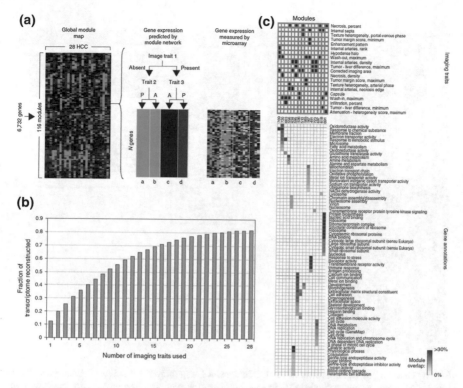

Fig. 7 Association map of imaging traits and global gene expression. **a** Overview of the association map. Each column is a sample, and each row is a module. For each module, a decision tree of imaging traits is associated with a variation in the expression level of the module's genes. A knowledge of the imaging traits thus allows an approximate reconstruction of the gene expression pattern. **b** Dense encoding of gene expression variation by imaging traits. Shown is the cumulative fraction of gene expression variation across the transcriptome that is reconstructed by the number of imaging traits in the model. **c** Matrix of modules, associated with imaging traits, and their enriched GO annotations. Only modules and annotations with significant enrichment (false discovery rate <0.05 after accounting for multiple hypothesis testing) are shown [147]

2.3.1 Detection and Segmentation

The accurate segmentation of lung lesions by an automatic method is also difficult because of the heterogeneity of the lesions, including the detection of the lung lesion. As shown in Fig. 9, because of the diversity of lung lesions, the current segmentation accuracy is inadequate. The shape, intensity and location of lung lesions change greatly because of the spatial genetic heterogeneity of various lesions. The intensity of lung lesions is sometimes close to the intensity of vessels, fissures, or the chest wall (Fig. 9a(1)–a(3)). However, at other times, it is close to the intensity of the lung field such as the ground-glass opacity (GGO) (Fig. 9c(1)–c (3)), which is a nonspecific finding on CT scans that indicates a partial filling of air spaces by exudate or transudate, as well as the interstitial thickening or partial

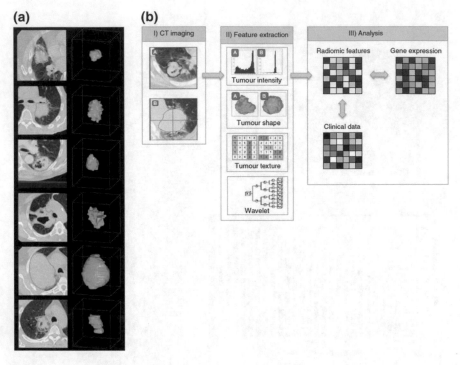

Fig. 8 General process of radiomics on CT images. **a** Lung tumors are different. Examples of CT images of lung cancer patients. CT images with tumor contours are shown on the left, and three-dimensional visualizations are shown on the right. Please note the strong phenotypic differences that can be captured with routine CT imaging, such as the intratumor heterogeneity and tumor shape. **b** Strategy for extracting radiomics data from images. (I) Experienced physicians contour the tumor areas on all the CT slices. (II) Features are extracted from within the defined tumor contours in the CT images, quantifying the tumor intensity, shape, texture, and wavelet texture. (III) In the analysis, the radiomics features are compared with clinical data and gene-expression data [147]

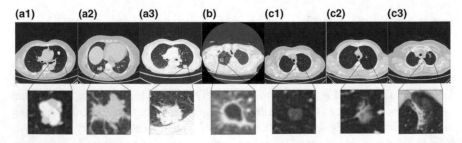

Fig. 9 Different types of lung lesions: (**a1**)–(**a3**): solid nodule, (**a1**): solitary nodule, (**a2**): juxta-vascular, (**a3**): juxta-pleural, (**b**): cavity, (**c1**)–(**c3**): GGO–(**c1**): solitary, (**c2**): juxta-vascular, (**c3**): juxta-pleural [154]

collapse of lung alveoli. Moreover, the influence of inherent noise in CT images can also be significant. All of these factors make it is very challenging to achieve the precise delineation of lung lesions automatically.

Based on the CT data for lungs, many researchers have done relevant studies on pulmonary parenchyma, airways [17, 24, 94], and lung lesion segmentation. Campos et al. [22] proposed a supervised lung nodule segmentation method via a volumetric shape index, convergence index filter, and k-nearest neighbor (k-NN) regression to gain three coarse segmentation results. A feature-based two-layer supervised learning method for nodule classification was used simultaneously. Then, a refining method by an artificial neural network (ANN) was used to segment the lung nodules. The results showed a 12% relative volume error for GGO. However, the three preliminary segmentations they used to obtain a feature set were time-consuming. Another problem was that their segmentation needed human interaction for the initial seed point. Diciotti et al. divided the lesions into "well circumscribed" and "juxta-vascular" groups in [39], and obtained a detection sensitivity of 85.3% using the Lung Image Database Consortium (LIDC-IDRI) dataset, which contained 23 lesions at that time. The dataset has since been expanded to 1010 cases [7], and is widely used to evaluate lung lesion segmentation methods, as an internationally recognized lung lesion database. In [38], a local shape analysis method for small lung nodule segmentation was used on juxta-vascular and juxta-pleural lesions, and a detection sensitivity of 88.5% was reported on 157 lesions from the LIDC-IDRI database. In Wu and Lu's work [176], a system based on a conditional random field model that integrated the texture, grayscale, shape, and curvature was constructed to provide a reasonable segmentation input for the subsequent classification. The authors also used probability response maps and pairwise probability co-occurrence maps to find the contextual correlation of nodules. However, the co-occurrence matrix emphasizes the image texture among pixels rather than the pixel intensity information itself. As a result, it is not applicable to weak texture lesions. A novel level set approach for lung nodule segmentation was proposed in [47], and a detection sensitivity of 94.3% was obtained using a dataset that included 742 lung lesions. Another method that concentrated on juxta-vascular lesion segmentation based on the flow entropy and geodesic distance was represented in [156], and obtained a detection sensitivity of 91.7% on 157 lesions from the LIDC-IDRI database. Recently, an automated delineation method of lung tumors using the single click ensemble segmentation approach (SCES) was applied to solid tumor extraction [67]. The work was based on a lung tumor analysis tool [16] within the Definiens Cognition Network Technology developed by Definiens AG [10] and Merck & Co., Inc., which could provide a fast and easy annotation of lung lesions or other user-defined ROIs. Compared with manual segmentation, an accuracy of 78.72% was obtained using SCES, although one human interaction was needed. A new dynamic programming and multi-direction fusion technique was presented in [171]. The first dataset (23 lesions) and second dataset (64 lesions) from the LIDC-IDRI were both used to verify the new approach, and a 75% segmentation accuracy was obtained. Another research method for lung lesion segmentation was proposed by Kubota [86].

A convexity model with a morphological method was used to deal with the intensity heterogeneity in lung lesions. To evaluate the algorithm, 105 lesions from the LIDC-IDRI database were used, and a 69% segmentation accuracy was obtained. In [106], the authors tried to present a new pathological lung segmentation approach to detect all abnormal imaging patterns such as consolidations, nodules, ground-glass opacities, and honeycombs. In this research, the fuzzy connectedness and rib cage were used to estimate the lung volume. This study could delineate most types of lung lesions. However, the authors only presented the accuracy of lung field segmentation; the similarity of their lesion segmentation results with the published manual segmentation standard was not discussed.

In order to make lung lesion segmentation fully automatic, it is necessary to develop an automatic and accurate method for the seed point selection. As the precursor of lesion detection, methods for 3D lung volume segmentation were provided in [9, 73], where the measurement error was less than a pixel when compared with human analysis. In addition, accuracies of 90% for lung volume segmentation and 89% for lesion detection sensitivity were reported in [8, 81, 103], which used pixel intensity features and texture features. Recently, a large-scale lung cancer screening study including more than 3000 lesions was used for pulmonary nodule detection in [116]. The lesion curvedness and phenotype descriptors were used for seed point selection in each lesion cluster. Then, K-NN clustering with multiple features was applied to reduce false positives. In [110], lesion candidate masks were extracted from 15 thresholds with the opening operation. Then, phenotypical features were used for pulmonary nodule recognition. However, the latter segmentation only achieved an accuracy of 63%, which is relatively poor. A nodule detection method using isosurface triangulation with varying thresholds and phenotypical features was presented to detect lesions in [63]. Based on self-organizing maps (SOMs) and artificial neural networks (ANNs) classification, this method obtained a detection sensitivity of 80% on CT images from the LIDC-IDRI. Divergence and multi-scale enhancement filters for nodule clustering were used in [158]. A genetic algorithm and ANNs were the final classifiers for false positive elimination, and a detection sensitivity of 87.5% with an average of four false positives per scan was achieved. Recently, a method has been proposed for automatic lung lesion segmentation, and better segmentation of ground glass opacity was obtained compared with other methods [154], as shown in Fig. 10.

2.3.2 Extraction and Quantification

Phenotypical feature extraction from CT images is the key to a prognostic analysis, and characteristics with valuable prognostic information always play a decisive role in the subsequent analysis. Therefore, the feature extraction method should be comprehensive, with a high degree of recognition and the ability to reduce the redundant features. In general, a complete feature set needs to be set up in the first place. In one study [8] to find the relationship between the phenotype characteristics and survival in NSCLC, the authors divided the lung cancer phenotype

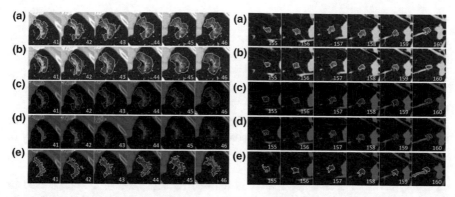

Fig. 10 Representative segmentation results of two GGOs from two patients' CT images:
a method proposed by [154], **b** radiologist 1, **c** radiologist 2, **d** level set, and **e** skeleton graph cut
[154]

characteristics of the CT image into the following parts: the shape, texture feature, and 'wavelet' [153], as shown in Fig. 11. This classification method is basically identical to the method proposed in [73]. Strictly speaking, the Gabor is a kind of texture, because the Gabor feature works well in areas such as face recognition; it is classified as an independent group by itself. Concise descriptions of the four categories are presented as follows.

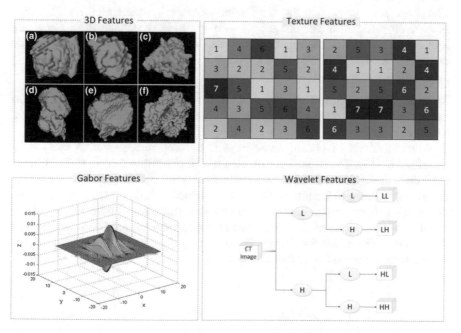

Fig. 11 Groups of phenotypical characteristics. Normally, the radiographic features include 3D features, texture features, Gabor features, and wavelet features [153]

Group 1: Texture

1. Run-length

The run-length is a metric that is used to quantify the gray-level runs in an image. Because consecutive pixels with the same gray-level value in one direction can be measured, the gray-level run is defined as the length measured in pixels. In a gray-level run length matrix $M(i,j|\theta)$, the (i,j) th element describes the number of times the gray level j appears i times consecutively in the direction specified by θ.

2. Gray-level co-occurrence

The gray-level co-occurrence matrix is defined as $M(i,j,D,\theta)$, a matrix used to describe the gray-level distribution by a distance of D pixels in direction θ of an image with a size of $N(g) \times N(g)$, where the (i,j)th element represents the number of times the combination of intensity levels occurs in two pixels in the image.

Group 2: Gabor

The Gabor filter, named after Dennis Gabor, is a linear filter used for edge detection, which is usually used in the field of face recognition. It can select valuable image information in different directions and different scales. Therefore, the visual characteristics of a lung lesion could be well described by Gabor filters. The Gabor feature could be extracted in multiple scales and directions.

Group 3: Shape

The shape features present the distribution of voxel intensities in the CT image. A three-dimensional tumor image is X with N voxels. V denotes the volume, and A is the surface area of the volume of interest. The shape group could consist of the compactness, skewness, kurtosis and sphericity.

Group 4: Wavelet

The wavelet transform effectively decouples the textural information by decomposing the original image, in a manner similar to a Fourier analysis, using low and high frequencies.

A complete set of phenotype features is the key to a prognosis analysis, as described in [13]. The authors constructed a feature set that contained 329 features (219 three-dimensional and 110 two-dimensional) for feature selection, These were statistically filtered to identify a subset of reproducible and non-redundant features. A test-retest concordance correlation coefficient method was used to identify the stability of the characteristics. After this selection method, the "test-retest concordance correlation coefficient" and "dynamic range" of the 29 key features were significantly different from other features.

2.3.3 Statistics and Prognosis

Data analysis is the core of computer aided diagnosis, and it is the final step in radiomics to realize personalized medicine. For different clinical applications, selecting appropriate machine learning methods to obtain corresponding clinical results is the basic direction of the current radiomics research. This includes using the support vector machine (SVM) method for aided prediction to distinguish between benign and malignant tumors, using a neural network algorithm based on a big data analysis to achieve the aided prognosis of lung cancer using the hierarchical clustering method to obtain clinical recommendations for advanced lung cancer or lung cancer in the early stage, and using computer aided analysis software (R, SPSS, SAS) to predict the overall survival of NSCLC patients.

Studies have proved that the clinical prediction results of NSCLC can be obtained by appropriate radiomics methods. For example in reference [1, 2], using the unsupervised clustering method, 1019 patients were grouped into three categories according to 440 features. The research also found that the clinical staging and pathological staging of NSCLC presented a high correlation with the groups. As shown in Fig. 12, the radiomics' signature proposed by this study divided the patients into low- and high-risk groups. The preference of this signature was validated using a validation data set and proved its prognostic value.

In addition, deep learning is a hot spot in the field of radiomics research; a recent study found that according to the imaging characteristics, a convolutional neural network could obtain higher classification results for lung cancer [148] compared with traditional methods. A classification method based on a convolutional neural network could reduce the influence of the ROI segmentation and the time cost of lung tumor segmentation. The framework of a convolutional neural network is described in Fig. 13.

In addition, researchers have proved that quantitative imaging using radiomics may have predictive power for certain phenotypes according to specific genetic mutations. As reported in reference [57], a radiogenomics' strategy using quantitative image features was used to evaluate the association between the tumor phenotype and clusters of co-expressed genes (metagenes). This radiogenomics' strategy was applied to a cohort of 26 patients with NSCLC for whom gene expression and 180 image features from CT and PET/CT images were available. The prognostic significance of the predicted image features was evaluated using a public gene expression data set with survival outcomes. They found that there were 243 statistically significant pairwise correlations between the image features and metagenes of NSCLC, and the accuracy of the prediction of metagenes by image features was acceptable. Moreover, the prognostic significance of various image features was found, including the tumor size, edge shape, and sharpness, which ranked the highest when the predicted image features were mapped to a public gene expression data set with survival outcomes. Thereby, it could be concluded that using quantitative image features to identify imaging biomarkers may enable a more rapid evaluation of novel imaging modalities, thereby accelerating their translation to personalized medicine.

290

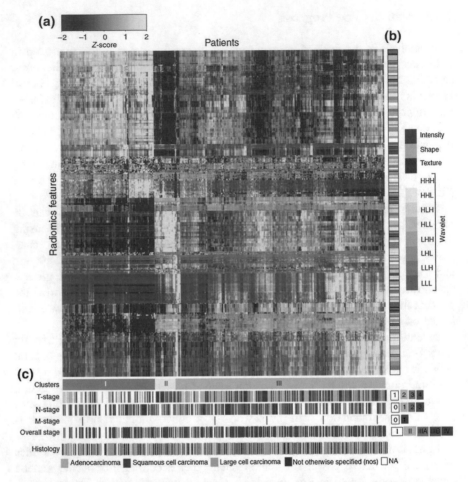

Fig. 12 Radiomics heat map for classification. **a** Unsupervised clustering of 422 lung cancer patients on the y axis and 440 radiomics feature expressions on the x axis, revealing clusters of patients with similar radiomics expression patterns. **b** Clinical patient parameters showing significant association of the radiomics expression patterns in the primary tumor stage, overall stage, and histology. **c** Correspondence of radiomics feature groups with the clustered expression patterns [147]

2.4 Future of Radiomics in Lung Cancer

The application of radiomics, as previously described, predicts benign or malignant tumors using a computed classifier. It uses survival analysis methods for the overall survival prediction, and based on the patient's score, determines a suitable treatment [99]. The results of radiomics could also provide a clinician with valuable suggestion about where to biopsy or resect in the clinical cases that are difficult to diagnose. As with therapies motivated by molecular biology, radiomics offers great

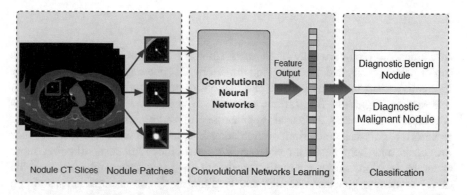

Fig. 13 Multi scale CNN for lung cancer classification. This approach first extracted multiple nodule patches to capture the wide range of nodule variability from input CT images. The obtained patches were then fed into three networks simultaneously to compute discriminative features. Finally, our approach applied a classier to label the input nodule malignancy [148]

potential to accelerate precision medicine [59]. However, radiomics research faces various problems. The first involves data; as a big-data-driven method, the use of various data acquisition mechanisms and data protection method by different research institutes increases the difficulty of radiomics becoming a standard, open and stable mechanism. Second, data mining technology is always changing. There is no internationally recognized computer algorithm for using radiomics as an auxiliary cancer prognostic method. This is a challenge in radiomics for the long-term goal of precision medicine, but it is also an opportunity for its development. In addition, the emergence of radiomics not only brings new ideas to modern medicine, but also changes the way radiologists work. Traditionally, radiologists have utilized with picture archiving and communication system software to identify, segment, and extract features from ROIs based on pattern changes. If studies on tumor segmentation and feature extraction are universally available, the ROIs will be automatically identified by the reading software. As part of the reading, a complete feature dataset will be automatically extracted and uploaded to a shared database and algorithmically compared with prior images to enable more precise diagnoses [59]. These ideas are not far from reality, as most picture archiving and communication systems have the capability to co-register current images with standard images and perform user-interactive segmentation. For the foreseeable future, the field of radiomics research will concentrate on improving classifier models to provide the most accurate possible diagnoses and, hence, better patient care and outcomes.

2.5   Summary

In conclusion, radiomics may be the next frontier in clinical decision making. As tumor heterogeneity is depicted and quantified by CT, phenotypical descriptors may indirectly reflect tumor prognosis. The numerous studies previously mentioned in this section suggested that further research on quantitative imaging features is warranted, with more advanced applications of radiomics used for treatment monitoring, outcome prediction, or biomarker imaging. The identification of a poor prognosis may help avoid unnecessary drug toxicities and cost, allowing more accurate decisions about alternative treatment regimens that might improve the clinical outcome. Because effective and credible prediction is important to plan a subsequent definitive treatment, quantitative radiomics-related studies could provide better prognostic information about cancers.

3   Radiomics in MRI Imaging

3.1   Introduction

3.1.1   What Is MRI?

Basic Principles of MRI [61]

MRI is an important modality in medical imaging. Measurement techniques and applications have been developed for nearly 30 years after the initial clinical scanners were invented.

MRI is a measurement technique that is used to examine atoms and molecules. It is based on the interaction between an applied magnetic field and a particle that possesses spin. Electrons and other subatomic particles which are able to spin can be examined using MRI techniques. An MRI experiment can be conducted in terms of energy transfer. During the measurement process, the patient or sample is exposed to energy at frequency that can be absorbed. A short time later, this energy is reemitted, at which time it can be detected and processed. The process by which the protons release the energy that they absorbed from the Radio frequency (RF) pulse is known as relaxation. Relaxation is a fundamental aspect of MR, as essential as energy absorption, and provides the primary mechanism for the MRI image. It is a time-dependent process and is characterized by a rate constant known as the relaxation time, which is measured for the entire sample of spin.

3.1.2 What Is GBM?

Introduction

GBM (World Health Organization [WHO] grade IV astrocytoma) is the most common malignant primary brain tumor, accounting for 45.2% of malignant primary brain tumors and about 15.6% of all primary brain tumors [101, 132]. The best current standard of care for GBM includes surgical resection, followed by adjuvant local radiotherapy and systemic chemotherapy with temozolomide (TMZ) [155].

Despite these aggressive multiple treatments, the relative survival of GBM is low; less than 5% of patients survived for 5 years after-diagnosis [132]. The median overall survival duration for patients ranges from 12.2 to 15.9 months [155]. This is thought to be attributed to the high invasiveness and heterogeneity exhibited by GBM on the molecular and genomic levels, which lead to differences in individual treatment responses and prognoses [167]. Approximately 90% of GBM tumors recur at the site of surgical resection because of invasive tumor cells that were left behind after resection and managed to avert radiation therapy [3].

Genetic biomarker of GBM

Most malignant tumors are now associated with changes in the expressions of multiple genes rather than a single gene [142]. This diversity in genetic alterations renders identification of certain predictive and prognostic genetic biomarkers for GBM a great challenge. During the last decade, the use of microarray-based high output sequencing methods has allowed the simultaneous measurement of many genes and their products, and a further quantitative analysis of entire gene networks has deepened the insight into the processes underlying the development of GBM. A thorough analysis of the Cancer Genome Atlas (TCGA) data concluded that GBM harbors more than 60 genetic alterations including genetic mutations and chromosomal aberrations [15]. TCGA, which began in 2006, is a publicly available large-scale multi-institutional collaborative effort funded by the National Cancer Institute and the National Human Genome Research Institute to establish a better understanding of the molecular alterations of cancer associated with pathological and radiological features and the response to therapy. GBM was the first cancer examined by TCGA. By identifying the specific genetic mutations and microRNA expressions in nearly 500 tumor samples, TCGA-driven studies have increased our awareness of the significance of genetic and molecular pathways in the pathogenesis of GBM and the identification of potential novel molecular therapeutic targets [3]. The typical identified alterations include mutations affecting the epidermal growth factor receptor (EGFR), protein 53 (P53), cyclin-dependent kinase inhibitor 2a, cyclin-dependent kinase 4, retinoblastoma 1, and phosphatase and tensin homolog (PTEN) genes, along with deletions on several chromosomal arms including 1p, 9p, 10p, 10q, 13q, 17p, 19q, and 22 [145]. Some of the most significant GBM genetic biomarkers that have been identified include the EGFR, O6-methylguanine–DNA methyltransferase (MGMT)-promoter methylation, isocitrate dehydrogenase-1 (IDH1) mutation, 1p/19q co-deletion, and P53 mutation.

Prognostic biomarkers provide information about a patient's probable long-term outcome (overall survival), either untreated or with a standard treatment [151].

3.2 Automated Brain Tumor Segmentation

Brain tumor detection or segmentation is an important topic for measuring tumor progression and the clinical response to therapy [100]. Conventional methods have relied on manual labeling by experts, but this approach is labor-intense and involves inter-variability among radiologists. To accelerate the process of tum-or delineation, there is a rich body of literature on automated brain tumor segmentation using MRI. It has become an interdisciplinary area that includes artificial intelligence knowledge [30], medical physics [82] and computer vision [182]. The problem is challenging because it is impossible to segment a tumor using a simple thresholding technique because of the presence of tumor heterogeneity [35]. For example, as a visual reflection of the underlying tumor heterogeneity, the MRI phenotype visually exhibits ambiguous tissue appearances, which makes the segmentation process difficult. Machine learning is challenging primarily because of: (a) the complex nature of the brain tumor data and (b) the hurdle of translating learning knowledge into a series of generalized operations. This section briefly reviews brain tumor segmentation approaches.

Numerous comprehensive reviews have summarized the brain tumor segmentation techniques. Thus this section highlights the fundamental concepts in developing automated tumor segmentation approaches. A more detailed introduction to brain tumor segmentation can be found in (see three references below). [(1) State of the art survey on MRI brain tumor segmentation, (2) Review of brain MRI image segmentation methods, (3) Survey of MRI-based medical image analysis for brain tumor studies.]

A. Segmentation with multi-modality MRI

A successful segmentation heavily relies on an understanding of the underlying structure of the brain tumor imaging data and machine learning model. As a rule of thumb, the segmentation process is typically viewed as a binary classification problem, i.e., segmenting the gross tumor from healthy brain tissues. Given the variety of brain tumor imaging techniques, different tumor segmentation approaches have been proposed. One study [168] used multiparametric imaging sequences to quantify the brain neoplasm by combining structural MRI and diffusion tensor imaging (DTI). In [35], only T2W MRI images were used to detect tumor and edema regions with an outlier detection scheme. Four MRI modalities (T1W, T1CE, T2W and FLAIR) were used in [64] for the joint segmentation and deformable registration of a brain tumor.

Beyond the strategy of binary segmentation, multiple subclasses exist for brain tumors. GBM typically consists of different sub-regions (e.g., active cells, necrosis, and edema). They often present different visual properties including various shapes and appearances, with irregular boundaries between the necrosis and active areas, and different spatial locations for tumors. Thus, numerous approaches have been proposed to define tumor segmentation as a multi-classes segmentation problem. These have emphasized tumor shape segmentation and explored specific tissue segmentation (e.g., the active region and edema). This is a more challenging task because the potential multiple classes turn the problem into one involving more precise sub-structures. For instance, studies [168, 187, 188] classified three relevant tissues: active cells, necrotic core and edema. Another study [35] mainly considered gross tumor and edema tissue segmentation.

B. Machine learning in brain tumor segmentation

In the context of automated brain tumor segmentation, machine-learning approaches are the principle techniques and generally include two types: generative approaches and discriminative approaches [120]. Consider a classic binary classification problem, where $x \in R^d$, and θ_i, $i = [150]$. A classifier is designed to find a solution to an optimization problem:

$$\theta = \arg\max_{\theta_i} p(\theta_i | x) \tag{3.1}$$

A generative model typically describes observations based on a Bayesian probabilistic model. Given likelihood $p(x\theta|_i)$ and prior probability $p(\theta_i)$, $p(\theta_i|x)$ can be inferred:

$$p(\theta_i|x) \frac{p(x|\theta_i)p(\theta_i)}{p(x)} \tag{3.2}$$

An optimal decision boundary can be further made using a log likelihood ratio:

$$l_{Gen}(x) = \frac{p(\theta_1|x)}{p(\theta_2|x)} \tag{3.3}$$

As opposed to a generative model, a discriminative model directly searches for the optimal decision boundary (e.g., hyperplane) between classes. By means of optimizing parameters, the discriminant function is given below, where the parameter set [w, α] can be fit through minimizing the training error.

$$l_{Dis}(x) = \sum_{i=1}^{n} \omega_i x_i \alpha \tag{3.4}$$

(1) Generative approach: Generative probabilistic models have shown their effectiveness in brain tumor segmentation because they exhibit a good generalization for unknown data [109, 138]. Corso et al. [35] proposed an integrated Bayesian

model, i.e., an integrated multilevel segmentation approach with a weighted aggregation algorithm. Similarly, another study [64] designed an expectation maximization (EM) algorithm, as a classic probabilistic theory, to split the normal brain atlas into tissue and tumor growth model. Conditional random fields (CRFs) [14] is another probabilistic model used to estimate the joint distribution of a discrete label configuration and take into account the neighborhood pixel relationships. Following this idea, one study [168] used CRFs that incorporated spatial constraints to show a notable improvement over discriminative classifiers. Cobzas et al. [31] embedded CRFs in a level set framework—the CRFs could be efficiently estimated and led to a discriminative property for the brain tumor segmentation task. More recently, Menze et al. [31] introduced a generative probabilistic model that made full use of multi-modal MRI volumes by estimating the tumor boundary of each modality.

They showed that the delineation of the tumor area in each of these modalities individually was highly preferred for the subsequent quantitative analysis of the tumor shape and evolution.

(2) Discriminative approach: Discriminative classifiers learn a decision boundary directly by learning input data x with class labels. A large number of studies on brain tumor segmentation were derived with this approach [48, 144, 183]. Because of its powerful generalization property, the SVM method has been widely applied in supervised problems. For instance, one study [96] used SVM for the brain tumor segmentation task. However, SVM typically does not consider the correlation between the adjacent voxels, which limits its performance for the segmentation problem. Another study [187, 188] used the random forest classifier as an alternative discriminative multi-class classification method to determine a predicted class for each input pixel.

Both generative and discriminative models have their own challenges. Discriminative approaches are sensitive to the missing data, and often require sufficient training data to preserve a stable performance. In addition, they mainly couple with voxel-based samples, i.e., it is relatively hard for discriminative models to capture the anatomical or topology structure. Generative models may directly generalize to multichannel observations [139], but they do not allow for modeling the differences between the biological processes observed in different modalities [109]. There are works that made efforts to combine the benefits of these models [96, 173, 187, 188]. For instance, a unifying framework was proposed in: initial class probabilities (tumor or non-tumor) were estimated based on the likelihood from training Gaussian mixture models (GMMs). Then, the feature vector was formed by concatenating probabilistic values with pre-defined context features. Finally, the classification was performed using the discriminative classifier.

C. Atlas-based segmentation approaches

The brain atlas—a referenced image template, was created by averaging manual segmentations of normal brain tissues and registering them using an affine transformation [139]. The brain tumor detection problem can be simplified using this atlas, because the atlas provides a statistical construction of MRI scans that aids the analysis and understanding of brain tumor locations [64]. Researchers have utilized an atlas reference model for the tumor segmentation task [19, 91, 173]. Atlases are mainly used for locating the tumor region with respect to healthy tissue. For example, the spatial locations of anatomical structures were derived from a registered anatomical atlas [91]. Using such additional knowledge, a fully auto-mated segmentation tool can be developed for ventricle and brain tumor segmen-tation. In general, the use of an atlas, as an extra spatial constraint, is usually combined with other machine learning schemes for the tumor segmentation task. Additionally, as mentioned in [12], in an atlas-based scheme, the spatial prior knowledge gives a more smooth deformation, with the potential to produce gen-eralized segmentation outcomes.

3.3 GBM: Feature Extraction

Feature extraction is a very important step in the "radiomics" flow path, which has the goal of obtaining image-derived features to implement the prediction classifi-cation, prognostic analysis or gene-related analysis in the following stages of "ra-diomics". For GBM, multimodal MRI sequences usually contain T1, T1-contrast, T2 and FLAIR. We separately extracted features from each sequence using the same set of features. Here, we will demonstrate the detailed formulas of two kinds of features: textural and non-textural features.

3.3.1 Non-textural Features

Non-textural features include shape and size features and intensity features.

- **Shape and size features**:

  These features describe the shape and size of the tumor region. We used V to denote the volume and A to denote the surface area of the volume of interest. The definitions of the features are as follows:

Compactness 1	$\text{compactness } 1 = \dfrac{V}{\sqrt{\pi}A^{\frac{2}{3}}}$
Compactness 2	$\text{compactness } 2 = 36\pi \dfrac{V^2}{A^3}$
Spherical disproportion	$\text{spherical disproportion} = \dfrac{A}{4\pi R^2}$ where R is the radius of a sphere with the same volume as the tumor
Sphericity	$\text{sphericity} = \dfrac{\pi^{\frac{1}{3}}(6V)^{\frac{2}{3}}}{A}$

(continued)

(continued)

Surface area	The surface area is calculated by triangulation (i.e. dividing the surface into connected triangles) and is defined as follows: $$A = \sum_{i=1}^{N} \frac{1}{2} |a_i b_i \times a_i c_i|$$ where N is the total number of triangles covering the surface and a, b and c are edge vectors of the triangles
Surface to volume ratio	surface to volume ratio $= \frac{A}{V}$
Maximum 3D diameter	The maximum three-dimensional tumor diameter is measured as the largest pairwise Euclidean distance between voxels on the surface of the tumor volume

- **Intensity features**:

Intensity features are extracted from the histogram of the tumor region, and describe the distribution of voxel intensities within the MRI image. We use X to denote the image matrix with N voxels as the total. P represents the first-order histogram with N_l discrete intensity levels. The definitions of the intensity features are as follows:

Energy	$$energy = \sum_{i}^{N} X(i)^2$$
Entropy	$$entropy = \sum_{i=1}^{N_l} P(i) \log_2 P(i)$$ *Measures texture randomness or irregularity
Kurtosis	$$kurtosis = \frac{\frac{1}{N}\sum_{i=1}^{N}(X(i)-\bar{x})^4}{\left(\sqrt{\frac{1}{N}\sum_{i=1}^{N}(X(i)-\bar{x})^2}\right)^2}$$ where $\bar{X}$ is the mean of X *Describes "peakedness" of a distribution Kurtosis > 3: sharper than a normal distribution, with values concentrated around the mean and thicker tails. This means high probability for extreme values Kurtosis < 3: flatter than a normal distribution with a wider peak. The probability for extreme values is less than for a normal distribution, and the values are spread more widely around the mean Kurtosis = 3: normal distribution
Maximum	The maximum intensity value of X
Mean	$$mean = \frac{1}{N}\sum_{i}^{N} X(i)$$
Mean absolute deviation	The mean of the absolute deviations of all the voxel intensities around the mean intensity value
Median	The median intensity value of X

(continued)

(continued)

Minimum	The minimum intensity value of X
Range	The range of intensity values of X
Root mean square (RMS)	$RMS = \sqrt{\dfrac{\Sigma_i^N X(i)^2}{N}}$
Skewness	$skewness = \dfrac{\frac{1}{N}\Sigma_{i=1}^N (X(i)-\bar{x})^3}{\left(\sqrt{\frac{1}{N}\Sigma_{i=1}^N (X(i)-\bar{x})^2}\right)^3}$ where X^- is the mean of X *Asymmetry and deviation from a normal distribution Skewness > 0: right skewed, most values concentrated on the left of the mean Skewness < 0: left skewed, most values concentrated on the right of the mean Skewness $= 0$: symmetrical distribution around the mean
Standard deviation	$standard\ deviation = \left(\frac{1}{N-1}\sum_{i=1}^N (X(i)-\bar{X})^2\right)^{1/2}$ where X^- is the mean of X *Quantify the amount of variation or dispersion of a set of data values. Std close to 0 indicates that the data points tend to be very close to the mean of the set, while a high standard deviation indicates that the data points are spread out over a wider range of values
Uniformity	$uniformity = \sum_{i=1}^{N_t} P(i)^2$
Variance	$variance = \frac{1}{N-1}\sum_{i=1}^N (X(i)-\bar{X})^2$ where $\bar{X}$ is the mean of X.

3.3.2 Textural Features

Textural features are extracted based on four matrices: the gray-level co-occurrence matrix (GLCM) [20], gray-level run-length matrix (GLRLM) [18, 36, 50, 160, 161], gray-level size zone matrix (GLSZM) [18, 36, 50, 160, 161] and neighborhood gray-tone difference matrix (NGTDM) [5]. These could be constructed using a 3D analysis of a tumor region with 26-voxel connectivity, where 6 voxels are at a distance of one, 12 voxels are at a distance of $\sqrt{2}$, and 8 voxels are at a distance of $\sqrt{3}$ around the center voxel. These voxels at different distances are treated differently in the calculation of the GLCM, whereas the GLRLM and NGTDM take into account the discretization length differences. Before constructing these matrices, it is necessary to discretize the ROI of the MRI image. The voxel intensities should be resampled into equally spaced bins. This discretization step could reduce image noise. It could also normalize the intensities for all patients. Next, we will show how the features are extracted from these four matrices.

Fig. 14 Example of calculation of co-occurrence matrix for 4 × 4 image with 4 gray levels

Image

Gray Level (i)	Cooccurrences (j)			
	1	2	3	4
1	0	1	1	3
2	1	4	2	0
3	1	2	0	2
4	3	0	2	2

```
1  2  3  4   =>
1  3  4  4
3  2  2  2
4  1  4  1
```

- **GLCM**

Here, we use P(i, j; δ, α) to represent the GLCM matrix, the size of which is N × N, where N represents the number of discrete gray-level intensities, the (i, j)th element represents the number of times that intensity levels i and j occur adjacently in the image, and the distance between them is δ in direction α. Figure 14 shows an example of the calculation of a co-occurrence matrix [160, 161]:

The following specific features are derived from the GLCM:

Preliminary Definitions
P(i, j) is the co-occurrence matrix for an arbitrary δ and α
Ng is the number of discrete intensity levels in the image
μ is the mean of P(i, j)
$\rho_x(i) = \sum_{j=1}^{N_g} P(i,j)$ depicts the marginal row probabilities
$\rho_y(i) = \sum_{i=1}^{N_g} P(i,j)$ depicts the marginal column probabilities
μx is the mean of ρx
μy is the mean of ρy
σx is the standard deviation of ρx
σy is the standard deviation of ρy
$\rho_{x+y}(k) = \sum_{i=1}^{N_g}\sum_{j=1}^{N_g} P(i,j), i+j = k, k = 2, 3,..., 2\,N_g$
$\rho_{x-y}(k) = \sum_{i=1}^{N_g}\sum_{j=1}^{N_g} P(i,j), i+j = k, k = 2, 3,..., 2\,N_g$
$HX = -\sum_{i=1}^{N_g} \rho_x(i) \log_2[\rho_x(i)]$ is the entropy of ρx
$HY = -\sum_{i=1}^{N_g} \rho_y(i) \log_2\left[\rho_y(i)\right]$ is the entropy of ρy
$H = -\sum_{i=1}^{N_g}\sum_{j=1}^{N_g} P(i,j) \log_2[P(i,j)]$ is the entropy of P(i, j)

(continued)

(continued)

Preliminary Definitions
$HXY1 = -\sum_{i=1}^{N_g}\sum_{lj=1}^{N_g} P(i,j)\log\left(\rho_x(i)\rho_y(j)\right)$
$\mathbf{HXY2} = -\sum_{i=1}^{N_g}\sum_{lj=1}^{N_g}\rho_x(i)\rho_y(j)\log\left(\rho_x(i)\rho_y(j)\right)$

GLCM Features	
Autocorrelation	$\text{autocorrelation} = \sum_{i=1}^{N_g}\sum_{lj=1}^{N_g} ijP(i,j)$
Cluster Prominence	$\text{cluster prominence} = \sum_{i=1}^{N_g}\sum_{lj=1}^{N_g}\left(i+j-\mu_x(i)-\mu_y(j)\right)^4 P(i,j)$
Cluster Shade	$\text{cluster shade} = \sum_{i=1}^{N_g}\sum_{lj=1}^{N_g}\left(i+j-\mu_x(i)-\mu_y(j)\right)^3 P(i,j)$
Cluster Tendency	$\text{cluster tendency} = \sum_{i=1}^{N_g}\sum_{lj=1}^{N_g}\left(i+j-\mu_x(i)-\mu_y(j)\right)^2 P(i,j)$
Contrast	$\text{contrast} = \sum_{i=1}^{N_g}\sum_{lj=1}^{N_g}|i-j|^2 P(i,j)$ *Measures contrast or local intensity variation and favors contributions away from the diagonal
Correlation	$\text{correlation} = \frac{\sum_{i=1}^{N_g}\sum_{j=1}^{N_g} ijP(i,j) - \mu_i(i)\mu_j(j)}{\sigma_x(i)\sigma_y(j)}$ *Reflects the grey-level linear dependencies
Difference Entropy	$\text{difference entropy} = \sum_{i=0}^{N_g-1} P_{x-y}(i)\log_2\left[P_{x-y}(i)\right]$
Dissimilarity	$\text{dissimilarity} = \sum_{i=1}^{N_g}\sum_{j=1}^{N_g}|i-j|P(i,j)$ *Reflects the difference between elements in the matrix
Energy	$\text{energy} = \sum_{i=1}^{N_g}\sum_{j=1}^{N_g} P(i,j)^2$ *Reflects the homogeneity of the gray-level distribution, the small value means the strong homogeneity
Entropy (H)	$\text{entropy} = -\sum_{i=1}^{N_g}\sum_{j=1}^{N_g} P(i,j)\log_2[P(i,j)]$ *Measures texture randomness or irregularity
Homogeneity 1	$\text{homogeneity 1} = \sum_{i=1}^{N_g}\sum_{j=1}^{N_g}\frac{P(i,j)}{1+|i-j|}$ *Measures the closeness of the distribution of elements in the matrix to the diagonal
Homogeneity 2	$\text{homogeneity 2} = \sum_{i=1}^{N_g}\sum_{j=1}^{N_g}\frac{P(i,j)}{1+|i-j|^2}$

(continued)

(continued)

GLCM Features	
Information measure of correlation 1 (IMC1)	$IMC1 = \dfrac{HXY - HXY_1}{\max\{HX, HY\}}$
Information measure of correlation 2 (IMC2)	$IMC2 = \sqrt{1 - e^{-2(HXY2 - HXY)}}$
Inverse Difference Moment Normalized (IDMN)	$IDMN = \sum\limits_{i=1}^{N_g} \sum\limits_{j=1}^{N_g} \dfrac{P(i,j)}{1 + \left(\dfrac{\|i-j\|^2}{N^2}\right)}$ *Measures the local heterogeneity, the large IDM means the coarse texture
Inverse Difference Normalized (IDN)	$IDN = \sum\limits_{i=1}^{N_g} \sum\limits_{j=1}^{N_g} \dfrac{P(i,j)}{1 + \left(\dfrac{\|i-j\|}{N}\right)}$
Inverse variance	$\text{inverse variance} = \sum\limits_{i=1}^{N_g} \sum\limits_{j=1}^{N_g} \dfrac{P(i,j)}{\|i-j\|^2}, i \neq j$
Maximum Probability	$\text{maximum probability} = \max\{P(i,j)\}$
Sum average	$\text{sum average} = \sum\limits_{i=2}^{2N_g} \left[i P_{x+y}(i)\right]$ *Reflects the average intensities of the image
Sum entropy	$\text{sum entropy} = -\sum\limits_{i=2}^{2N_g} P_{x+y}(i) \log_2\left[P_{x+y}(i)\right]$
Sum variance	$\text{sum variance} = \sum\limits_{i=2}^{2N_g} (i - SE)^2 P_{x+y}(i)$
Variance	$\text{variance} = \sum\limits_{i=1}^{N_g} \sum\limits_{j=1}^{N_g} (i - \mu)^2 P(i,j)$ *Quantify the amount of variation or dispersion

- **GLRLM**

The gray level run-length represents a series of consecutive pixels with the same gray-level value. $P(i, j|\theta)$ is used to represent the gray level run-length matrix, where the (i, j)th element describes gray-level i which consecutively appears j times in the

Fig. 15 Example of calculation of a run length matrix for 4 × 4 image with 4 gray levels

Image

1	2	3	4
1	3	4	4
3	2	2	2
4	1	4	1

=>

Gray Level (i)	Run Length (j)			
	1	2	3	4
1	4	0	0	0
2	1	0	1	0
3	3	0	0	0
4	3	1	0	0

ROI in the direction θ. Figure 15 shows an example of the calculation of a run length matrix [5]:

The following specific features are derived from the GLRLM:

Preliminary Definitions
$\rho(i, j\|\theta)$ is the (i, j)th entry in the given run-length matrix ρ for a direction θ
Ng is the number of discrete intensity values in the image
Nr is the number of different run lengths
$\rho_x(i) = \sum\limits_{j=1}^{N_g} P(i, j)$ depicts the marginal row probabilities

GLRLM Features	
Short Run Emphasis (SRE)	$$SRE = \frac{\sum_{i=1}^{N_g} \sum_{j=1}^{N_r} \left[\frac{\rho(i,j\|\theta)}{j^2}\right]}{\sum_{i=1}^{N_g} \sum_{j=1}^{N_r} \rho(i,j\|\theta)}$$ *Measures the distribution of short runs. It depends on the occurrence of short runs. The large value corresponds to the fine texture
Long Run Emphasis (LRE)	$$LRE = \frac{\sum_{i=1}^{N_g} \sum_{j=1}^{N_r} j^2 \rho(i,j\|\theta)}{\sum_{i=1}^{N_g} \sum_{j=1}^{N_r} \rho(i,j\|\theta)}$$ *Measures the distribution of long runs. It depends on the occurrence of long runs. The large value corresponds to the coarse texture
Gray Level Non-Uniformity (GLN)	$$GLN = \frac{\sum_{i=1}^{N_g} \left[\sum_{j=1}^{N_r} \rho(i,j\|\theta)\right]^2}{\sum_{i=1}^{N_g} \sum_{j=1}^{N_r} \rho(i,j\|\theta)}$$ *Measures the similarity of grey level values throughout the image. If the grey level values are similar, the value is small
Run Length Non-Uniformity (RLN)	$$RLN = \frac{\sum_{j=1}^{N_r} \left[\sum_{i=1}^{N_g} \rho(i,j\|\theta)\right]^2}{\sum_{i=1}^{N_g} \sum_{j=1}^{N_r} \rho(i,j\|\theta)}$$ *Measures the similarity of the length of runs throughout the image. If the length of runs are similar, the value is small
Run Percentage (RP)	$$RP = \sum_{i=1}^{N_g} \sum_{j=1}^{N_r} \frac{\rho(i,j\|\theta)}{N_\rho}$$ *Measures the homogeneity and the distribution of runs of an image in a specific direction. It is largest when the length of runs is 1 for all grey levels in a specific direction
Low Gray Level Run Emphasis (LGLRE)	$$LGLRE = \frac{\sum_{i=1}^{N_g} \sum_{j=1}^{N_r} \left[\frac{\rho(i,j\|\theta)}{i^2}\right]}{\sum_{i=1}^{N_g} \sum_{j=1}^{N_r} \rho(i,j\|\theta)}$$ *Measures the distribution of low gray level values. The LGRE is expected large for the image with low gray level values.
High Gray Level Run Emphasis (HGLRE)	$$HGLRE = \frac{\sum_{i=1}^{N_g} \sum_{j=1}^{N_r} i^2 \rho(i,j\|\theta)}{\sum_{i=1}^{N_g} \sum_{j=1}^{N_r} \rho(i,j\|\theta)}$$

(continued)

(continued)

	*Measures the distribution of high gray level values. The HGRE is expected large for the image with high gray level values
Short Run Low Gray Level Emphasis (SRLGLE)	$$SRLGLE = \frac{\sum_{i=1}^{N_g} \sum_{j=1}^{N_r} \left[\frac{\rho(i,j|\theta)}{i^2 j^2} \right]}{\sum_{i=1}^{N_g} \sum_{j=1}^{N_r} \rho(i,j|\theta)}$$ *Measures the joint distribution of short runs and low gray level values. The SRLGE is expected large for the image with many short runs and lower gray level values
Short Run High Gray Level Emphasis (SRHGLE)	$$SRHGLE = \frac{\sum_{i=1}^{N_g} \sum_{j=1}^{N_r} \left[\frac{\rho(i,j|\theta) i^2}{j^2} \right]}{\sum_{i=1}^{N_g} \sum_{j=1}^{N_r} \rho(i,j|\theta)}$$ *Measures the joint distribution of short runs and high gray level values. The SRHGE is expected large for the image with many short runs and high gray level values
Long Run Low Gray Level Emphasis (LRLGLE)	$$LRLGLE = \frac{\sum_{i=1}^{N_g} \sum_{j=1}^{N_r} \left[\frac{\rho(i,j|\theta) j^2}{i^2} \right]}{\sum_{i=1}^{N_g} \sum_{j=1}^{N_r} \rho(i,j|\theta)}$$ *Measures the joint distribution of long runs and low gray level values. The LRLGE is expected large for the image with many long runs and low gray level values
Long Run High Gray Level Emphasis (LRHGLE)	$$LRHGLE = \frac{\sum_{i=1}^{N_g} \sum_{j=1}^{N_r} \rho(i,j|\theta) i^2 j^2}{\sum_{i=1}^{N_g} \sum_{j=1}^{N_r} \rho(i,j|\theta)}$$ *Measures the joint distribution of long runs and high gray level values. The LRHGE is expected large for images with many long runs and high gray level values

- **GLSZM**

The GLSZM describes the size of each area with pixels of the same gray level value. The definition of GLSZM is similar to the GLRLM principle. The (i, j)th element represents gray-level j in the areas of size i, and the value of the matrix is the number of the (i, j)th element. Figure 16 shows an example of the calculation of a size zone matrix [5]:

The following specific features (13 features in total) are derived from the GLSZM:

Fig. 16 Example of calculation of Size Zone Matrix for 4 × 4 image with 4 gray levels

Image

1	2	3	4	=>
1	3	4	4	
3	2	2	2	
4	1	4	1	

Gray Level (i)	Size Zone (j)			
	1	2	3	4
1	2	1	0	0
2	1	0	1	0
3	0	0	1	0
4	2	0	1	0

Short Zone Emphasis (SZE)	$SZE = \dfrac{\sum_i \sum_j \frac{P(i,j)}{j^2}}{\sum_i \sum_j P(i,j)}$ *Measures the distribution of small zones. It depends on the occurrence of small zone. The large value corresponds to the fine texture
Long Zone Emphasis (LZE)	$LZE = \dfrac{\sum_i \sum_j j^2 P(i,j)}{\sum_i \sum_j P(i,j)}$ *Measures the distribution of large zones. It depends on the occurrence of large zones. The large value corresponds to the coarse texture
Gray-Level Non-uniformity for Zone (GLNZ)	$GLNZ = \dfrac{\sum_i \left(\sum_j P(i,j)\right)^2}{\sum_i \sum_j P(i,j)}$ *Measures the similarity of grey level values throughout the image. If the grey level values are similar, the value is small
Zone Length Non-uniformity (ZLN)	$ZLN = \dfrac{\sum_j \left(\sum_i P(i,j)\right)^2}{\sum_i \sum_j P(i,j)}$ *Measures the similarity of the size of zones throughout the image. If the size of zones is similar, the value is small
Zone Percentage (ZP)	$ZP = \dfrac{\sum_i \sum_j P(i,j)}{\sum_i \sum_j (j \cdot P(i,j))}$ *Measures the homogeneity and the distribution of zones of an image. It is largest when the size of zones is 1 for all grey levels
Low Gray-Level Zone Emphasis (LGZE)	$LGZE = \dfrac{\sum_i \sum_j \frac{P(i,j)}{i^2}}{\sum_i \sum_j P(i,j)}$ *Measures the distribution of low gray level values. The LGZE is expected large for the image with low gray level values
High Gray-Level Zone Emphasis (HGRE)	$HGRE = \dfrac{\sum_i \sum_j P(i,j)}{\sum_i \sum_j P(i,j)}$ *Measures the distribution of high gray level values. The HGZE is expected large for the image with high gray level values
Short Zone Low Gray-Level Emphasis (SZLGE)	$SZLGE = \dfrac{\sum_i \sum_j \frac{P(i,j)}{i^2 \cdot j^2}}{\sum_i \sum_j P(i,j)}$ *Measures the joint distribution of small size zones and low gray level values. The SZLGE is expected large for the image with many small size zone and lower gray level values
Short Zone High Gray-Level Emphasis (SZHGE)	$SZHGE = \dfrac{\sum_i \sum_j \frac{i^2 \cdot P(i,j)}{j^2}}{\sum_i \sum_j P(i,j)}$ *Measures the joint distribution of small size zones and high gray level values. The SZRHGE is expected large for the image with many small size zones and high gray level values

(continued)

(continued)

Long Zone Low Gray-Level Emphasis (LZLGE)	$LZLGE = \dfrac{\sum_i \sum_j \frac{j^2 \cdot P(i,j)}{j^2}}{\sum_i \sum_j P(i,j)}$ *Measures the joint distribution of large size zones and low gray level values. The LRLGE is expected large for the image with many large size zones and low gray level values
Long Zone High Gray-Level Emphasis (LZHGE)	$LZHGE = \dfrac{\sum_i \sum_j \left(i^2 \cdot j^2 \cdot P(i,j) \right)}{\sum_i \sum_j P(i,j)}$ *Measures the joint distribution of large size zones and high gray level values. The LRHGE is expected large for images with many large size zones and high gray level values
Gray-Level Variance (GLV)	$Var_I = \sqrt{\dfrac{1}{I \times J} \sum_{i=1}^{I} \sum_{j=1}^{J} \left(i \times P(i,j) - \mu_I \right)^2}$ with $\mu_I = \dfrac{1}{I \times J} \sum_{i=1}^{I} \sum_{j=1}^{J} i \times P(i,j)$
Zone-Size Variance (ZSV)	$Var_J = \sqrt{\dfrac{1}{I \times J} \sum_{i=1}^{I} \sum_{j=1}^{J} \left(i \times P(i,j) - \mu_J \right)^2}$ with $\mu_J = \dfrac{1}{I \times J} \sum_{i=1}^{I} \sum_{j=1}^{J} j \times P(i,j)$

- **NGTDM**

The NGTDM extracts features based on the visual properties of an image. It is a column matrix formed by the absolute value of the pixel being observed minus the average of the pixels in its neighborhood. Figure 17 shows an example of an NGTDM calculation result [5].

Fig. 17 a Sample image. b NGTDM for the sample image

(a)

1	1	4	3	1
3	4	0	1	1
5	4	2	2	2
2	1	1	4	4
0	2	2	5	1

(b)

i	s(i)
0	2.750
1	4.125
2	0.250
3	0.000
4	4.875

In the indicated square in Fig. 17, there are two pixels with gray tone = 2. Thus, for this image:

$$s(2) = \left| 2 - \frac{17}{8} \right| + \left| 2 - \frac{15}{8} \right| = 0.250$$

The following specific features are derived from the NGTDM:

Coarseness	$\text{coarseness} = \frac{1}{\sum_i p_i \cdot S(i)}$ *Based on differences between each voxel and the neighboring voxels in adjacent image planes, it measures the granularity within an image. Described as the most fundamental property of texture
Contrast	$\text{contrast} = \left(\frac{1}{N_L(N_L-1)} \sum_i \sum_j p_i p_j (i-j)^2 \right) \left(\frac{1}{(N-2d)^2} \sum_i S(i) \right)$ *This value increases with the amount of local variation in intensity. An image is said to have a high level of contrast if areas of different intensity levels are clearly visible. Thus, a high contrast means that the intensity difference between neighboring regions is large. This is usually the case when the dynamic range of the grey scale is large or when it is stretched
Busyness	$\text{Busyness} = \frac{\sum_i (p_i . S(i))}{\sum_i \sum_j (i p_i - j p_j)}$. *A busy texture is one in which there are rapid changes in intensity from one pixel to its neighbor; that is the spatial frequency of intensity changes is very high. A higher value of busyness would tend to emphasize the frequency of spatial changes in intensity values
Complexity	$\sum_i \sum_j \left(|i-j|/n^2 \left(p_i + p_j \right) \right) \left(p_i S(i) + p_j S(j) \right),$ $p_i \neq 0, p_j \neq 0$ *A texture has high complexity if the information content is high and there are many grey values present. Complexity is the sum of pairs of normalized differences between intensity values
Strength	$\sum_i \sum_j \left(\left(p_i + p_j \right)(i-j)^2 \right) / \sum_i S(i), p_i \neq 0, p_j \neq 0$ *Emphasize the boldness or distinctiveness of the primitives. And a high value corresponds to a strong texture

3.4 GBM Prediction

Prediction of GBM using molecular biomarkers

GBM is the most common primary malignant neoplasm in adults, with a median survival of one year [125]. Recently, there has been progress in understanding the molecular basis of the tumor's aggressiveness and heterogeneity. Various molecular subclassifications have been proposed on the basis of the genetic makeup of these tumors with the hope that a better understanding of the origin of tumor cells and molecular pathogenesis may predict the response to targeted therapies. Verhaak et al. [167] subclassified GBM into four subtypes–classic, mesenchymal, proneural, and neural–based on the similarity to defined genomic expression signatures. Phillips et al. subclassified high-grade glioma into three subtypes–proneural, proliferative, and mesenchymal. They found that the subtypes of malignant gliomas could provide prognostic information. There was a trend toward longer survival for patients with a proneural GBM in a combined analysis of TCGA and validation samples for all subtypes relative to Proneural. Yan et al. [179] used high-throughput microarrays to measure the miRNA expression levels in 116 samples from different progression stages of glioma. They found that five-miRNA signature types (two protective miRNAs: miR-767-5p, miR-105; and three risky miRNAs: miR-584, miR-296-5p and miR-196a) could identify patients with a high risk of an unfavorable outcome for anaplastic gliomas regardless of the histology type.

Prediction of GBM by using MRI

Jain et al. [78] correlated the tumor blood volume, measured using dynamic susceptibility contrast material–enhanced T2*-weighted MR perfusion studies, with patient survival and determined its association with molecular subclasses of GBM. They found that the rCBVmax measurements could be used to predict the patient's overall survival independent of the molecular subclasses of GBM; increased rCBV measures were associated with poor overall survival for GBM. Verhaak [167] classifiers provided additional information, suggesting that molecular markers could be used in combination with hemodynamic imaging biomarkers in the future.

Regional variations in the tumor blood flow and necrosis are commonly observed in cross-sectional imaging of clinical cancers. Radiologically-defined regional variations in tumor characteristics can be used to define distinct "habitats" that reflect the underlying evolutionary dynamics. Zhou et al. [186] used an experimental framework to extract spatially-explicit variations in tumor features (habitats) from multiple MRI sequences performed on patients with GBM. They found that the heterogeneity of GBM measured through distance features (DF) could be used as a strong predictor of the survival time. In an initial cohort of 16 cases, slowly progressing tumors had lower DF values (were less heterogeneous) compared to those with fast progression and short survival times.

3.5   *Radiogenomics in GBM*

Radiogenomics in GBM, an emerging field in translational brain cancer research, investigates the association between imaging features and genomics signatures. In clinical routine, MRI has been a major healthcare tool to monitor and quantify the observable characteristics of GBM, providing anatomical information in both the temporal and spatial dimensions. In parallel, the rapid development of genomic signatures has resulted in a deeper understanding of complex molecular events in GBM. For example, the MGMT promoter methylation has been found to strongly correlate to the chemotherapy agent of temozolomide, which can be viewed as an independent prognostic factor for patients suffering from GBM [72]. As defined by radiogenomics, a central focus is placed on establishing a link between the cross-domain knowledge at the imaging and molecular levels. It shows promise in non-invasive molecular tumor assessment, which was previously only available through biological genetic testing. For example, when the identification of non-invasive imaging feature surrogates the relevant molecular events such as EGFR gene mutation in GBM, the transitional value of radiogenomics can be readily seen from non-invasive imaging characteristics. In particular, the growing volumes of clinical MRI and available genomic data for patients fuel the shift in radiogenomics studies from hypothesis-driven to data-driven analytics that enable a rapid synergistic knowledge transition between imaging and genomics.

The field of radiogenomics for GBM is quickly-evolving in numerous research directions. In view of definition of molecular information, recent studies have addressed molecular expression in terms of two representative fronts. First, a pre-defined set of molecular signatures (e.g., EGFR, IDH1, RB1, and NF1) are typically selected for the association evaluation. Second, gene-expression modules are presented to enable shared functional themes in a group or cluster of genes. A typical approach involves an unsupervised hierarchical clustering to partition the high-dimensional gene expression data into co-expressed gene modules.

3.5.1 Radiogenomics Research with Pre-defined Molecular Signatures

The identification of explicit molecular factors is essential in revealing the signaling pathways that are highly expressed in GBM. This has shown promise for improving the understanding of the disease sub-type classification [167] and the prognostic performance in patients [43]. A priority of radiogenomics is identifying the surrogate imaging variables that measure the typical molecular signatures found in GBM.

Another study [68] correlated the genetic mutation, gene expression and copy number to imaging features in GBM using a TCGA cohort. More specifically, EGFR, ERBB2, IDH1, NF1, PDGFRA, PIK3CA, PIK3R1, PTEN, RB1, and TP53 were selected for evaluation. A set of VASARI MR image features (from T1-w, T2-w, and FLAIR scans) were used to quantify the proposition of abnormal tissues (i.e., contrast-enhanced tumor, necrosis, edema and non-enhanced tumor). A major finding showed that EGFR mutant GBMs were significantly larger on T2-w FLAIR images (P < 0.05) while TP53 mutant GBMs were smaller than the wild type on T2-w FLAIR images [102]. Despite its preliminary results on a limited cohort, the exploratory analysis provided proof-of-concept evidence for GBM radiogenomics. In addition to specific gene mutation studies, predicting the molecular subtype of GBM using computational imaging features presents a unique avenue to non-invasively study the molecularly defined GBM sub-types. A recent study [102] proposed a machine-learning framework to predict typical GBM sub-types on 99 GBM tumors including classical, mesenchymal, proneural, and neural subtypes that were well defined in [136]. An overall accuracy of 75.67% was achieved in predicting these four-classes of molecular sub-types from 120-dimensional computational image features. The results indicated the predictive power of high-dimensional imaging features in differentiating molecular events in a GBM that is conventionally defined using genomic data.

In addition to identify the molecular sub-types, messenger RNA (mRNA) and DNA copy number variation have been incorporated into radiogenomics research on GBM [118]. It was reported that six MR imaging features showed strong correlation ($P < 0.05$) with concordant variations in the gene dose and mRNA expression of 34 genes. The major findings elucidated that multi-level radiogenomic association maps could be created given the mRNA expression and DNA copy number variation profiles of GBM patients. As a result, to glean insight into the molecular biology of tumors, leveraging multi-scale omics data with imaging features is particularly demanding for the future research in radiogenomics for GBM.

3.5.2 Radiogenomics Research with Gene-Expression Modules

Gene-expression modules, also known as co-expressed genes, represent a set of molecular data that shares functional themes in the form of groups or clusters. A major motivation of module definition is to simplify the multi-modality molecular data and find shared gene functions or signaling pathways using clustering techniques. It is particularly helpful when dealing with complex, high-dimensional biological data.

Exploratory evidence [128] has shown that gene-expression modules, integrating gene expression, DNA methylation, and copy number data, have significantly correlated ($P < 0.05$) with quantitative image features for GBM. The defining modules come with a gene regulatory program that connects driver genes and their downstream targets [128]. Similarly, the identification of imaging surrogates for gene-expression modules has been studied, revealing that tumor contrast enhancement in MRI can predict the hypoxia gene-expression program [107]. A recent study [189] presented the result of a comprehensive investigation using large-scale gene- and microRNA expression data in GBM and linking them to quantitative MRI features. A functional microRNA network was created as clusters for ingenuity pathway identification. A major finding was that MRI-FLAIR modality could be used as a key detector for characterizing cellular migration and invasion in GBM. It should be noted that, defining highly differentiated gene-expression modules is a difficult task because the biological data is heterogeneous, and clustering approaches may not be able to explicitly reveal distinct modules for specific disease diagnoses. Advanced bioinformatic techniques to identify functional modules are needed for radiogenomic studies in GBM. Thus, finding the imaging-to-genomic association at a cluster level would enable a direct link between functional molecular pathways and phenotypic clusters in GBM. A recent study [77] showed that three distinct imaging clusters were found from high-dimensional quantitative image features, revealing a unique set of molecular signaling pathways in GBM.

3.5.3 Role of Radiomics in Radiogenomics

The recent development of radiomics has given rise to new opportunities in radiogenomics studies. The radiomic strategy [59, 88, 92] generates a large number of quantitative image features using high-throughput techniques. In contrast to conventional radiological features, which rely heavily on the judgment of human experts, radiomics builds upon data-driven analytics, with the extraction of high-dimensional image features empowering medical decision making by identifying novel biomarkers. Typically, large-scale radiomic data extraction relies on computer vision and image processing techniques. Low-level image feature descriptors are the principle approaches used to define the tumor shapes, sharpness, compactness, and visual appearances of tumor. Therefore, the vast quantity of radiomic data makes it possible to realize cross-domain medical data integration, which would otherwise be difficult to achieve in conventional radiology. Genomics methods, including RNA sequencing, DNA copy numbers, DNA methylation, and microarrays, present a variety of molecules at tissue scales. On the other hand, by translating cross-sectional imaging arrays into minable quantitative features, has paved the way for a radiogenomics framework to integrate cross-domain knowledge and thereby draw causal inferences between different types of knowledge.

The rapid development of radiomics offers a unique channel to assess the underlying molecular events in tumor biology. As discussed in prior sections, pioneering studies [189] have illustrated that radiomic data can be used to surrogate or mimic important molecular features in a tumor. These radiomic studies have primarily concentrated on conventional imaging modalities including postcontrast T1-w, FLAIR, and T2-w sequences. Yet a variety of advanced imaging acquisitions have not been explicitly addressed. For example, MR perfusion and diffusion data were particularly useful in understanding the antiangiogenic therapy mechanism for a brain tumor [75]. Currently, these imaging-specific studies are largely limited to clinically-relevant imaging descriptions without emphasizing high-throughput techniques in radiomics. Incorporating the radiomic strategy into advanced imaging would facilitate a molecular functional understanding of a tumor with a specific therapy. In particular, it will offer an opportunity to understand the tumor evolutionary biology of a tumor (e.g., identifying consistent molecular pathways) by quantitatively assessing its imaging characteristic over time

Interpretation and consistency are two key factors in studying radiogenomics. It is notable that large volumes of radiomic data pose a challenge to clinical interpretation and its association to genomics. In this regard, the creation of a semantic feature database will be appreciated because it will define high-level tumor imaging characteristics that are easily interpretable in a clinic. In addition, new types of benchmark radiomic data are needed to construct precise and meaningful imaging-to-genomic links in radiogenomics research. For example, enriched radiomic data, collected from diagnostic timelines from pre-treatment to post-treatment, will enhance our understanding of tumor biology and hold potential to draw prognostic inference from time-sensitive imaging data, which will allow that the found imaging-to-genomic links to be repeatedly examined and verified.

3.5.4 Discussion

The radiogenomics studies of GBM have incorporated new translational values in treating this lethal disease (examples in Table 3.1). The outcomes of radiogenomics aim at revealing causal relationships between radiomic data and genomic information for GBM that were previously unknown. The additional evidence gained from lung cancer [57], breast cancer [149] and related studies [1, 2, 83] has reaffirmed the existence of underlying links between imaging features and genomic signatures. With the growing number of new therapeutic methods available, insights into such data-driven integrated analytics would definitely help explore the intratumoral heterogeneity of GBM and thereby accelerate translational care in personalized treatment planning and management [89].

Despite its promise in rapid translational healthcare, technical challenges remain in mining the links between high-dimensional radiomic data and genomic data. Currently, univariate and multivariate feature assessments are the primary metrics for evaluating imaging-genomic relationships. However, these metrics cannot be able to reveal the structured relationships between two databases that underpin the feature subset relationships. For example, it is well recognized that, instead of an entire gene network, only a proposition of genes (i.e., driver genes) and their regulator genes make significant contributions in response to cancer therapies. Likewise, comparing image textures, tumor shapes, image histograms, and filter-based responses (e.g., gabor filters), it is very possible that only a propositional number of image features strongly indicate disease prognosis. The challenges include how to define number-reduced sets of radiomic or genomic data and how to statistically determine such image-to-genomic causality in a reduced feature space that is more manageable from a computational perspective. Meeting these challenges will broaden the scope of current radiogenomics studies, not only on GBM but also for a wide spectrum of computer-assisted cancer research.

In addition to elucidating novel imaging-genomics associations, external validation is urgently needed to realize reproducibility, which is crucial in cancer translational research. However, the current quantitative approaches are largely restrained by limited cohorts with little study at scale. Related studies have primarily leveraged the TCGA and TCIA public cohorts for genomic and imaging data respectively. The advent of high-variety and high-volume GBM cohorts will be a major hurdle for finding meaningful feature correlations. Thus, to meet the goal of capturing disease features from the growing volume of health data, developing scalable approaches will become an integral part of a radiogenomics framework. In addition, such scalable techniques, under the theme of a big data strategy, are particularly useful in validating the generalized performance of the underlying relationships between image features and genomic signatures.

The use of radiogenomics for GBM empowers a bidirectional medical knowledge translation from imaging to genomics. Building upon the causal links between imaging features and genomic signatures, a non-invasive assessment can be readily made from imaging alone to identify, associate, and predict the underlying molecular events and disease pathways. The strategy of radiogenomics, towards unraveling the interrelationships between in the growing quantity of radiomics data, will continue to seek new evidence for better diagnosis, prognosis and therapeutic planning for patients with GBM and other cancers.

4 Radiomics in PET Imaging

The analysis process of radiomics in PET is similar to that of other imaging modalities, including tumor segmentation, feature extraction and the application of informatics analysis and data mining [32]. As is well known, the intra- and inter-tumoral genetic heterogeneity both within and between patients is one of the principles of radiomics. Specifically, malignant tumors correspond to cellular and molecular characteristics such as high cellular proliferation, necrosis, fibrosis, regions with angiogenesis, and the presence of specific receptors [27]. These characteristics show different metabolic characteristics. For example, cellular proliferation and angiogenesis indicate a strong metabolism, while necrosis and fibrosis indicate a weak metabolism. Compared to other imaging modalities, PET is famous for its ability to reflect the metabolic characteristics of tumors at the molecular level. Therefore, the heterogeneity could be well reflected in PET images, and a radiomics' analysis in PET has attracted much attention from scholars. Recently, a series of relevant studies has been published aiming at different cancers, including lung cancer [33, 164, 166], head and neck cancer [26, 46], cervical cancer [46, 114, 115, 180], esophageal cancer [42, 159, 162], sarcomas [44, 123, 124, 127], and other cancers [26, 172]. In this section, we will focus on the study of cervical cancer.

4.1 Cervical Cancer

According to the latest world cancer report published in 2014, cervical cancer was the third most common cancer with a high incidence rate (0.14‰), and the fourth most common cause of cancer death with a high mortality rate (0.068‰) among women worldwide in 2012 [23]. It is the most common cancer among women in 39 of 184 countries worldwide, and it is the leading cause of cancer death in women in 45 countries.

Cervical cancer originates at the site between the columnar epithelium of the endocervix and the squamous epithelium of the ectocervix, which is continuously changing. Human papillomavirus (HPV) infection in the epithelium, which is the most common sexually transmitted infection worldwide, may cause the development of precancerous lesions, a small part of which may deteriorate to invasive cervical cancer over a period of 10–20 years [23]. In addition, sexual activity starting at a young age (<16 years), having more than four sexual partners, continuous genital warts, and cigarette smoking (or exposure to passive smoke) all increase the risk of developing cervical cancer [152, 169].

Over 90% of cervical cancers are squamous cell carcinomas, and originate in the surface epithelium of the cervix. Approximately 5–9% of cervical cancers are adenocarcinomas that originate in the cervical glandular tissue. About 2–5% of cervical cancers are adenosquamous carcinoma, which is much less common. The remainder includes cervical sarcomas and small cell carcinoma of the cervix [170].

Once diagnosed with an invasive carcinoma, the patient should be staged immediately according to the FIGO staging system [129] (Table 2). Usually, the stage is determined clinically based primarily on the size of the tumor in the cervix and its extension into the pelvis at the time of the primary diagnosis, and should never be changed. The clinical stage is a reliable prognostic indicator for cervical cancer victims. Patients at stage IA have a 100% 5-year survival rate, with a rate of nearly 70–85% for patients at stage IB1. The 5-year disease-free survival is 50–70% for patients with tumors in stages IB2 and IIB, 30–50% for patients with tumors in stages III, and 5–15% for patients with tumors in stage IV [169]. In addition, accurate staging plays an important role in treatment planning. Patients receive different treatments according to the stage, as listed in Table 1. However, some quality-of-life issues should also be considered during the design of the treatment, and the assessment of the quality of life will be a particularly important part compared to radiotherapy with surgery alone or combined surgery and radiotherapy [65, 146].

A genetic analysis of cervical tumors has also been conducted [175], and validated mutations were detected in 60% of the cervical tumors (60%). The PIK3CA, KRAS, and EGFR genes had the highest mutation rates. In addition, KRAS mutations were identified only in adenocarcinomas (17.5% vs. 0%), a novel EGFR mutation was detected only in squamous cell carcinomas (0% vs. 7.5%), and PIK3CA mutations were associated with shorter survival.

4.2   Tumor Segmentation of Cervical Cancer

Compared to other tumors, cervical tumor segmentation faces more challenges. On the one hand, the tumor appears iso-attenuating to the normal cervical stroma on CT images [134], which means it is difficult to recognize the tumor from CT images. On the other hand, the urine in the adjacent bladder has a signal intensity similar to the tumor (or even higher than the tumor) on PET images [174], which means it is also difficult to isolate the tumor region from the effect of the bladder on PET images, as shown in Fig. 18.

Table 1 Treatment method for cervical cancer [169]

Stage	Description
0	Carcinoma-in-situ, intraepithelial carcinoma
I	The carcinoma is strictly confined to the cervix (extension to the uterine corpus should be disregarded)
IA	Invasive cancer identified only microscopically. (All gross lesions even with superficial invasion are stage IB cancers). Invasion is limited to measured stromal invasion with a maximum depth of 5 mm and a width no greater than 7 mm
IA1	Measured invasion of stroma ≤ 3 mm in depth and ≤ 7 mm in width
IA2	Measured invasion of stroma >3 mm and <5 mm in depth and ≤ 7 mm in width
IB	Clinical lesions confined to the cervix, or preclinical lesions greater than stage IA
IB1	Clinical lesions no greater than 4 cm in size
IB2	Clinical lesions >4 cm in size
II	The carcinoma extends beyond the uterus, but has not extended onto the pelvic wall or to the lower third of the vagina
IIA	The carcinoma extends beyond the uterus, but has not extended onto the pelvic wall or to the lower third of the vagina
IIA1	Clinically visible lesion ≤ 4 cm
IIA2	Clinically visible lesion >4 cm
IIB	Obvious parametrial involvement but not onto the pelvic sidewall
III	The carcinoma has extended onto the pelvic sidewall. On rectal examination, there is no cancer free space between the tumor and pelvic sidewall. The tumor involves the lower third of the vagina. All cases of hydronephrosis or non-functioning kidneys should be included unless they are known to be due to other causes
IIIA	Involvement of the lower vagina but no extension onto the pelvic sidewall
IIIB	Extension onto the pelvic sidewall, or hydronephrosis/non-functioning kidneys
IV	The carcinoma has extended beyond the true pelvis or has clinically involved the mucosa of the bladder and/or rectum
IVA	Spread to adjacent pelvic organs
IVB	Spread to distant organs

In most of the literature, the segmentation of the cervical tumor is based on traditional fixed-threshold-based segmentation techniques, and the commonly used thresholds is 40% of the SUVmax (the maximum SUV of the ROI) [119]. For cases where the segmentation results include the bladder, manual bladder elimination was needed [111].

Because that manual segmentation is subjective and time consuming, which is not suitable for the following feature extraction, many scholars have tried to develop an automatic or semiautomatic method to segment a cervical tumor.

Roman-Jimenez et al. [141] used the region-growing adaptive threshold (RGAT) method to obtain the likely tumoral region (LTR), which includes the bladder in many cases. Then, a fusion-and Gaussian-mixture-based classification (FGMC) method was proposed to separate the bladder and tumor. For each voxel selected in the LTR, three features were taken into consideration: the standard uptake value

Table 2 FIGO staging system for cervical cancer [129]

Stage	Clinical features	Treatment
IA1	Invasion ≤3 mm in depth	If patient desires fertility, conization of the cervix If she does not, simple hysterectomy (abdominal or vaginal)
	With lymph vascular space invasion	Hysterectomy with or without pelvic lymphadenectomy
IA2	3–5 mm invasion, ≤7 mm lateral spread	Radical hysterectomy with pelvic lymphadenectomy Radiotherapy
IB1	Tumor 4 cm or less	Radical hysterectomy with pelvic lymphadenectomy plus chemoradiotherapy for poor prognostic surgical-pathological factors* Radiotherapy
IB2	Tumor bigger than 4 cm	Radical hysterectomy with pelvic lymphadenectomy plus chemoradiotherapy for poor prognostic surgical and pathological factors* Chemoradiotherapy Chemoradiotherapy plus adjuvant hysterectomy
IIA	Upper-two-thirds vaginal involvement	Radical hysterectomy with pelvic lymphadenectomy Chemoradiotherapy
IIB	With parametrial extension	Chemoradiotherapy
IIIA	Low-third vaginal involvement	Chemoradiotherapy
IVA	Local extension with pelvis	Chemoradiotherapy Primary pelvic exenteration
IVB	Distant metastases	Palliative chemotherapy Chemoradiotherapy

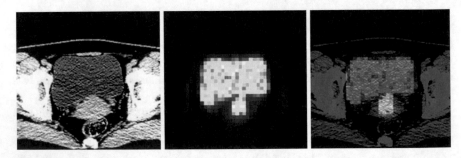

Fig. 18 CT, PET and their fusion images of cervical cancer

(SUV) on PET images, the Hounsfield unity value (HU) on CT images and a tumor membership probability (TMP). They defined TMP as follows:

$$TMP(x_i) = 1 - \frac{d(x_i, s)}{\max_i d(x_i, s)}$$

(4.1)

where $d(x_i, s)$ is the Euclidean distance of voxel x_i from seed s. A smaller TMP is associated with a lower probability of the voxel belonging to the tumor, based on the assumption that a voxel far away from the reference does not belong to the tumor. Then, using the Gaussian mixture model GMM, the LTR could be separated into two clusters, the bladder and tumor. It was necessary to decide whether to perform FGMC visually for each case when using this method and the chosen reference voxel seed, which was important because it may affect the final segmentation results.

Arbones et al. [25] applied a level set method based on the Chan-Vese (CV) model to delineate heterogeneous PET-positive areas. Then through iterative erosion with an increasing kernel shape and backtracking the kernel size process, the bladder could be detected and removed under the hypothesis that the bladder is the largest object [6]. It is worth noting that this method obtained better segmentation results for images with a high resolution.

Mu et al. [114, 115] proposed an automatic segmentation method based on tissue specificity and an improved level set method. First, a hyper-image represented by three features was constructed. The first feature was the SUV normalized to the maximum SUV in PET images. The second feature was the Hounsfield unit (HU) density values normalized to the maximum HU values in CT images, and the third feature was the product of the above two features. Then, according to the tissue specificity, this hyper-image could be divided into four parts, and the initial tumor could be extracted. Finally, a new evolution equation was constructed as follows:

$$\frac{\partial \phi(x)}{\partial t} = \left\{ -\lambda (I_\sigma - c_1)^2 + (I_\sigma - c_2)^2 \right\} \cdot \tanh \left(\cot <\nabla\phi(x), \nabla I_\sigma> \right) \cdot sgn(\delta_{\varepsilon_1}(\phi))$$

(4.2)

where I_σ represents the Gaussian filtered PET images using a Gaussian kernel with a standard deviation σ, $\lambda > 0$, $< * >$ stands for the angle between the two vectors (within the range of 0 to π), and $| * |$ stands for the magnitude of the vector. The definition of c_1 and c_2 can be represented as follows:

$$\begin{cases} c_1(\phi) = \dfrac{\int_\Omega I_\sigma(x, y, z) \cdot H_\varepsilon(\phi(x, y, z)) dxdydz}{\int_\Omega H_\varepsilon(\phi(x, y, z)) dxdydz} \\ c_2(\phi) = \dfrac{\int_\Omega I_\sigma(x, y, z) \cdot (1 - H_\varepsilon(\phi(x, y, z))) dxdydz}{\int_\Omega (1 - H_\varepsilon(\phi(x, y, z))) dxdydz} \end{cases}$$

(4.3)

This evolution guaranteed the accurate segmentation of a tumor without introducing the effect of the bladder.

So far, there is no certain segmentation method, and accurate cervical segmentation is still an open problem, which deserves a deeper investigation.

4.3 Tumor Characterization of Cervical Cancer

4.3.1 Standardized Uptake Value (SUV) Analysis

As most commonly used in clinical practice, SUV indices including the SUVmax, SUVmean and SUVpeak, which are measured for tumor volumes while normalizing the decay-corrected injected activity and the patient's weight on the PET examination date. To be more specific, SUVmax is obtained from one voxel with the maximum SUVvalue in the delineated tumor region, SUVmean represents the average SUV in the tumor region, and SUVpeak represents the local average within a small region (i.e. 26 neighbors in three dimensions) centered on the voxel with SUVmax.

The obvious disadvantage of SUVmax is that it could not characterize the total activity for the entire tumor, since a single voxel cannot reflect the heterogeneity of the entire tumor [140]. In addition, SUV is very sensitive to many different factors, such as the dependency on the time interval between injection and scanning, the image acquisition settings and the tumor segmentation methods [163].

4.3.2 Metabolic Tumor Volume (MTV) and Total Lesion Glycolysis (TLG) Analysis

In addition to SUV indices, the MTV and TLG (calculated as SUVmean × MTV) [93] have been widely reported in the literature. Based on their experiments, both of these indices performed much better in discrimination, prediction and prognostic evaluation than SUV alone [28, 76, 84, 104, 143]. However, the clinical significance of these parameters has not been established, and more prospective and large scale studies are required [140].

4.3.3 Textural Analysis

Recently, a large number of parameters for describing the heterogeneity of a tumor have also been proposed and validated. These could provide additional information associated with disease progression, response to therapy and the malignant behavior of a tumor compared to simple SUV-based measurements alone. In medical imaging, tumor heterogeneity is recorded as spatial variations in the intensity, which could be analyzed by using textural analysis.

The method for measuring heterogeneity could be divided into global, regional and local textural features representing the relationships between adjacent voxel intensities, and have long been used in other medical imaging files like CT and MRI files (parts 2 and 3). However their introduction to PET imaging was relatively late. The most commonly used statistical methods include first-order (one voxel), second-order (two voxel) and high-order (three or more voxels) parameters. Given that PET images are 3D images, we changed the traditional 2D texture features into 3D texture features.

First order features, calculated from the histogram, are the simplest global features. They only consider the statistical distribution of the intensity of each pixel and ignore the spatial relationships between voxels. The representative features include the mean, minimum, maximum, standard deviation (std), skewness, kurtosis and entropy.

Second order features describe local textural features that reflect the spatial relation of two adjacent pixels, and can be calculated using a spatial gray-level co-occurrence matrix (GLCM) [70]. For an n × m × p gray-level image I, the GLCM C could be defined as follows:

$$C_d(i,j,k) = \sum_{x=1}^{n} \sum_{y=1}^{m} \sum_{z=1}^{p} \begin{cases} 1 & \text{if } I(x,y,z) = i \text{ and } I(x+d_x, y+d_y, z+d_z) = j \\ 0 & \text{otherwise} \end{cases} \quad (4.4)$$

where d is the offset vector. GLCM has an important characteristic in that it is independent of the intensity transform [113]. The commonly used features based on GLCM include the average, variance, contrast, correlation, energy, entropy, homogeneity, intensity, dissimilarity and inverse difference moment (IDM). The 3D features of 3D images could be calculated similarly, and all of these features were the average value calculated from the GLCMs at 26 different directions.

High-order parameters can be calculated from the gray-level run length matrix (GLRLM) [50, 177], gray level size zone matrix (GLSZM) [160, 161] and neighborhood gray tone difference matrix (NGTDM) [5].

The GLRLM describes regional textural features. The element (i, j) of the GLRLM is defined as the number of runs with voxels of gray level i and run length j in the given direction. For 3D images, there are 26 directions in total. The commonly used features based on the GLRLM include the short run emphasis (SRE), long run emphasis (LRE), gray-level non-uniformity for run (GLNR), run length non-uniformity (RLN), run percentage (RP), low gray-level run emphasis (LGRE), high gray-level run emphasis (HGRE), short run low gray-level emphasis (SRLGE), short run high gray-level emphasis (SRHGE), long run low gray-level emphasis (LRLGE), and long run high gray-level emphasis (LRHGE). All of these features were the average values calculated from the GLRLMs at 26 different directions.

The GLSZM describes the flat zones, which are the connected regions of constant intensity in the image. The element (i, j) of the GLSZM is given by the number of the flat zones of size i and gray level j. Compared to the GLRLM, the

GLSZM does not require calculations in different directions. The commonly used features based on the GLSZM include the short zone emphasis (SZE), long zone emphasis (LZE), gray-level non-uniformity for zone (GLNZ), zone length non-uniformity (ZLN), zone percentage (ZP), low gray-level zone emphasis (LGZE), high gray-level zone emphasis (HGRE), short zone low gray-level emphasis (SZLGE), short zone high gray-level emphasis (SZHGE), long zone low gray-level emphasis (LZLGE), and long zone high gray-level emphasis (LZHGE).

The NGTDM reflects the amount of local intensity variation and intensity difference relative to the nearby voxels. For an n × m × p gray-level image I, the ith entry of NGTDM S could be calculated as the sum of the differences between the intensity i and the average intensity A_i over the neighboring pixels centered on the voxel with intensity i:

$$S(i) = \begin{cases} \sum |i - A_i| & \text{for } i \in N_i \text{ if } N_i \neq 0 \\ 0 & \text{otherwise} \end{cases} \tag{4.5}$$

where $\{N_i\}$ is the set of all pixels with gray level i, and

$$A_i = A(x, y, z) = \frac{1}{W - 1} \left[\sum_{m=-d}^{d} \sum_{n=-d}^{d} \sum_{p=-d}^{d} I(x+m, y+n, z+p) \right] \quad (m, n, p) \neq (0, 0, 0) \tag{4.6}$$

where d is the size of the neighborhood and $W = (2d + 1)^3$. The commonly used features based on the NGTDM include the coarseness, contrast, busyness, complexity and strength.

In addition to the previously mentioned statistical texture methods, other methods, such as the model-based method represented by the Markov random field (MRF) [71] and local binary pattern (LBP) [126], still exist and have some application.

4.4 Application of Informatics Analysis and Data Mining in Cervical Cancer

So far, the application of PET radiomics to cervical cancer has mainly focused on the treatment outcome prediction [46], cancer staging [114, 115], prognostic evaluation [112] and temporal analysis [180].

Usually, a statistical analysis is performed on the obtained features. Through a correlation analysis, the features could be divided into several groups, where the indices in the same group have high correlation coefficients and the indices in different groups are uncorrelated or have low correlation coefficients. This process of grouping helps us reduce redundant features in the following analysis.

The capacity of each feature at the baseline to distinguish patients with respect to the treatment outcome, cancer stage or survival could be investigated using the Receiver-operating-characteristic (ROC) Curves Analysis or ANOVA test.

Then, a series of multi-dimensional feature vectors could be constructed with different combinations of the selected optimal indices, and could be automatically classified by a trained SVM classifier [157] or other classifiers. Therefore, we could realize the automatic treatment outcome predication, cancer staging, etc.

Finally, for the prognostic evaluation and temporal analysis, the Kaplan-Meier method was used with the statistical significance assessed by using the log-rank test. It is worth noting that the best cutoff value for the Kaplan-Meier analysis could use the upper-left corner of the ROC.

Generally, the texture features perform much better in treatment outcome prediction, cancer staging, prognostic evaluation and temporal analysis compared to SUV alone.

4.5 Influencing Factors

It's worth mentioning some factors which may affect the final results need to be paid attention to during the process of radiomics analysis in PET images.

First, different textural features have been found to vary with the acquisition method (2D vs. 3D), matrix size (128 × 128 vs. 256 × 256), reconstruction algorithm, reconstruction settings and post-reconstruction filter. Galavis et al. found that the entropy, energy, maximal correlation coefficient and LGLRE exhibited small variations in analyses of adrenal gland carcinoma, lung, epiglottis, and esophageal cancer under different acquisition modes and reconstruction parameters [49]. Yan et al. found that the entropy, IDM, LGRE, HGRE and LGZE were the most robust features based on the analysis of different iteration numbers, FWHMs, and grid sizes using with lung cancer PET/CT images [178]. So far, there have been few studies on the synthetic assessment of all of the texture features for each kind of cancer under different acquisition methods, matrix sizes, reconstruction algorithms, reconstruction settings, and post-reconstruction filters, which play important roles in radiomics with PET. In addition, more robust features are desired.

Second, the discretization of SUV may also affect the texture feature. Leijienaar et al. compared the texture features calculated from discretized SUV using a fixed intensity resolution in SUV units with a fixed number of bins, and found that the manner of SUV discretization had a crucial effect on the resulting textural features [97]. Therefore, the robustness validation SUV discretization of different texture features is very important.

In addition, the image noise, test-retest reproducibility and reliability should also be considered in a radiomics' analysis of PET images.

References

1. Aerts, H.J., Velazquez, E.R., Leijenaar, R.T., Parmar, C., Grossmann, P., Cavalho, S., Bussink, J., Monshouwer, R., Haibe-Kains, B., Rietveld, D.: Decoding tumour phenotype by noninvasive imaging using a quantitative radiomics approach. Nat. Commun. **5** (2014)
2. Aerts, H.J., Velazquez, E.R., Leijenaar, R.T., Parmar, C., Grossmann, P., Cavalho, S., Bussink, J., Monshouwer, R., Haibe-Kains, B., Rietveld, D., Hoebers, F., Rietbergen, M.M., Leemans, C.R., Dekker, A., Quackenbush, J., Gillies, R.J., Lambin, P.: Decoding tumour phenotype by noninvasive imaging using a quantitative radiomics approach. Nat. Commun. **5**, 4006 (2014)
3. Agnihotri, S., Burrell, K.E., Wolf, A., Jalali, S., Hawkins, C., Rutka, J.T., Zadeh, G.: Glioblastoma, a brief review of history, molecular genetics, animal models and novel therapeutic strategies. Archivum Immunologiae Et Therapiae Experimentalis **61**(1), 25–41 (2013)
4. Al Gindi, A., Rashed, E., Sami, M.: Development and Evaluation of a computer-aided diagnostic algorithm for lung nodule characterization and classification in chest radiographs using multiscale wavelet transform. J. Am. Sci. **10**(2) (2014)
5. Amadasun, M., King, R.: Textural features corresponding to textural properties. IEEE Trans. Syst. Man Cybern. **19**(5), 1264–1274 (1989)
6. Arbonès, D.R., Jensen, H.G., Jakobsen, A.L., af Rosenschöld, P.M., Hansen, A.E., Igel, C., Darkner, S.: Automatic FDG-PET-based tumor and metastatic lymph node segmentation in cervical cancer. In: SPIE Medical Imaging. International Society for Optics and Photonics (2014)
7. Armato III, S.G., McLennan, G., Bidaut, L., McNitt-Gray, M.F., Meyer, C.R., Reeves, A.P., Zhao, B., Aberle, D.R., Henschke, C.I., Hoffman, E.A.: The lung image database consortium (LIDC) and image database resource initiative (IDRI): a completed reference database of lung nodules on CT scans. Med. Phys. **38**(2), 915–931 (2011)
8. Armato, S.G., Giger, M.L., MacMahon, H.: Automated detection of lung nodules in CT scans: preliminary results. Med. Phys. **28**(8), 1552–1561 (2001)
9. Armato, S.G., Sensakovic, W.F.: Automated lung segmentation for thoracic CT: impact on computer-aided diagnosis. Acad. Radiol. **11**(9), 1011–1021 (2004)
10. Athelogou, M., Schmidt, G., Schäpe, A., Baatz, M., Binnig, G.: Cognition Network Technology—A Novel Multimodal Image Analysis Technique for Automatic Identification and Quantification of Biological Image Contents. Springer, Berlin (2006)
11. Auffray, C., Sieweke, M.H., Geissmann, F.: Blood monocytes: development, heterogeneity, and relationship with dendritic cells. Annu. Rev. Immunol. **27**, 669–692 (2009)
12. Bach Cuadra, M., De Craene, M., Duay, V., Macq, B., Pollo, C., Thiran, J.P.: Dense deformation field estimation for atlas-based segmentation of pathological MR brain images. Comput. Methods Programs Biomed. **84**(2–3), 66–75 (2006)
13. Balagurunathan, Y., Gu, Y., Wang, H., Kumar, V., Grove, O., Hawkins, S., Kim, J., Goldgof, D.B., Hall, L.O., Gatenby, R.A., Gillies, R.J.: Reproducibility and prognosis of quantitative features extracted from CT images. Transl. Oncol. **7**(1), 72–87 (2014)
14. Bauer, S., Nolte, L.-P., Reyes, M.: Fully automatic segmentation of brain tumor images using support vector machine classification in combination with hierarchical conditional random field regularization. In: Fichtinger, G., Martel, A., Peters, T. (eds.) Medical Image Computing and Computer-Assisted Intervention—MICCAI 2011: 14th International Conference, Toronto, Canada, 18–22 Sept 2011, Proceedings, Part III, pp. 354–361. Springer, Berlin (2011)
15. Belden, C.J., Valdes, P.A., Ran, C., Pastel, D.A., Harris, B.T., Fadul, C.E., Israel, M.A., Paulsen, K., Roberts, D.W.: Genetics of glioblastoma: a window into its imaging and histopathologic variability. Radiographics **31**(6), 1717–1740 (2011)

16. Bendtsen, C., Kietzmann, M., Korn, R., Mozley, P.D., Schmidt, G., Binnig, G.: X-ray computed tomography: semiautomated volumetric analysis of late-stage lung tumors as a basis for response assessments. Int. J. Biomed. Imaging **2011**, 361589 (2011)

17. Bian, Z., Tan, W., Yang, J., Liu, J., Zhao, D.: Accurate airway centerline extraction based on topological thinning using graph-theoretic analysis. Biomed. Mater. Eng. **24**(6), 3239–3249 (2014)

18. Bocchino, C., Carabellese, A., Caruso, T., Della Sala, G., Ricart, S., Spinella, A.: Use of gray value distribution of run lengths for texture analysis. Pattern Recogn. Lett. **11**(6), 415–419 (1990)

19. Brett, M., Leff, A.P., Rorden, C., Ashburner, J.: Spatial normalization of brain images with focal lesions using cost function masking. NeuroImage **14**(2), 486–500 (2001)

20. by Haralick, R.M., Dinstein, I., Shanmugam, K.: Textural features for image classification. IEEE Trans. Syst. Man Cybern. (2012)

21. Cameron, A., Khalvati, F., Haider, M., Wong, A.: MAPS: A Quantitative Radiomics Approach for Prostate Cancer Detection (2015)

22. Campos, D.M., Simões, A., Ramos, I., Campilho, A.: Feature-Based Supervised Lung Nodule Segmentation **42**, 23–26 (2014)

23. Cancer, I. A. f. R. o.: World Cancer Report 2014. Lyon, International Agency for Research on Cancer Press (2014)

24. Candemir, S., Jaeger, S., Palaniappan, K., Musco, J.P., Singh, R.K., Zhiyun, X., Karargyris, A., Antani, S., Thoma, G., McDonald, C.J.: Lung segmentation in chest radiographs using anatomical atlases with nonrigid registration. IEEE Trans. Med. Imaging **33**(2), 577–590 (2014)

25. Chan, T.F., Vese, L.A.: Active contours without edges. IEEE Trans. Image Process. **10**(2), 266–277 (2001)

26. Cheng, N.-M., Fang, Y.-H.D., Chang, J.T.-C., Huang, C.-G., Tsan, D.-L., Ng, S.-H., Wang, H.-M., Lin, C.-Y., Liao, C.-T., Yen, T.-C.: Textural features of pretreatment 18F-FDG PET/CT images: prognostic significance in patients with advanced T-stage oropharyngeal squamous cell carcinoma. J. Nucl. Med. **54**(10), 1703–1709 (2013)

27. Chicklore, S., Goh, V., Siddique, M., Roy, A., Marsden, P.K., Cook, G.J.: Quantifying tumour heterogeneity in 18F-FDG PET/CT imaging by texture analysis. Eur. J. Nucl. Med. Mol. Imaging **40**(1), 133–140 (2013)

28. Choi, E.-S., Ha, S.-G., Kim, H.-S., Ha, J.H., Paeng, J.C., Han, I.: Total lesion glycolysis by 18F-FDG PET/CT is a reliable predictor of prognosis in soft-tissue sarcoma. Eur. J. Nucl. Med. Mol. Imaging **40**(12), 1836–1842 (2013)

29. Clark, K., Vendt, B., Smith, K., Freymann, J., Kirby, J., Koppel, P., Moore, S., Phillips, S., Maffitt, D., Pringle, M.: The Cancer Imaging Archive (TCIA): maintaining and operating a public information repository. J. Digit. Imaging **26**(6), 1045–1057 (2013)

30. Clark, M.C., Hall, L.O., Goldgof, D.B., Velthuizen, R., Murtagh, F.R., Silbiger, M.S.: Automatic tumor segmentation using knowledge-based techniques. IEEE Trans. Med. Imaging **17**(2), 187–201 (1998)

31. Cobzas, D., Schmidt, M.: Increased discrimination in level set methods with embedded conditional random fields. In: IEEE Conference on Computer Vision and Pattern Recognition, 2009. CVPR 2009 (2009)

32. Cook, G.J., Siddique, M., Taylor, B.P., Yip, C., Chicklore, S., Goh, V.: Radiomics in PET: principles and applications. Clin. Transl. Imaging **2**(3), 269–276 (2014)

33. Cook, G.J., Yip, C., Siddique, M., Goh, V., Chicklore, S., Roy, A., Marsden, P., Ahmad, S., Landau, D.: Are pretreatment 18F-FDG PET tumor textural features in non-small cell lung cancer associated with response and survival after chemoradiotherapy? J. Nucl. Med. **54**(1), 19–26 (2013)

34. Coroller, T.P., Grossmann, P., Hou, Y., Velazquez, E.R., Leijenaar, R.T., Hermann, G., Lambin, P., Haibe-Kains, B., Mak, R.H., Aerts, H.J.: CT-based radiomic signature predicts distant metastasis in lung adenocarcinoma. Radiother. Oncol. **114**(3), 345–350 (2015)

35. Corso, J.J., Sharon, E., Dube, S., El-Saden, S., Sinha, U., Yuille, A.: Efficient multilevel brain tumor segmentation with integrated Bayesian model classification. IEEE Trans. Med. Imaging **27**(5), 629–640 (2008)
36. Dasarathy, B.V., Holder, E.B.: Image characterizations based on joint gray level—run length distributions. Pattern Recogn. Lett. **12**(8), 497–502 (1991)
37. de Carvalho Filho, A.O., de Sampaio, W.B., Silva, A.C., de Paiva, A.C., Nunes, R.A., Gattass, M.: Automatic detection of solitary lung nodules using quality threshold clustering, genetic algorithm and diversity index. Artif. Intell. Med. **60**(3), 165–177 (2014)
38. Diciotti, S., Lombardo, S., Falchini, M., Picozzi, G., Mascalchi, M.: Automated segmentation refinement of small lung nodules in CT scans by local shape analysis. IEEE Trans. Biomed. Eng. **58**(12), 3418–3428 (2011)
39. Diciotti, S., Picozzi, G., Falchini, M., Mascalchi, M., Villari, N., Valli, G.: 3-D segmentation algorithm of small lung nodules in spiral CT images. IEEE Trans. Inf. Technol. Biomed. **12** (1), 7–19 (2008)
40. Doi, K.: Computer-aided diagnosis in medical imaging: historical review, current status and future potential. Comput. Med. Imaging Graph. **31**(4), 198–211 (2007)
41. Doi, K.: Current status and future potential of computer-aided diagnosis in medical imaging. Br. J. Radiol. (2014)
42. Dong, X., Xing, L., Wu, P., Fu, Z., Wan, H., Li, D., Yin, Y., Sun, X., Yu, J.: Three-dimensional positron emission tomography image texture analysis of esophageal squamous cell carcinoma: relationship between tumor 18F-fluorodeoxyglucose uptake heterogeneity, maximum standardized uptake value, and tumor stage. Nucl. Med. Commun. **34**(1), 40–46 (2013)
43. Dunn, G.P., Rinne, M.L., Jill, W., Giannicola, G., Quayle, S.N., Dunn, I.F., Agarwalla, P.K., Chheda, M.G., Benito, C., Alan, W.: Emerging insights into the molecular and cellular basis of glioblastoma. Genes Dev. **26**(8), 756–784 (2012)
44. Eary, J.F., O'Sullivan, F., O'Sullivan, J., Conrad, E.U.: Spatial heterogeneity in sarcoma 18F-FDG uptake as a predictor of patient outcome. J. Nucl. Med. **49**(12), 1973–1979 (2008)
45. El-Baz, A., Nitzken, M., Khalifa, F., Elnakib, A., Gimel'farb, G., Falk, R., El-Ghar, M.A.: 3D shape analysis for early diagnosis of malignant lung nodules. In: Information Processing in Medical Imaging. Springer (2011)
46. El Naqa, I., Grigsby, P., Apte, A., Kidd, E., Donnelly, E., Khullar, D., Chaudhari, S., Yang, D., Schmitt, M., Laforest, R.: Exploring feature-based approaches in PET images for predicting cancer treatment outcomes. Pattern Recogn. **42**(6), 1162–1171 (2009)
47. Farag, A.A., Abd El Munim, H.E., Graham, J.H., Farag, A.A.: A novel approach for lung nodules segmentation in chest CT using level sets. IEEE Trans. Image Process. **22**(12), 5202–5213 (2013)
48. Görlitz, L., Menze, B.H., Weber, M.-A., Kelm, B.M., Hamprecht, F.A.: Semi-supervised tumor detection in magnetic resonance spectroscopic images using discriminative random fields. In: Hamprecht, F.A., Schnörr, C., Jähne, B. (eds.) Pattern Recognition: 29th DAGM Symposium, Heidelberg, Germany, 12–14 Sept 2007. Proceedings, pp. 224–233. Springer, Berlin (2007)
49. Galavis, P.E., Hollensen, C., Jallow, N., Paliwal, B., Jeraj, R.: Variability of textural features in FDG PET images due to different acquisition modes and reconstruction parameters. Acta Oncol. **49**(7), 1012–1016 (2010)
50. Galloway, M.M.: Texture analysis using gray level run lengths. Comput. Graph. Image Process. **4**(2), 172–179 (1975)
51. Ganesan, K., Acharya, U., Chua, C.K., Min, L.C., Abraham, K.T., Ng, K.B.: Computer-aided breast cancer detection using mammograms: a review. IEEE Rev. Biomed. Eng. **6**, 77–98 (2013)
52. Ganeshan, B., Goh, V., Mandeville, H.C., Ng, Q.S., Hoskin, P.J., Miles, K.A.: Non-small cell lung cancer: histopathologic correlates for texture parameters at CT. Radiology **266**(1), 326–336 (2013)

53. Ganeshan, B., Panayiotou, E., Burnand, K., Dizdarevic, S., Miles, K.: Tumour heterogeneity in non-small cell lung carcinoma assessed by CT texture analysis: a potential marker of survival. Eur. Radiol. **22**(4), 796–802 (2012)
54. Ganeshan, B., Skogen, K., Pressney, I., Coutroubis, D., Miles, K.: Tumour heterogeneity in oesophageal cancer assessed by CT texture analysis: preliminary evidence of an association with tumour metabolism, stage, and survival. Clin. Radiol. **67**(2), 157–164 (2012)
55. Gatenby, R.A., Grove, O., Gillies, R.J.: Quantitative imaging in cancer evolution and ecology. Radiology **269**(1), 8–14 (2013)
56. Gerlinger, M., Rowan, A.J., Horswell, S., Larkin, J., Endesfelder, D., Gronroos, E., Martinez, P., Matthews, N., Stewart, A., Tarpey, P., Varela, I., Phillimore, B., Begum, S., McDonald, N.Q., Butler, A., Jones, D., Raine, K., Latimer, C., Santos, C.R., Nohadani, M., Eklund, A.C., Spencer-Dene, B., Clark, G., Pickering, L., Stamp, G., Gore, M., Szallasi, Z., Downward, J., Futreal, P.A., Swanton, C.: Intratumor heterogeneity and branched evolution revealed by multiregion sequencing. N. Engl. J. Med. **366**(10), 883–892 (2012)
57. Gevaert, O., Xu, J., Hoang, C.D., Leung, A.N., Xu, Y., Quon, A., Rubin, D.L., Napel, S., Plevritis, S.K.: Non-small cell lung cancer: identifying prognostic imaging biomarkers by leveraging public gene expression microarray data–methods and preliminary results. Radiology **264**(2), 387–396 (2012)
58. Giger, M., MacMahon, H.: Image processing and computer-aided diagnosis. Radiol. Clin. North Am. **34**(3), 565–596 (1996)
59. Gillies, R.J., Kinahan, P.E., Hricak, H.: Radiomics: images are more than pictures, they are data. Radiology 151169 (2015)
60. Glasser, O., Tucker, J.C., Boveri, M.: Wilhelm Conrad Röntgen and the Early History of the Roentgen Rays. C. C. Thomas, Springfield, IL (1934)
61. Glover, G.H.: Abstract: MRI: basic principles and future potential. Comput. Aided Surg. **5** (2), 132 (2000)
62. Goh, V., Ganeshan, B., Nathan, P., Juttla, J.K., Vinayan, A., Miles, K.A.: Assessment of response to tyrosine kinase inhibitors in metastatic renal cell cancer: CT texture as a predictive biomarker. Radiology **261**(1), 165–171 (2011)
63. Golosio, B., Masala, G.L., Piccioli, A., Oliva, P., Carpinelli, M., Cataldo, R., Cerello, P., De Carlo, F., Falaschi, F., Fantacci, M.E., Gargano, G., Kasae, P., Torsello, M.: A novel multithreshold method for nodule detection in lung CT. Med. Phys. **36**(8), 3607–3618 (2009)
64. Gooya, A., Pohl, K.M., Bilello, M., Biros, G., Davatzikos, C.: Joint segmentation and deformable registration of brain scans guided by a tumor growth model. In: Fichtinger, G., Martel, A., Peters, T. (eds.) Medical Image Computing and Computer-Assisted Intervention —MICCAI 2011: 14th International Conference, Toronto, Canada, 18–22 Sept 2011, Proceedings, Part II, pp. 532–540. Springer, Berlin (2011)
65. Greimel, E., Thiel, I., Peintinger, F., Cegnar, I., Pongratz, E.: Prospective assessment of quality of life of female cancer patients. Gynecol. Oncol. **85**(1), 140–147 (2002)
66. Grove, O., Berglund, A.E., Schabath, M.B., Aerts, H.J., Dekker, A., Wang, H., Velazquez, E.R., Lambin, P., Gu, Y., Balagurunathan, Y.: Quantitative computed tomographic descriptors associate tumor shape complexity and intratumor heterogeneity with prognosis in lung adenocarcinoma. PloS one **10**(3) (2015)
67. Gu, Y., Kumar, V., Hall, L.O., Goldgof, D.B., Li, C.-Y., Korn, R., Bendtsen, C., Velazquez, E.R., Dekker, A., Aerts, H.: Automated delineation of lung tumors from CT images using a single click ensemble segmentation approach. Pattern Recogn. **46**(3), 692–702 (2013)
68. Gutman, D.A., Cooper, L.A.D., Hwang, S.N., Holder, C.A., Jingjing, G., Aurora, T.D., Dunn, W.D., Lisa, S., Tom, M., Rajan, J.: MR imaging predictors of molecular profile and survival: multi-institutional study of the TCGA glioblastoma data set. Radiology **267**(2), 560–569 (2013)
69. Han, F., Wang, H., Zhang, G., Han, H., Song, B., Li, L., Moore, W., Lu, H., Zhao, H., Liang, Z.: Texture feature analysis for computer-aided diagnosis on pulmonary nodules. J. Digit. Imaging **28**(1), 99–115 (2015)

70. Haralick, R.M., Shanmugam, K., Dinstein, I.H.: Textural Features for Image Classification. IEEE Trans. Syst. Man Cybern. **SMC-3**(6), 610–621 (1973)
71. Hassner, M., Sklansky, J.: The use of Markov random fields as models of texture. Comput. Graph. Image Process. **12**(4), 357–370 (1980)
72. Hegi, M.E.: MGMT gene silencing and benefit from temozolomide in glioblastoma. Dkgest World Latest Med. Inf. **352**(10), 997–1003 (2005)
73. Hu, S.Y., Hoffman, E.A., Reinhardt, J.M.: Automatic lung segmentation for accurate quantitation of volumetric X-ray CT images. IEEE Trans. Med. Imaging **20**(6), 490–498 (2001)
74. Hu, Z., Zou, J., Gui, J., Rong, J., Zhang, Q., Xia, D., Zheng, H.: geometric calibration based on identification of ellipse parameters of a micro-CT system for small-animal imaging. Sens. Lett. **9**(5), 1938–1942 (2011)
75. Huang, R.Y., Neagu, M.R., Reardon, D.A., Wen, P.Y.: Pitfalls in the neuroimaging of glioblastoma in the era of antiangiogenic and immuno/targeted therapy—detecting illusive disease, defining response. Front. Neurol. **6**, 33 (2015)
76. Hyun, S.H., Ahn, H.K., Kim, H., Ahn, M.-J., Park, K., Ahn, Y.C., Kim, J., Shim, Y.M., Choi, J.Y.: Volume-based assessment by 18F-FDG PET/CT predicts survival in patients with stage III non-small-cell lung cancer. Eur. J. Nucl. Med. Mol. Imaging **41**(1), 50–58 (2014)
77. Itakura, H., Achrol, A.S., Mitchell, L.A., Loya, J.J., Liu, T., Westbroek, E.M., Feroze, A.H., Rodriguez, S., Echegaray, S., Azad, T.D.: Magnetic resonance image features identify glioblastoma phenotypic subtypes with distinct molecular pathway activities. Sci. Trans. Med. **7**(303) (2015)
78. Jain, R., Poisson, L., Narang, J., Gutman, D., Scarpace, L., Hwang, S.N., Holder, C., Wintermark, M., Colen, R.R., Kirby, J., Freymann, J., Brat, D.J., Jaffe, C., Mikkelsen, T.: Genomic mapping and survival prediction in glioblastoma: molecular subclassification strengthened by hemodynamic imaging biomarkers. Radiology **267**(1), 212–220 (2013)
79. Jalalian, A., Mashohor, S.B., Mahmud, H.R., Saripan, M.I.B., Ramli, A.R.B., Karasfi, B.: Computer-aided detection/diagnosis of breast cancer in mammography and ultrasound: a review. Clin. Imaging **37**(3), 420–426 (2013)
80. Jiang, Y., Nishikawa, R.M., Schmidt, R.A., Metz, C.E., Giger, M.L., Doi, K.: Improving breast cancer diagnosis with computer-aided diagnosis. Acad. Radiol. **6**(1), 22–33 (1999)
81. Kakar, M., Olsen, D.R.: Automatic segmentation and recognition of lungs and lesion from CT scans of thorax. Comput. Med. Imaging Graph. **33**(1), 72–82 (2009)
82. Kapur, T., Grimson, W.E.L., Wells Iii, W.M., Kikinis, R.: Segmentation of brain tissue from magnetic resonance images. Med. Image Anal. **1**(2), 109–127 (1996)
83. Karlo, C.A., Pier Luigi, D.P., Joshua, C., Ari, H.A., Irina, O., Paul, R., Hedvig, H., Robert, M., Hsieh, J.J., Oguz, A.: Radiogenomics of clear cell renal cell carcinoma: associations between CT imaging features and mutations. Radiology **270**(2), 464–471 (2014)
84. Klabatsa, A., Chicklore, S., Barrington, S.F., Goh, V., Lang-Lazdunski, L., Cook, G.J.: The association of 18F-FDG PET/CT parameters with survival in malignant pleural mesothelioma. Eur. J. Nucl. Med. Mol. Imaging **41**(2), 276–282 (2014)
85. Krizhevsky, A., Sutskever, I., Hinton, G.E.: Imagenet classification with deep convolutional neural networks. Adv. Neural Inf. Process. Syst. (2012)
86. Kubota, T., Jerebko, A.K., Dewan, M., Salganicoff, M., Krishnan, A.: Segmentation of pulmonary nodules of various densities with morphological approaches and convexity models. Med. Image Anal. **15**(1), 133–154 (2011)
87. Kumar, D., Shafiee, M.J., Chung, A.G., Khalvati, F., Haider, M.A., Wong, A.: Discovery Radiomics for Computed Tomography Cancer Detection. arXiv preprint arXiv:1509.00117 (2015)
88. Kumar, V., Gu, Y., Basu, S., Berglund, A., Eschrich, S.A., Schabath, M.B., Forster, K., Aerts, H.J., Dekker, A., Fenstermacher, D.: Radiomics: the process and the challenges. Magn. Reson. Imaging **30**(9), 1234–1248 (2012)

89. Kuo, M.D., Neema, J.: Behind the numbers: decoding molecular phenotypes with radiogenomics–guiding principles and technical considerations. Radiology 270(2), 320–325 (2014)

90. Kuo, W.-J., Chang, R.-F., Chen, D.-R., Lee, C.C.: Data mining with decision trees for diagnosis of breast tumor in medical ultrasonic images. Breast Cancer Res. Treat. 66(1), 51–57 (2001)

91. Kyriacou, S.K., Davatzikos, C., Zinreich, S.J., Bryan, R.N.: Nonlinear elastic registration of brain images with tumor pathology using a biomechanical model [MRI]. IEEE Trans. Med. Imaging 18(7), 580–592 (1999)

92. Lambin, P., Rios-Velazquez, E., Leijenaar, R., Carvalho, S., van Stiphout, R.G., Granton, P., Zegers, C.M., Gillies, R., Boellard, R., Dekker, A.: Radiomics: extracting more information from medical images using advanced feature analysis. Eur. J. Cancer 48(4), 441–446 (2012)

93. Larson, S.M., Erdi, Y., Akhurst, T., Mazumdar, M., Macapinlac, H.A., Finn, R.D., Casilla, C., Fazzari, M., Srivastava, N., Yeung, H.W.: Tumor treatment response based on visual and quantitative changes in global tumor glycolysis using PET-FDG imaging: the visual response score and the change in total lesion glycolysis. Clin. Positron Imaging 2(3), 159–171 (1999)

94. Lassen, B., van Rikxoort, E.M., Schmidt, M., Kerkstra, S., van Ginneken, B., Kuhnigk, J.M.: Automatic segmentation of the pulmonary lobes from chest CT scans based on fissures, vessels, and bronchi. IEEE Trans. Med. Imaging 32(2), 210–222 (2013)

95. LeCun, Y., Bottou, L., Bengio, Y., Haffner, P.: Gradient-based learning applied to document recognition. Proc. IEEE 86(11), 2278–2324 (1998)

96. Lee, C.-H., Schmidt, M., Murtha, A., Bistritz, A., Sander, J., Greiner, R.: Segmenting brain tumors with conditional random fields and support vector machines. In: Liu, Y., Jiang, T., Zhang, C. (eds.) Computer Vision for Biomedical Image Applications: First International Workshop, CVBIA 2005, Beijing, China, 21 Oct 2005. Proceedings, pp. 469–478. Springer, Berlin (2005)

97. Leijenaar, R.T., Nalbantov, G., Carvalho, S., van Elmpt, W.J., Troost, E.G., Boellaard, R., Aerts, H.J., Gillies, R.J., Lambin, P.: The effect of SUV discretization in quantitative FDG-PET Radiomics: the need for standardized methodology in tumor texture analysis. Sci. Rep. 5 (2015)

98. Li, M., Zhou, Z.-H.: Improve computer-aided diagnosis with machine learning techniques using undiagnosed samples. IEEE Trans. Syst. Man Cybern. Part A: Syst. Hum. 37(6), 1088–1098 (2007)

99. Liang, W., Zhang, L., Jiang, G., Wang, Q., Liu, L., Liu, D., Wang, Z., Zhu, Z., Deng, Q., Xiong, X., Shao, W., Shi, X., He, J.: Development and validation of a nomogram for predicting survival in patients with resected non-small-cell lung cancer. J. Clin. Oncol. 33(8), 861–869 (2015)

100. Liu, J., Udupa, J.K., Odhner, D., Hackney, D., Moonis, G.: A system for brain tumor volume estimation via MR imaging and fuzzy connectedness. Comput. Med. Imaging Graph. 29(1), 21–34 (2005)

101. Louis, D.N., Ohgaki, H., Wiestler, O.D., Cavenee, W.K., Burger, P.C., Jouvet, A., Scheithauer, B.W., Kleihues, P.: The 2007 WHO classification of tumours of the central nervous system. Acta Neuropathol. 114(2), 97–109 (2007)

102. Macyszyn, L., Akbari, H., Pisapia, J.M., Da, X., Attiah, M., Pigrish, V., Bi, Y., Pal, S., Davuluri, R.V., Roccograndi, I.: 135 imaging patterns predict patient survival and molecular subtype in glioblastoma using machine learning techniques. Neurosurgery 62 (Suppl 1) (2015). Clinical Neurosurgery

103. Madabhushi, A., Metaxas, D.N.: Combining low-, high-level and empirical domain knowledge for automated segmentation of ultrasonic breast lesions. IEEE Trans. Med. Imaging 22(2), 155–169 (2003)

104. Maffione, A.M., Ferretti, A., Grassetto, G., Bellan, E., Capirci, C., Chondrogiannis, S., Gava, M., Marzola, M.C., Rampin, L., Bondesan, C.: Fifteen different 18F-FDG PET/CT qualitative and quantitative parameters investigated as pathological response predictors of

locally advanced rectal cancer treated by neoadjuvant chemoradiation therapy. Eur. J. Nucl. Med. Mol. Imaging **40**(6), 853–864 (2013)

105. Mandeville, H.C., Ng, Q.S., Daley, F.M., Barber, P.R., Pierce, G., Finch, J., Burke, M., Bell, A., Townsend, E.R., Kozarski, R., Vojnovic, B., Hoskin, P.J., Goh, V.: Operable non-small cell lung cancer: correlation of volumetric helical dynamic contrast-enhanced CT parameters with immunohistochemical markers of tumor hypoxia. Radiology **264**(2), 581–589 (2012)

106. Mansoor, A., Bagci, U., Xu, Z.Y., Foster, B., Olivier, K.N., Elinoff, J.M., Suffredini, A.F., Udupa, J.K., Mollura, D.J.: A generic approach to pathological lung segmentation (vol. 33, p. 2293, 2014). IEEE Trans. Med. Imaging **34**(1), 354–354 (2015)

107. Maximilian, D., Christine, N., Wang, D.S., Susan, M.G., Mahesh, J., Yu, L., Kenneth, A., Soonmee, C., Kuo, M.D.: Identification of noninvasive imaging surrogates for brain tumor gene-expression modules. Proc. Natl. Acad. Sci. U.S.A. **105**(13), 5213–5218 (2008)

108. McNitt-Gray, M.F., Armato, S.G., Meyer, C.R., Reeves, A.P., McLennan, G., Pais, R.C., Freymann, J., Brown, M.S., Engelmann, R.M., Bland, P.H.: The Lung Image Database Consortium (LIDC) data collection process for nodule detection and annotation. Acad. Radiol. **14**(12), 1464–1474 (2007)

109. Menze, B.H., Leemput, K., Lashkari, D., Weber, M.-A., Ayache, N., Golland, P.: A generative model for brain tumor segmentation in multi-modal images. In: Jiang, T., Navab, N., Pluim, J.P.W., Viergever, M.A.: Medical Image Computing and Computer-Assisted Intervention—MICCAI 2010: 13th International Conference, Beijing, China, 20–24 Sept 2010, Proceedings, Part II, pp. 151–159. Springer, Berlin (2010)

110. Messay, T., Hardie, R.C., Rogers, S.K.: A new computationally efficient CAD system for pulmonary nodule detection in CT imagery. Med. Image Anal. **14**(3), 390–406 (2010)

111. Miller, T.R., Grigsby, P.W.: Measurement of tumor volume by PET to evaluate prognosis in patients with advanced cervical cancer treated by radiation therapy. Int. J. Radiat. Oncol. Biol. Phys. **53**(2), 353–359 (2002)

112. Miller, T.R., Pinkus, E., Dehdashti, F., Grigsby, P.W.: Improved prognostic value of 18F-FDG PET using a simple visual analysis of tumor characteristics in patients with cervical cancer. J. Nucl. Med. **44**(2), 192–197 (2003)

113. Mohamed, S., Youssef, A., El-Saadany, E., Salama, M.M.: Prostate tissue characterization using TRUS image spectral features, pp. 589–601. Springer, Image Anal. Recogn. (2006)

114. Mu, W., Chen, Z., Liang, Y., Shen, W., Yang, F., Dai, R., Wu, N., Tian, J.: Staging of cervical cancer based on tumor heterogeneity characterized by texture features on 18F-FDG PET images. Phys. Med. Biol. **60**(13), 5123 (2015)

115. Mu, W., Chen, Z., Shen, W., Yang, F., Liang, Y., Dai, R., Wu, N., Tian, J.: A Segmentation Algorithm for Quantitative Analysis of Heterogeneous Tumors of the Cervix with 18F-FDG PET/CT (2015)

116. Murphy, K., van Ginneken, B., Schilham, A.M.R., de Hoop, B.J., Gietema, H.A., Prokop, M.: A large-scale evaluation of automatic pulmonary nodule detection in chest CT using local image features and k-nearest-neighbour classification. Med. Image Anal. **13**(5), 757–770 (2009)

117. Nair, V.S., Gevaert, O., Davidzon, G., Napel, S., Graves, E.E., Hoang, C.D., Shrager, J.B., Quon, A., Rubin, D.L., Plevritis, S.K.: Prognostic PET 18F-FDG uptake imaging features are associated with major oncogenomic alterations in patients with resected non-small cell lung cancer. Cancer Res. **72**(15), 3725–3734 (2012)

118. Neema, J., Maximilian, D., Markus, B., Kuo, M.D.: Illuminating radiogenomic character-istics of glioblastoma multiforme through integration of MR imaging, messenger RNA expression, and DNA copy number variation. Radiology **270**(1), 212–222 (2014)

119. Nestle, U., Kremp, S., Grosu, A.-L.: Practical integration of [18F]-FDG-PET and PET-CT in the planning of radiotherapy for non-small cell lung cancer (NSCLC): the technical basis, ICRU-target volumes, problems, perspectives. Radiother. Oncol. **81**(2), 209–225 (2006)

120. Ng, A.Y., Jordan, M.I.: On discriminative vs. generative classifiers: a comparison of logistic regression and naive Bayes. Adv. Neural. Inf. Process. Syst. **28**(3), 169–187 (2001)

121. Ng, F., Ganeshan, B., Kozarski, R., Miles, K.A., Goh, V.: Assessment of primary colorectal cancer heterogeneity by using whole-tumor texture analysis: contrast-enhanced CT texture as a biomarker of 5-year survival. Radiology 266(1), 177–184 (2013)
122. Nishizuka, Y.: The molecular heterogeneity of protein kinase C and its implications for cellular regulation. Nature 334(6184), 661–665 (1988)
123. O'Sullivan, F., Roy, S., O'Sullivan, J., Vernon, C., Eary, J.: Incorporation of tumor shape into an assessment of spatial heterogeneity for human sarcomas imaged with FDG-PET. Biostatistics 6(2), 293–301 (2005)
124. O'Sullivan, F., Wolsztynski, E., O'Sullivan, J., Richards, T., Conrad, E., Eary, J.: A statistical modeling approach to the analysis of spatial patterns of FDG-PET uptake in human sarcoma. IEEE Trans. Med. Imag. 30(12), 2059–2071 (2011)
125. Ohgaki, H., Kleihues, P.: Population-based studies on incidence, survival rates, and genetic alterations in astrocytic and oligodendroglial gliomas. J. Neuropathol. Exp. Neurol. 64(6), 479–489 (2005)
126. Ojala, T., Pietikäinen, M., Mäenpää, T.: Multiresolution gray-scale and rotation invariant texture classification with local binary patterns. IEEE Trans. Pattern Anal. Mach. Intell. 24 (7), 971–987 (2002)
127. Okazumi, S., Dimitrakopoulou-Strauss, A., Schwarzbach, M., Strauss, L.G.: Quantitative, dynamic 18F-FDG-PET for the evaluation of soft tissue sarcomas: relation to differential diagnosis, tumor grading and prediction of prognosis. Hellenic J. Nucl. Med. 12(3), 223–228 (2008)
128. Olivier, G., Mitchell, L.A., Achrol, A.S., Jiajing, X., Sebastian, E., Steinberg, G.K., Cheshier, S.H., Sandy, N., Greg, Z., Plevritis, S.K.: Glioblastoma multiforme: exploratory radiogenomic analysis by using quantitative image features. Radiology 276(1), 168–174 (2015)
129. Oncology, F. C. o. G.: FIGO staging for carcinoma of the vulva, cervix, and corpus uteri. Int. J. Gynecol. Obstet. 125(2), 97–98 (2014)
130. Oransky, I.: Sir Godfrey N. Hounsfield. Lancet 364(9439), 1032 (2004)
131. Orban, G., Horvath, G.: Lung nodule detection on digital tomosynthesis images: a preliminary study. In: 2014 IEEE 11th International Symposium on Biomedical Imaging (ISBI). IEEE (2014)
132. Ostrom, Q.T., Gittleman, H., Farah, P., Ondracek, A., Chen, Y.W., Wolinsky, Y., Stroup, N. E., Kruchko, C., Barnholtz-Sloan, J.S.: CBTRUS statistical report: primary brain and central nervous system tumors diagnosed in the United States in 2006–2010. Neuro Oncol. 15, 1–56 (2013)
133. Ozkan, E., West, A., Dedelow, J.A., Chu, B.F., Zhao, W., Yildiz, V.O., Otterson, G.A., Shilo, K., Ghosh, S., King, M.: CT gray-level texture analysis as a quantitative imaging biomarker of epidermal growth factor receptor mutation status in adenocarcinoma of the lung. Am. J. Roentgenol. 205(5), 1016–1025 (2015)
134. Pannu, H.K., Corl, F.M., Fishman, E.K.: CT evaluation of cervical cancer: spectrum of disease 1. Radiographics 21(5), 1155–1168 (2001)
135. Parmar, C., Leijenaar, R.T., Grossmann, P., Velazquez, E.R., Bussink, J., Rietveld, D., Rietbergen, M.M., Haibe-Kains, B., Lambin, P., Aerts, H.J.: Radiomic feature clusters and prognostic signatures specific for lung and head & neck cancer. Sci. Rep. 5 (2015)
136. Phillips, H.S., Kharbanda, S., Chen, R., Forrest, W.F., Soriano, R.H., Wu, T.D., Misra, A. Nigro, J.M., Colman, H., Soroceanu, L., Williams, P.M., Modrusan, Z., Feuerstein, B.G., Aldape, K.: Molecular subclasses of high-grade glioma predict prognosis, delineate a pattern of disease progression, and resemble stages in neurogenesis. Cancer Cell 9(3), 157–173 (2006)
137. Pignon, J.P., Tribodet, H., Scagliotti, G.V., Douillard, J.Y., Shepherd, F.A., Stephens, R.J., Dunant, A., Torri, V., Rosell, R., Seymour, L., Spiro, S.G., Rolland, E., Fossati, R., Aubert, D., Ding, K., Waller, D., Le Chevalier, T., L. C. Group: Lung adjuvant cisplatin evaluation: a pooled analysis by the LACE Collaborative Group. J. Clin. Oncol. 26(21), 3552–3559 (2008)

138. Pohl, K.M., Fisher, J., Levitt, J.J., Shenton, M.E., Kikinis, R., Grimson, W.E.L., Wells, W. M.: A unifying approach to registration, segmentation, and intensity correction. In: Duncan, J.S., Gerig, G. (eds.) Medical Image Computing and Computer-Assisted Intervention— MICCAI 2005: 8th International Conference, Palm Springs, CA, USA, 26–29 Oct 2005, Proceedings, Part I, pp. 310–318. Springer, Berlin (2005)

139. Prastawa, M., Bullitt, E., Moon, N., Van Leemput, K., Gerig, G.: Automatic brain tumor segmentation by subject specific modification of atlas priors. Acad. Radiol. **10**(12), 1341–1348 (2003)

140. Rahim, M.K., Kim, S.E., So, H., Kim, H.J., Cheon, G.J., Lee, E.S., Kang, K.W., Lee, D.S.: Recent trends in PET image interpretations using volumetric and texture-based quantification methods in nuclear oncology. Nucl. Med. Mol. Imaging **48**(1), 1–15 (2014)

141. Roman-Jimenez, G., Leseur, J., Devillers, A., David, J.: Segmentation and characterization of tumors in 18F-FDG PET-CT for outcome prediction in cervical cancer radio-chemotherapy. In: Image-Guidance and Multimodal Dose Planning in Radiation Therapy: A MICCAI Workshop, vol. 17 (2012)

142. Rutman, A.M., Kuo, M.D.: Radiogenomics: creating a link between molecular diagnostics and diagnostic imaging. Eur. J. Radiol. **70**(2), 232–241 (2009)

143. Ryu, I.S., Kim, J.S., Roh, J.-L., Cho, K.-J., Choi, S.-H., Nam, S.Y., Kim, S.Y.: Prognostic significance of preoperative metabolic tumour volume and total lesion glycolysis measured by 18F-FDG PET/CT in squamous cell carcinoma of the oral cavity. Eur. J. Nucl. Med. Mol. Imaging **41**(3), 452–461 (2014)

144. Schmidt, M., Levner, I., Greiner, R., Murtha, A., Bistritz, A.: Segmenting brain tumors using alignment-based features. In: Fourth International Conference on Machine Learning and Applications, 2005. Proceedings (2005)

145. Schmidt, M.C., Antweiler, S., Urban, N., Mueller, W., Kuklik, A., Meyer-Puttlitz, B., Wiestler, O.D., Louis, D.N., Fimmers, R., von Deimling, A.: Impact of genotype and morphology on the prognosis of glioblastoma. J. Neuropathol. Exp. Neurol. **61**(4), 321–328 (2002)

146. Schover, L.R.: Quality counts: the value of women's perceived quality of life after cervical cancer. Gynecol. Oncol. **76**(1), 3–4 (2000)

147. Segal, E., Sirlin, C.B., Ooi, C., Adler, A.S., Gollub, J., Chen, X., Chan, B.K., Matcuk, G.R., Barry, C.T., Chang, H.Y., Kuo, M.D.: Decoding global gene expression programs in liver cancer by noninvasive imaging. Nat. Biotechnol. **25**(6), 675–680 (2007)

148. Shen, W., Zhou, M., Yang, F., Yang, C., Tian, J.: Multi-scale convolutional neural networks for lung nodule classification. In: Information Processing in Medical Imaging. Springer (2015)

149. Shota, Y., Maki, D.D., Korn, R.L., Kuo, M.D.: Radiogenomic analysis of breast cancer using MRI: a preliminary study to define the landscape. Am. J. Roentgenol. **199**(3), 654–663 (2012)

150. Siegel, R., Naishadham, D., Jemal, A.: Cancer statistics, 2013. CA Cancer J. Clin. **63**(1), 11–30 (2013)

151. Simon, R.: Clinical trial designs for evaluating the medical utility of prognostic and predictive biomarkers in oncology. Personalized Med. **7**(1), 33–47 (2010)

152. Slattery, M.L., Robison, L.M., Schuman, K.L., French, T.K., Abbott, T.M., Overall, J.C., Gardner, J.W.: Cigarette smoking and exposure to passive smoke are risk factors for cervical cancer. JAMA **261**(11), 1593–1598 (1989)

153. Song, J., Liu, Z., Zhong, W., Huang, Y., Ma, Z., Dong, D., Liang, C., Tian, J.: Non-small cell lung cancer: quantitative phenotypic analysis of CT images as a potential marker of prognosis. Sci. Rep. **6** (2016)

154. Song, J.D., Yang, C.Y., Fan, L., Wang, K., Yang, F., Liu, S.Y., Tian, J.: Lung lesion extraction using a toboggan based growing automatic segmentation approach. IEEE Trans. Med. Imaging **35**(1), 337–353 (2016)

155. Stupp, R., Mason, W.P., van den Bent, M.J., Weller, M., Fisher, B., Taphoorn, M.J., Belanger, K., Brandes, A.A., Marosi, C., Bogdahn, U., Curschmann, J., Janzer, R.C.,

Ludwin, S.K., Gorlia, T., Allgeier, A., Lacombe, D., Cairncross, J.G., Eisenhauer, E., Mirimanoff, R.O.: Radiotherapy plus concomitant and adjuvant temozolomide for glioblastoma. N. Engl. J. Med. **352**(10), 987–996 (2005)

156. Sun, S.S., Guo, Y.: Juxta-vascular nodule segmentation based on the flowing entropy and geodesic distance feature. J. Invest. Med. **61**(4), S8–S8 (2013)

157. Suykens, J.A., Vandewalle, J.: Least squares support vector machine classifiers. Neural Process. Lett. **9**(3), 293–300 (1999)

158. Tan, M., Deklerck, R., Jansen, B., Bister, M., Cornelis, J.: A novel computer-aided lung nodule detection system for CT images. Med. Phys. **38**(10), 5630–5645 (2011)

159. Tan, S., Kligerman, S., Chen, W., Lu, M., Kim, G., Feigenberg, S., D'Souza, W.D., Suntharalingam, M., Lu, W.: Spatial-temporal [18 F] FDG-PET features for predicting pathologic response of esophageal cancer to neoadjuvant chemoradiation therapy. Int. J. Radiat. Oncol.* Biol.* Phys. **85**(5), 1375–1382 (2013)

160. Thibault, G., Fertil, B., Navarro, C., Pereira, S., Cau, P., Levy, N., Sequeira, J., Mari, J.: Texture Indexes and Gray Level Size Zone Matrix Application to Cell Nuclei Classification (2009)

161. Thibault, G., Fertil, B., Navarro, C., Pereira, S., Levy, N., Sequeira, J., Mari, J.L.: Texture indexes and gray level size zone matrix application to cell nuclei classification. In: Pattern Recognition and Information Processing (PRIP) (2009)

162. Tixier, F., Le Rest, C.C., Hatt, M., Albarghach, N., Pradier, O., Metges, J.-P., Corcos, L., Visvikis, D.: Intratumor heterogeneity characterized by textural features on baseline 18F-FDG PET images predicts response to concomitant radiochemotherapy in esophageal cancer. J. Nucl. Med. **52**(3), 369–378 (2011)

163. Tomasi, G., Turkheimer, F., Aboagye, E.: Importance of quantification for the analysis of PET data in oncology: review of current methods and trends for the future. Mol. Imag. Biol. **14**(2), 131–146 (2012)

164. Vaidya, M., Creach, K.M., Frye, J., Dehdashti, F., Bradley, J.D., El Naqa, I.: Combined PET/CT image characteristics for radiotherapy tumor response in lung cancer. Radiother. Oncol. **102**(2), 239–245 (2012)

165. van Ginneken, B., Setio, A.A., Jacobs, C., Ciompi, F.: Off-the-shelf convolutional neural network features for pulmonary nodule detection in computed tomography scans. In: 2015 IEEE 12th International Symposium on Biomedical Imaging (ISBI). IEEE (2015)

166. van Velden, F.H., Cheebsumon, P., Yaqub, M., Smit, E.F., Hoekstra, O.S., Lammertsma, A. A., Boellaard, R.: Evaluation of a cumulative SUV-volume histogram method for parameterizing heterogeneous intratumoural FDG uptake in non-small cell lung cancer PET studies. Eur. J. Nucl. Med. Mol. Imaging **38**(9), 1636–1647 (2011)

167. Verhaak, R.G.W., Hoadley, K.A., Purdom, E., Wang, V., Qi, Y., Wilkerson, M.D., Miller, C.R., Ding, L., Golub, T., Mesirov, J.P., Alexe, G., Lawrence, M., O'Kelly, M., Tamayo, P., Weir, B.A., Gabriel, S., Winckler, W., Gupta, S., Jakkula, L., Feiler, H.S., Hodgson, J.G., James, C.D., Sarkaria, J.N., Brennan, C., Kahn, A., Spellman, P.T., Wilson, R.K., Speed, T. P., Gray, J.W., Meyerson, M., Getz, G., Perou, C.M., Hayes, D.N.: Integrated genomic analysis identifies clinically relevant subtypes of glioblastoma characterized by abnormalities in PDGFRA, IDH1, EGFR, and NF1. Cancer Cell **17**(1), 98–110 (2010)

168. Verma, R., Zacharaki, E.I., Ou, Y., Cai, H., Chawla, S., Lee, S.-K., Melhem, E.R., Wolf, R., Davatzikos, C.: Multiparametric tissue characterization of brain neoplasms and their recurrence using pattern classification of MR images. Acad. Radiol. **15**(8), 966–977 (2008)

169. Waggoner, S.E.: Cervical cancer. Lancet **361**(9376), 2217–2225 (2003)

170. Wahl, R.L., Wagner, H.N., Beanlands, R.S.: Principles and Practice of PET and PET/CT. Lippincott Williams & Wilkins Philadelphia, PA (2009)

171. Wang, Q., Song, E.M., Jin, R.C., Han, P., Wang, X.T., Zhou, Y.Y., Zeng, J.C.: Segmentation of lung nodules in computed tomography images using dynamic programming and multidirection fusion techniques. Acad. Radiol. **16**(6), 678–688 (2009)

172. Watabe, T., Tatsumi, M., Watabe, H., Isohashi, K., Kato, H., Yanagawa, M., Shimosegawa, E., Hatazawa, J.: Intratumoral heterogeneity of F-18 FDG uptake differentiates between

gastrointestinal stromal tumors and abdominal malignant lymphomas on PET/CT. Ann. Nucl. Med. **26**(3), 222–227 (2012)

173. Wels, M., Carneiro, G., Aplas, A., Huber, M., Hornegger, J., Comaniciu, D.: A discriminative model-constrained graph cuts approach to fully automated pediatric brain tumor segmentation in 3-D MRI. In: Metaxas, D., Axel, L., Fichtinger, G., Székely, G. (eds.) Medical Image Computing and Computer-Assisted Intervention—MICCAI 2008: 11th International Conference, New York, NY, USA, 6–10 Sept 2008, Proceedings, Part I, pp. 67–75. Springer, Berlin (2008)

174. Wong, K.-P., Zhang, X., Huang, S.-C.: Improved derivation of input function in dynamic mouse [18F] FDG PET using bladder radioactivity kinetics. Mol. Imag. Biol. **15**(4), 486–496 (2013)

175. Wright, A.A., Howitt, B.E., Myers, A.P., Dahlberg, S.E., Palescandolo, E., Hummelen, P., MacConaill, L.E., Shoni, M., Wagle, N., Jones, R.T.: Oncogenic mutations in cervical cancer. Cancer **119**(21), 3776–3783 (2013)

176. Wu, D.J., Lu, L., Bi, J.B., Shinagawa, Y., Boyer, K., Krishnan, A., Salganicoff, M.: Stratified Learning of Local Anatomical Context for Lung Nodules in CT Images. In: 2010 IEEE Conference on Computer Vision and Pattern Recognition (Cvpr), pp. 2791–2798 (2010)

177. Xiaoou, T.: Texture information in run-length matrices. IEEE Trans. Image Process. **7**(11), 1602–1609 (1998)

178. Yan, J., Chu-Shern, J.L., Loi, H.Y., Khor, L.K., Sinha, A.K., Quek, S.T., Tham, I.W., Townsend, D.: Impact of image reconstruction settings on texture features in 18F-FDG PET. J. Nucl. Med. **56**(11), 1667–1673 (2015)

179. Yan, W., Li, R., Liu, Y., Yang, P., Wang, Z., Zhang, C., Bao, Z., Zhang, W., You, Y., Jiang, T.: MicroRNA expression patterns in the malignant progression of gliomas and a 5-microRNA signature for prognosis. Oncotarget **5**(24), 12908–12915 (2014)

180. Yang, F., Thomas, M.A., Dehdashti, F., Grigsby, P.W.: Temporal analysis of intratumoral metabolic heterogeneity characterized by textural features in cervical cancer. Eur. J. Nucl. Med. Mol. Imaging **40**(5), 716–727 (2013)

181. Yankelevitz, D.F., Reeves, A.P., Kostis, W.J., Zhao, B., Henschke, C.I.: Small pulmonary nodules: volumetrically determined growth rates based on CT evaluation. Radiology **217**(1), 251–256 (2000)

182. Zacharaki, E.I., Shen, D., Lee, S.K., Davatzikos, C.: ORBIT: a multiresolution framework for deformable registration of brain tumor images. IEEE Trans. Med. Imaging **27**(8), 1003–1017 (2008)

183. Zhang, J., Ma, K.-K., Er, M.-H., Chong, V.: Tumor Segmentation from Magnetic Resonance Imaging by Learning via one-class support vector machine. In: International Workshop on Advanced Image Technology (IWAIT '04), Singapore (2004)

184. Zhao, B., James, L.P., Moskowitz, C.S., Guo, P., Ginsberg, M.S., Lefkowitz, R.A., Qin, Y., Riely, G.J., Kris, M.G., Schwartz, L.H.: Evaluating variability in tumor measurements from same-day repeat CT scans of patients with non-small cell lung cancer. Radiology **252**(1), 263–272 (2009)

185. Zhao, B., Schwartz, L.H., Moskowitz, C.S., Ginsberg, M.S., Rizvi, N.A., Kris, M.G.: Lung cancer: computerized quantification of tumor response–initial results. Radiology **241**(3), 892–898 (2006)

186. Zhou, M., Hall, L.O., Goldgof, D.B., Gillies, R.J., Gatenby, R.A.: Survival time prediction of patients with glioblastoma multiforme tumors using spatial distance measurement. In: Medical Imaging 2013: Computer-Aided Diagnosis **8670** (2013)

187. Zikic, D., Glocker, B., Konukoglu, E., Criminisi, A., Demiralp, C., Shotton, J., Thomas, O. M., Das, T., Jena, R., Price, S.J.: Decision forests for tissue-specific segmentation of high-grade gliomas in multi-channel MR. In: Ayache, N., Delingette, H., Golland, P., Mori, K. (eds.) Medical Image Computing and Computer-Assisted Intervention – MICCAI 2012: 15th International Conference, Nice, France, October 1–5, 2012, Proceedings, Part III, pp. 369–376. Springer, Berlin (2012)

188. Zikic, D., Glocker, B., Shotton, J., Criminisi, A., Thomas, O.M., Das, T., Konukoglu, E., Ye, D.H., Demiralp, C., Jena, R.: Context-sensitive Classification Forests for Segmentation of Brain Tumor Tissues. Miccai (2012)
189. Zinn, P.O., Bhanu, M., Bhanu, M., Pratheesh, S., Singh, S.K., Sadhan, M., Jolesz, F.A., Colen, R.R.: Radiogenomic mapping of edema/cellular invasion MRI-phenotypes in glioblastoma multiforme. Plos One **6**(10), e25451 (2011)

Part V
Computer-Aided Therapy and Surgery

Markerless Tumor Gating and Tracking for Lung Cancer Radiotherapy based on Machine Learning Techniques

Tong Lin and Yucheng Lin

Abstract The respiratory lung tumor motion poses great challenge for radiation therapy of lung cancer patients. Traditional methods leverage external surrogates or implanted markers to indicate the position of tumors, but these methods suffer from inaccuracies or the risk of pneumothorax. In this chapter fluoroscopic images are employed to indicate the tumor position. We show how machine learning techniques can be used for tumor gating and tracking. Experimental results demonstrate the effectiveness of this new method without external or implanted markers. We also discuss some problems about this new method and point out new promising research frontiers.

1 Introduction

Lung cancer, also known as lung carcinoma, is the leading cause of cancer-related death worldwide [37]. One of the common treatments is radiotherapy. A major difficulty in conformal lung cancer radiotherapy is respiratory organ motion, which may cause clinically significant targeting errors. Accordingly, there is an urgent need to locate the position of moving tumors accurately in the process of tumor gating and tracking. In this chapter, we demonstrate how machine learning techniques can be applied to tumor gating and tracking. Also the experimental results are reported for using these new methods.

T. Lin (✉) · Y. Lin
Key Laboratory of Machine Perception (MOE), School of EECS,
Peking University, 2201E, Science Building #2, Beijing 100871, China
e-mail: lintong@pku.edu.cn

Y. Lin
e-mail: xklyc@pku.edu.cn

© Springer International Publishing AG 2018
K. Suzuki and Y. Chen (eds.), *Artificial Intelligence in Decision Support Systems for Diagnosis in Medical Imaging*, Intelligent Systems Reference Library 140,
https://doi.org/10.1007/978-3-319-68843-5_12

1.1 Prior Work on Tumor Gating

A major uncertainty in treating lung cancer with radiation is the respiratory lung tumor motion, which can be clinically significant for some patients. Respiratory gated lung cancer radiotherapy holds promise to precisely deliver prescribed radiation dose to the tumor, while minimizing the incidence and severity of normal tissue complications [11]. Respiratory gating limits radiation exposure to a portion of the breathing cycle when the tumor is in a predefined gating window. Due to a reduced planning target volume, precise target localization in real time is particularly important for gated radiotherapy [12].

Several template-matching methods have been proposed for attacking the fluoroscopic markerless gating problem [4, 6]. However, template matching does not utilize the information outside the gating window in building templates, which could be important for improving the accuracy and robustness of the algorithm. Recently, the gating problem has been regarded as a binary classification problem that can be solved by support vector machine (SVM) [39] combined with a dimensionality reduction technique called principal components analysis (PCA). This method achieves slightly higher accuracies compared to the template matching methods at the price of significant amount of training time to search the optimal parameter set [7].

Dimensionality reduction and classification are two essential parts in machine learning algorithms. Selecting the right dimensionality reduction technique and classification algorithm could improve the final accuracies. In this work, we adopt the same binary classification framework as proposed previously [7]. Within this framework, we investigate four other dimensionality reduction techniques besides PCA, namely locally linear embedding (LLE), local tangent space alignment (LTSA), Laplacian eigenmap (LAP) and diffusion maps (DMAP) [18]. PCA is one of the most widely used dimensionality reduction techniques. It finds the best linear representation of the data in the mean-square sense. Unlike PCA, these four algorithms belong to "manifold learning" algorithms, which represent the latest nonlinear dimensionality reduction techniques. In the recent literature, these algorithms have demonstrated better performance than classical dimensionality reduction techniques such as PCA, especially on curved and nonlinear data sets [31]. Specifically, the benefit of any manifold learning method over classical methods was shown on the famous Swiss roll dataset, which is curved and nonlinear. Linear methods such as PCA often fail while most manifold learning methods can successfully model the Swiss roll dataset. In exploratory data analysis, the linearity assumption often does not hold. It is therefore also important to investigate nonlinear dimensionality reduction techniques despite their higher computational cost. For classification, in addition to SVM, we combine the dimensionality reduction techniques with a three-layer artificial neural network (ANN) for gated lung cancer radiotherapy. The performance of the proposed algorithms is evaluated in a retrospective fashion on ten fluoroscopic video sequences of nine patients. We will compare the performance of ANN with SVM when combined with the aforementioned five dimensionality reduction techniques.

1.2   Prior Work on Tumor Tracking

Lung cancer radiotherapy is challenging even for patients with localized disease limited to the thorax. In-field recurrences are common, despite the use of concurrent chemotherapy and increasing doses of radiation. While tumor biology likely influences the aggressive clinical course of most lung cancers, targeting inaccuracies may also cause geographical miss, resulting in poor locoregional control with radiotherapy. A major source of targeting inaccuracy is from the respiration-induced lung tumor motion [11].

Two major classes of techniques have been developed to manage respiratory tumor motion. The main idea for the first class of techniques is to allow the tumor to move freely relative to the treatment beams and try to integrate the motion effect into the treatment plan (geometrical or dosimetric). These techniques include: (1) patient population based internal margin; (2) patient specific internal margin; (3) internal target volume (ITV) method; (4) IMRT optimization using motion probability density function (PDF) [11, 38]. The main idea for the other class of techniques is to freeze? the tumor motion relative to the treatment beams, which roughly divides into two categories: (1) control the tumor motion, using techniques such as breath holding, forced shallow breathing, or abdominal compression; (2) allow free tumor motion but adjust the treatment equipment to maintain a constant target position in the beams eye view when the beam is on, through respiratory gating, beam tracking, or couch-based motion compensation [11].

The beam tracking technique follows the target dynamically with the radiation beam. It was first implemented in a robotic radiosurgery system [1, 22, 23, 26, 32]. For linac-based radiotherapy, tumor motion can be compensated for using a dynamic multi-leaf collimator (MLC) [13, 14, 24, 25, 27–29, 35, 40–42]. Beam tracking could be the best technique for stereotactic body radiation therapy (SBRT) due to its potentially high treatment efficiency and precision. Although there are still many technical challenges, one of which is how to track the tumor location in real time with high precision.

Previous tumor tracking approaches can be roughly grouped into three categories: (1) deriving the tumor position based on external surrogates, such as the patient abdominal surface or lung volume [11]. The relationship between the external surrogates and the internal tumor position can vary from day to day, and even during the treatment of the same day. Therefore, this approach is often considered to suffer from lack of accuracy. (2) Fluoroscopic tracking of radiopaque fiducial markers implanted inside or near the tumor [33, 36]. The accuracy of this technology is better than 1.5 mm for tracking moving targets [34], which is much higher than the external surrogates approach. Another implementation of marker tracking is based on non-ionizing electromagnetic fields, using small wireless transponders implanted in human tissue [3]. However, no matter how marker tracking is realized, as long as the percutaneous marker implantation is involved, the clinical implementation of this technology in lung cancer radiotherapy is limited due to the risk of pneumothorax [2, 9]. (3) Fluoroscopic tracking of the lung tumor without implanted fiducial markers.

Some conventional motion tracking methods commonly used in computer vision, such as template matching, optical flow, and active shape model [8, 43, 44] have been proposed for tumor tracking. These tracking methods achieve promising results when the tumor has reasonably high contrast and clear boundary in the images. However, these methods would fail when the image quality is poor and the tumor is hard to identify in the images (even by human eyes), which is often the case for lung cancer fluoroscopic images.

Tracking the lung tumor in fluoroscopic image sequences is a very challenging task because, compared to the colored video sequences that are often seen in the field of computer vision, the fluoroscopic image sequences have much less information (gray scale versus true color and less texture), and also in most cases the tumors do not have clear shape boundaries. Additionally, the image quality is poor in many situations. Therefore, traditional tracking algorithms developed for computer vision applications may not be applied to fluoroscopic tumor images. In this chapter we propose a novel tumor tracking algorithm to solve this problem by using some "surrogate" regions.

2 Tumor Gating

The goal of gated radiotherapy is to decide when to turn the beam on or off. Therefore, the gating problem can be reformulated as a binary classification problem. That is, the problem now becomes finding a decision boundary that will separate future fluoroscopic images into two classes: beam ON or beam OFF. The classification algorithms are employed to learn an optimal decision boundary based on a training data set.

2.1 Fluoroscopic Image Data

Prior to treatment, a sequence of fluoroscopic images are acquired for training the classifier. A region-of-interest (ROI) containing the tumor motion is selected on the training fluoroscopic images. Each ROI is manually labeled by human expert observers with either class beam ON or beam OFF based on the gating window size determined during treatment planning. In patients where the tumor was hard to identify visually in the fluoroscopic images, an anatomical structure nearby the tumor was used.

Figure 1 shows an example of a set of training fluoroscopic images and the selected ROIs. The first two ROIs are within the gating window and labeled as beam ON class, and the next four are outside the gating window and thus labeled as beam OFF class.

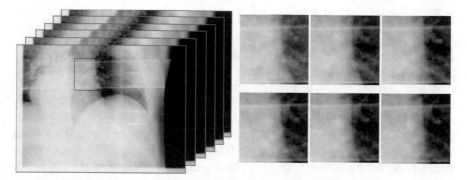

Fig. 1 A set of training fluoroscopic image sequence (left) and the selected ROI images (right)

2.2 Dimensionality Reduction Techniques

The purpose of dimensionality reduction is twofold. First, it can reduce the training sample size and therefore decrease the computational cost. A typical ROI size could be 100×100 pixels. This means that the dimensionality of a training sample would be $100 \times 100 = 10000$. Significant computational time and resources would be needed with these high dimensional samples. Clearly this is not practical for real-time gated radiotherapy. With dimensionality reduction, the dimensionalities of the training samples can be significantly reduced, and consequently much computational time and resource would be saved. Secondly, it can be regarded as extracting significant features of the ROI data automatically. A dimensionality reduction technique will automatically sort the information based on its importance and retain the most important components. For instance, PCA involves a mathematical procedure that transforms the original correlated variables into a small number of uncorrelated variables called principal components. The first principal component accounts for as much of the variability in the data as possible, and each succeeding component accounts for as much of the remaining variability as possible.

Besides PCA, four other dimensionality reduction techniques are investigated in this work, including LLE, LTSA, LAP and DMAP [18]. These four manifold learning methods find a nonlinear transformation by preserving neighborhood distances. Most manifold learning methods need two key parameters, one to describe the neighborhood size and one to describe the intrinsic dimension or output dimension. The results might be very different if these two parameters are varied. A detailed comparison of different dimensionality reduction techniques can be found in [18].

We first map each training ROI image into a 30-dimensional linear space using PCA. Then, we further reduce the dimensionality of the training ROI image to 10 using the five methods described above. These features lie in a significantly lower dimensional space compared with the original ROI image and will be fed later into the classification algorithms as the input.

2.3 *Artificial Neural Network (ANN)*

A neural network is an effective computational model for pattern classification and function approximation (or called regression analysis). It is inspired by the way the biological nervous system processes information. ANN is a massively parallel system with large numbers of interconnected simple processors, and it can solve many challenging computational problems. An ANN can learn any arbitrarily complex target function by adding neurons and layers to the network. A target function is learned by adjusting the weights of the network. These weights are tuned by minimizing a least-squares error optimization function through a back-propagation algorithm. For this gating problem, we employ a standard three-layer neural network with an error back-propagation algorithm. Figure 2 illustrates an example. In our gating system, the input layer has ten neurons to match the ten-dimensional input data after dimensionality reduction. There are five neurons in the hidden layer and only one neuron in the output layer.

A trained ANN can be thought of as an "expert" to analyze the training data. In our gated lung radiotherapy application, a trained ANN automatically processes the fluoroscopic images acquired during the simulated treatment and classify them into the beam ON or beam OFF class and then generate the corresponding gating signals.

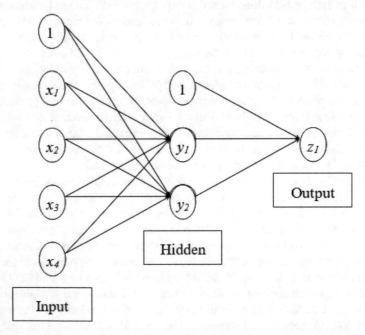

Fig. 2 A simple neural network with three-layer neurons. In this figure, there are 4 neurons in the input layer, 2 neurons in the hidden layer, and 1 neuron in the output layer

2.4   Simulated Treatment Delivery

During simulated treatment in this retrospective study, ROI at the same location in the training fluoroscopic images is automatically selected on each new fluoroscopic image acquired during simulated treatment. The same dimensionality reduction technique is applied on the newly coming ROIs. The trained ANN is then applied to automatically process each ROI with the reduced dimensionality and classifies it into either the beam ON or OFF class. Gating signals are then generated accordingly.

3   Tumor Tracking

3.1   Image Data

To develop and evaluate the proposed algorithm, fluoroscopic image sequences for 9 lung cancer patients were acquired at a speed of 15 frames per second using an on-board x-ray imaging (OBI) system (Varian Medical Systems, Palo Alto, CA, USA). One patient had tumors in both left and right lungs. Therefore, 10 fluoroscopic sequences were used retrospectively. Figure 3 shows the first frames of these 10 fluoroscopic image sequences. The average video length is about 40 s (i.e. 600 frames). For each patient, 15 s of fluoroscopic images (225 frames) at the beginning of the sequence are used as training data. The remaining data are used for testing the algorithm. The tumor positions are manually identified by human observers to serve as the "gold-standard" ground truth. All our algorithms are implemented in Matlab.

3.2   Outline of the Tracking Method

The proposed algorithm is based on the observation that the motion of some anatomic features in the images (called "surrogates") may be well correlated to the tumor motion. The correlation between the tumor position and the motion pattern of surrogates can be captured by regression analysis techniques. The proposed algorithm consists of four main steps: (1) selecting several surrogate windows; (2) extracting spatiotemporal patterns from the chosen surrogate windows; (3) establishing regression relations between the tumor position and the spatiotemporal patterns of surrogates; and (4) predicting the tumor location with the established regression model based on surrogate spatiotemporal patterns. The preceding three steps are done using training image data before the treatment, whereas the fourth step is done using image data acquired during the treatment delivery in real time.

A few surrogate windows are created in the first frame of the training image sequence, which are assumed to be more or less correlated with the tumor motion. In the remaining training frames, the location of a surrogate window is fixed while

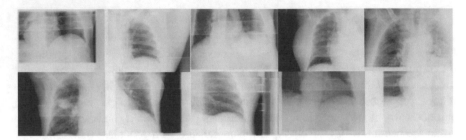

Fig. 3 First frames of 10 fluoroscopic image sequences used for testing the proposed tracking algorithm

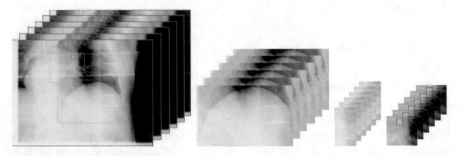

Fig. 4 Left: the selection of surrogate windows (green rectangular regions) on the first frame of the fluoroscopic image sequence. Note that the tumor area is marked in a red rectangle. Right: The selected three surrogate windows

the image content moves inside it. One window could be placed to contain the diaphragm, if visible in the image, which usually has a strong correlation with tumor motion in the superior-inferior (SI) direction (y-direction in the image coordinates). Other windows can contain any visible moving anatomic structures such as the lung boundary or even the tumor itself. In our preliminary experiments, only three surrogates are selected and placed on the diaphragm, the lung boundary, and the tumor itself, as shown in Fig. 4. The diaphragm is closely related to the tumor motion in y-direction, and the nearby lung wall correlates to the tumor motion in x-direction (lateral). If the image quality is acceptable and the tumor itself has clear shape, the surrogate window containing the tumor itself can also be helpful to predict the tumor position.

The images in the selected surrogate windows are not tracked directly. Instead, we use the principal component analysis (PCA) to map each surrogate window to a low-dimensional space to get a compact coordinate representation. In our experiments, based on the eigenvalues, we choose to use the most important three of principal components to represent a surrogate window. The coordinate representation of three surrogate windows are denoted as $(z_1, z_2, \ldots, z_9)$, where (z_1, z_2, z_3) is for the first window, (z_4, z_5, z_6) is for the second, and (z_7, z_8, z_9) is for the last. Figure 5 shows the 3D representations of the three surrogate windows in the PCA embedding space. We can

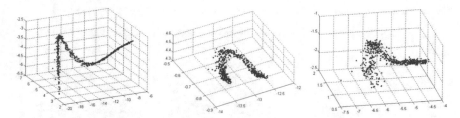

Fig. 5 3D representations of the three surrogate windows in the PCA embedding space. Left: the window containing the diaphragm. Middle: the window containing the lung boundary. Right: the window containing the tumor itself

Fig. 6 3D PCA embedding of the diaphragm images, and representative images are shown next to the red circled points at different locations in the trajectory

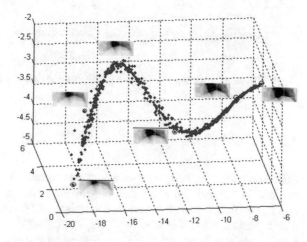

see that a surrogate window is reduced to a point in the 3D PCA space, which follows a well-defined trajectory. It also appears that the more clear the anatomic features in the window, the better defined the trajectory is. The location of a surrogate window selected on the first training frame is fixed for the remaining frames while the image content moves inside it, yielding the trajectory in PCA space. This is illustrated in Fig. 6, where representative images are shown next to red circled points at different parts of the trajectory in the 3D PCA space. As the diaphragm moves up and down, the corresponding point in 3D PCA space moves along the trajectory from one end to the other.

Figure 7 illustrates the curve representations of tumor positions (x, y) and 3D coordinates of three surrogate ROIs in PCA space. We can observe that there is a strong correlation between tumor positions and surrogate coordinates. The third step mentioned earlier is to build a regression model to predict the tumor position (x, y) based on the parametric representations of surrogate ROIs $(z_1, z_2, \ldots, z_9)$.

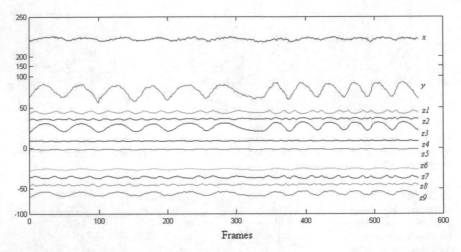

Fig. 7 Curve representations of tumor positions (x, y) and 3D coordinates of three surrogates $(z_1, z_2, \ldots, z_9)$ in PCA space

3.3 Principal Component Analysis (PCA)

PCA is a classic technique to reduce dimensionality with minimum loss of information. In our case, the original dimension is the size (or the number of pixels) in the ROIs. That is, if an ROI consists of 50×50 pixels, the dimension is $n = 50 \times 50 = 2500$. Let $\Sigma = \frac{1}{n} \sum_{i=1}^{n} (x_i - \bar{x})(x_i - \bar{x})^T$ be the $n \times n$ data covariance matrix, where x_i is an n-dimensional column vector of data point, and $\bar{x}$ is the sample mean. Specifically, x_i represents the image at time i in a fixed surrogate window with n pixels, and set $X = [x_1, \ldots, x_m]$ as the available m frames of images in the window. Let $U = [u_1, u_2, \ldots, u_d]$ be the unit eigenvectors corresponding to the d largest eigenvalues $(\lambda_1, \lambda_2, \ldots, \lambda_d)$ of the covariance matrix, such that $\Sigma U = U \Lambda$ where $\Lambda = diag[\lambda_1, \lambda_2, \ldots, \lambda_d]$. Then we obtain the PCA projection $Y = U^T \tilde{X}$, where $\tilde{X} = X(I - ee^T/k)$ is the zero mean version of the original data X, and Y is a $d \times m$ matrix representing the embedded results. Here e is a column vector of all ones. Geometrically, $U = [u_1, u_2, \ldots, u_d]$ forms a set of incomplete orthonormal basis for the data space, and the original data points have the largest diversity in these basis directions.

3.4 Regression Analysis

In order to predict the tumor position, a regression model should be established between the tumor position and the parametric representation of ROIs in the PCA space. Four regression methods are employed and compared for this end, including linear regression, two-degree polynomial regression, artificial neural network (ANN) and support vector machine (SVM). Note that ANN and SVM can be used for both regression and classification. In regression, target outputs can be any real numbers, whereas in classification target outputs have to be integers to indicate different discrete classes.

3.4.1 Linear Regression

Suppose we want to predict the target value y from an p-dimensional input vector $\mathbf{z} = [z_1, z_2, \ldots, z_p]$ with a linear model $y = a_0 + \sum_{i=1}^{p} a_i z_i$. This can be written as a matrix form: $\mathbf{y} = \mathbf{Z}\alpha + \varepsilon$, where $\mathbf{y}$ is an $m \times 1$ vector formed by m observations of target values, $\mathbf{Z}$ is an $m \times p$ matrix of input predictors, α is a $p \times 1$ vector of regression parameters, and ε is an $m \times 1$ vector of random noise. The parameter vector α can be computed by the least-squares solution $\alpha = (\mathbf{Z}^T\mathbf{Z})^{-1}\mathbf{Z}^T\mathbf{y}$, or $\alpha = (\mathbf{Z}^T\mathbf{Z} + \lambda\mathbf{I})^{-1}\mathbf{Z}^T\mathbf{y}$ for the regularized solution with a small scalar λ.

3.4.2 Two-Degree Polynomial Regression

In this case we predict the target y from an p-dimensional input vector $\mathbf{z} = [z_1, z_2, \ldots, z_p]$ with a two-degree polynomial model $y = a_0 + \sum_{i=1}^{p} a_i z_i + \sum_{i=1}^{p} \sum_{j \geq i}^{p} a_{ij} z_i z_j$. This can be treated as a linear predictor where the input vector changes to be

$$\tilde{\mathbf{z}} = [z_1, z_2, \ldots, z_p, z_1^2, z_1 z_2, \ldots, z_1 z_n, z_2^2, z_2 z_3, \ldots, z_2 z_p, \ldots, z_p^2].$$

The computation procedure is simply same as that in the linear regression model.

3.4.3 Artificial Neural Networks (ANN)

A typical neural network has three layers (with an example shown in Fig. 2): input layer, hidden layer and output layer. The output values of the output neurons represent target labels (discrete numbers) for classification or target values (real numbers) for regression. In our regression application, there are two output neurons to provide prediction results of the tumor position (x and y coordinates). The weights of this network are learned through the back-propagation method where the optimization problem can be efficiently solved by stochastic gradient descent (SGD).

3.4.4 Support Vector Machine (SVM)

SVM has become a standard tool for pattern classification in a variety of domains, and the popularity of the machine learning research is arguably attributed to the successful applications of SVM [39]. Given a set of data points $\{(x_1, y_1), (x_2, y_2), \ldots, (x_m, y_m)\}$, SVM can be used for classification ($y_i \in \{1, -1\}$) or regression ($y_i \in \mathbb{R}^1$). In classification applications, SVM seeks to maximize the margin between two classes of samples:

$$\max \frac{2}{\parallel w \parallel^2}, \quad \text{s.t. } y_i(w^T x_i + b) \geq 1, \; i = 1, 2, \ldots, m.$$

This is equivalent to the minimizing problem

$$\min \frac{\parallel w \parallel^2}{2}, \quad \text{s.t. } y_i(w^T x_i + b) \geq 1, \; i = 1, 2, \ldots, m.$$

In the case where the data is not linearly separable, the classification task can be solved by introducing some nonnegative slack variables:

$$\min \frac{\parallel w \parallel^2}{2} + C \sum_{i=1}^{n} \xi_i, \quad \text{s.t. } y_i(w^T x_i + b) \geq 1, \; \xi_i \geq 0, \; i = 1, 2, \ldots, m$$

where $C > 0$ is a penalty parameter. Furthermore, a "kernel trick" can be used to map the original data into a higher dimensional space by using a nonlinear kernel function $\phi(\cdot)$:

$$\min \frac{\parallel w \parallel^2}{2} + C \sum_{i=1}^{n} \xi_i, \quad \text{s.t. } y_i(w^T \phi(x_i) + b) \geq 1, \; \xi_i \geq 0, \; i = 1, 2, \ldots, m.$$

For regression tasks, the standard form of support vector regression becomes

$$\min_{w,b,\xi,\xi^*} \frac{\parallel w \parallel^2}{2} + C \sum_{i=1}^{n} \xi_i + C \sum_{i=1}^{n} \xi_i^*,$$

$$\text{s.t. } w^T \phi(z_i) + b - y_i \leq \varepsilon + \xi_i,$$

$$y_i - w^T \phi(z_i) - b \leq \varepsilon + \xi_i^*,$$

$$\xi_i \geq 0, \; \xi_i^* \geq 0, \; i = 1, 2, \ldots, m.$$

4 Experimental Results

4.1 Results on Tumor Gating

For this tumor gating study, ten fluoroscopic image sequences of nine lung cancer patients have been acquired at University of California San Diego (UCSD) using a Varian on-board imaging (OBI) system (Varian Medical Systems, Palo Alto, CA,

USA). The fluoroscopic image frequency is 15 Hz, and each image size is 1024×768 pixels. The average image sequence length is about 40 s (namely having around 600 frames). For each patient, 15 s of fluoroscopic images (225 frames) at the beginning of the sequence are used as training data. The rest of frames are used as testing data for validation purpose. We used CMUs ANN implementation in C (http://www.cs. cmu.edu/afs/cs/project/ai-repository/ai/areas/neural/bench/0.html) and Libsvm for SVM implementation [5] in C++. Both implementations were wrapped into DLLs that can be called from MatLab (MathWorks, Natick, MA, USA). All other proposed computational methods were implemented in MatLab.

We define the true positive (tp), false positive (fp), true negative (tn) and false negative (fn) in Table 1. Figure 8 shows an example of tp, fp, tn and fn. A sequence of fluoroscopic images are mapped onto three-dimensional space as shown in Fig. 8a, where the blue points are true beam ON class and red points are true beam OFF class. Figure 8b shows the classification results in terms of tp, fp, tn and fn, where different color represents different category. Figure 9 shows an example of gating signal generated by classification results. The corresponding tp, fp, tn and fn are displayed in the figure. The classification results are measured in terms of the classification accuracy (CA), the recall rate (RR), and the target coverage (TC), where $CA = (tp + tn)/all$, $RR = tp/(tp + fn)$ and $TC = tp/(tp + fp)$. Among these three metrics, TC is the most important one for our gating application. For instance, a TC of 80% means that 80% of the prescribed dose is delivered to the target and 20% delivered to the surrounding normal tissues. Besides TC, duty cycle (DC) was used as another evaluation metric defined as $DC = tp/all$ [7]. It is easy to see that given a particular data set with a ground truth gating signal, RR and DC are always proportional to each other independent of what algorithms are used. Thus, they can be considered as equivalent metrics for evaluation purpose.

The experimental results are reported in Tables 2 and 3. From Table 2, we can see that the RR for fluoroscopic sequences 1, 2, 3, 4 and 9 is markedly lower than the other sequences for most dimensionality reduction techniques (except LTSA, whose average RR is much lower than others). A similar pattern may also be observed for SVM-based results in Table 3. A low RR indicates a large number of false negatives compared with true positives, meaning that the radiation beam will be turned off more frequently when it should be on, leading to a prolonged treatment. From this perspective, we point out that the three evaluation metrics used here are not equally important in clinical sense. A false positive gating signal is much worse clinically than a false negative one. Therefore, when comparing with two results, TC should

Table 1 Categories of classification results

		Ground-truth	
		Beam ON	Beam OFF
Classification results	Beam ON	True positive	False positive
	Beam OFF	False negative	True negative

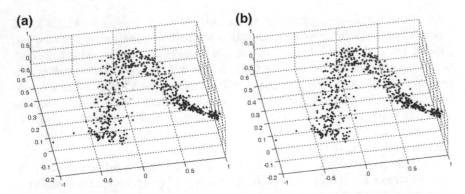

Fig. 8 **a** 3D representation of the original fluoroscopic images using PCA projection, where red and blue dots indicate ground truth of two classes. **b** Classification results: red (tp), blue (tn), cyan (fp), and yellow (fn)

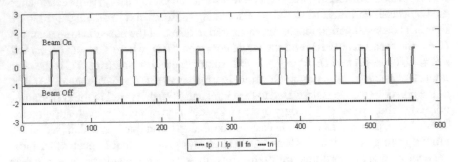

Fig. 9 An example of gating signal showing four kinds of classification results: true positive (tp), false positive (fp), false negative (fn), and true negative (tn)

be given more weight than RR. It is encouraging to see that in most cases TC is often larger than 90% although RR seldom reaches 90%.

The reason for a lower RR is very complicated. It might be the situation that the tumor cannot be seen clearly in the fluoroscopic images and the 'ground truth' itself is not accurate. There might exist shape and size changes in the tumor as well as interfering movements of other organs (particularly heart) during simulated treatment. These variations will be captured by PCA even if the tumor is in the same location. Another potential issue is the increase of breathing amplitude during simulated treatment over that of the training set. Since these new images are not represented in the training set, they might be mapped incorrectly in the PCA subspace.

From Table 2, the average CA and TC values of the ANN and PCA combination are greater than other combinations with the smallest standard deviation although the RR for PCA with ANN is slightly lower than several other manifold learning methods with ANN. Similarly, we can see from Table 3 that the SVM and PCA combination performs better than other combinations too. This suggests that for the gating

Table 2 Performance of ANN classification combined with various dimensionality reduction techniques. Three numbers in each cell represent the classification accuracy (CA), the recall rate (RR) and the target coverage (TC) in percentage

Data	PCA	LLE	LTSA	LAP	DMAP
1	94.5, 79.1, 100	92.0, 80.6, 89.3	88.7, 65.7, 88.9	94.2, 81.3, 96.9	92.6, 81.7, 91.3
2	95.4, 82.7, 98.2	90.6, 82.3, 82.0	89.3, 65.0, 88.8	94.0, 80.9, 94.3	93.4, 84.2, 90.1
3	95.3, 82.6, 97.9	92.5, 80.8, 88.8	88.8, 65.1, 86.5	93.3, 81.9, 91.5	94.4, 84.0, 93.2
4	95.5, 83.3, 97.8	92.9, 83.6, 87.8	89.4, 65.1, 88.6	93.8, 82.1, 92.5	93.4, 85.6, 89.2
5	97.9, 95.8, 98.3	93.1, 95.9, 86.7	73.8, 72.1, 62.3	91.3, 96.5, 82.9	92.4, 97.8, 84.6
6	97.3, 97.4, 97.4	98.1, 98.4, 97.9	62.6, 50.0, 68.3	97.8, 96.8, 98.9	97.8, 98.9, 96.9
7	98.0, 95.4, 98.3	96.9, 98.0, 93.3	77.1, 73.3, 63.1	93.6, 98.5, 85.4	93.8, 99.0, 85.4
8	98.9, 98.4, 99.2	98.6, 99.2, 97.7	55.5, 29.1, 50.7	98.9, 97.6, 100	98.6, 96.9, 100
9	95.8, 87.0, 97.7	96.0, 88.4, 96.7	83.5, 44.2, 93.3	96.0, 88.0, 97.4	96.0, 87.8, 97.7
10	94.6, 97.5, 93.5	92.9, 95.7, 92.4	70.0, 94.8, 67.5	93.6, 97.5, 92.2	96.8, 99.0, 95.7
Mean	96.3, 89.9, 97.8	94.4, 90.3, 91.3	77.9, 62.4, 75.8	94.7, 90.1, 93.2	94.9, 91.5, 92.4
±SD	±1.6, ±7.6, ±1.7	±2.8, ±7.9, ±5.3	±12, ±18, ±15	±2.3, ±7.9, ±5.6	±2.2, ±7.4, ±5.2

problem, a linear projection of the data using PCA might suffice for a good classification result with ANN or SVM.

Comparing Tables 2 with 3, we can see that when PCA is used for dimensionality reduction, there is a slight advantage of using ANN over SVM in all the three evaluation metrics. In order to quantitatively assess the performance gain (if any) of ANN over SVM when used with PCA, we performed a one-side paired t-test on three evaluation metrics for the ten fluoroscopic sequences. The reason why we used this particular t-test is that we are suspecting that ANN is better than SVM (hence one-side) and there is a one-to-one correspondence between each entry in Tables 2 and 3 since they came from the same sequence in the same patient (hence paired). We rejected the null hypothesis for CA and RR under the 0.05 significance level (p-value: 0.024 and 0.006, respectively). This means that the gain of ANN over SVM in terms of CA and RR is statistically significant. However, we cannot reject the null hypothesis for TC (p-value: 0.405). Combining these results with those of Cui et al.

Table 3 Performance of SVM classification combined with various dimensionality reduction techniques. Three numbers in each cell represent the classification accuracy (CA), the recall rate (RR), and the target coverage (TC) in percentage

Data	PCA	LLE	LTSA	LAP	DMAP
1	92.6, 74.6, 97.9	92.0, 71.9, 97.3	87.9, 56.8, 97.0	87.6, 64.7, 89.2	90.9, 76.9, 91.5
2	94.5, 78.0, 99.1	91.4, 68.1, 95.8	89.0, 60.3, 94.2	87.3, 62.5, 86.3	93.7, 76.5, 97.5
3	94.4, 78.9, 97.8	91.9, 71.1, 95.1	88.7, 57.2, 96.1	89.0, 60.0, 94.2	94.0, 81.6, 94.6
4	94.0, 77.0, 98.3	91.5, 67.9, 96.1	88.2, 54.8, 96.6	88.5, 61.8, 92.4	93.1, 75.0, 96.9
5	97.0, 94.4, 97.3	94.5, 93.4, 92.6	88.1, 80.1, 88.0	89.8, 95.6, 82.4	94.3, 94.6, 91.6
6	96.7, 92.4, 99.1	86.9, 66.8, 98.7	76.8, 41.6, 96.6	96.6, 92.1, 99.0	93.1, 82.9, 99.0
7	92.2, 77.2, 98.4	95.0, 89.5, 94.9	90.9, 89.4, 84.5	93.7, 94.4, 89.1	96.4, 90.8, 98.2
8	96.8, 93.9, 97.0	95.6, 90.4, 97.0	78.0, 40.9, 93.7	96.7, 93.2, 97.3	96.3, 92.2, 97.0
9	94.7, 84.2, 96.4	95.6, 89.0, 95.1	89.9, 69.1, 92.8	95.0, 83.6, 98.3	92.6, 75.5, 97.0
10	96.5, 98.4, 95.8	95.2, 97.8, 94.3	78.1, 90.3, 76.6	92.8, 96.8, 91.4	96.4, 99.2, 95.0
Mean	94.9, 84.9, 97.7	93.0, 80.6, 95.7	85.6, 64.1, 91.6	91.7, 80.5, 92.0	94.1, 84.5, 95.8
±SD	±1.7, ±9.0, ±1.1	±2.8, ±12, ±1.7	±5.6, ±18, ±6.7	±3.7, ±16, ±5.4	±1.8, ±9.0, ±2.6

[7], we can say that ANN with PCA is better than the template-based approach in terms of TC and RR (or DC).

Another important issue for real-time applications is the computational cost (or latency) in the system. Training an ANN is more efficient than training SVM since SVM needs a brute force search for the best combination of two parameters. The running time of training ANN ten times is about 0.1521 s on an Intel Core 2 Duo 2.66 GHz Machine, while it takes 2.6332 s on training SVM to search the best parameters and learn the SVM decision boundary. However, since the training process is done before treatment and only needs to be done once, the training time may be of secondary concern. What is more relevant here is the running time in the testing phase. For this particular data set, we estimated that the average running time for ANN in combination with PCA is about 6.7 ms for each frame. For SVM combined with PCA, it takes about 11 ms to process each frame. This is consistent with the previous literature in that SVM in general is slower in terms of running time than ANN for a similar generalization performance [10]. One of the reasons is that there is no control over the number of data samples selected by SVM for use as support vectors (during testing, the running time of SVM grows linearly with respect to the number of support vectors). This is in contrast to ANN, which has fixed computational complexity once a network architecture is selected. In this respect, ANN is more appealing than SVM for this application. At this stage, it seems that the system latency for both ANN and SVM when combined with PCA is acceptable for realtime gated radiotherapy.

4.2 Results on Tumor Tracking

We compare four regression methods for the tumor tracking scenario. Figure 10 shows a tracking example for Patient 1. We can see that all four methods perform better on the first 225 frames of training data than on the remaining testing data. The two-degree linear regression may suffer from the overfitting problem, as the tracking errors for the testing data are much higher than that of the training data. In contrast, we compute the mean tracking errors, $\bar{e}$ and the maximum tracking error at a 95% confidence level, e_{95}. Table 4 summarizes the tracking results of four regression methods on 10 fluoroscopic videos. We can see that the performance of all four regression methods is about on the same level, with ANN regression performing slightly better than others at $\bar{e} = 2.1$ pixels and $e_{95} = 4.6$ pixels (the pixel size is about 0.5 mm). It is worth noticing that ANN is also more robust than other methods, with the maximum e_{95} of 6.5 pixels, while for the other three methods the maximum e_{95} at least doubles this value.

We observed the time performance of our algorithm. For this study, three ROIs were selected with a total of 9794 pixels. The average time needed to project the ROIs onto the PCA space and to obtain the tumor position was 8.2 ms in a PC with

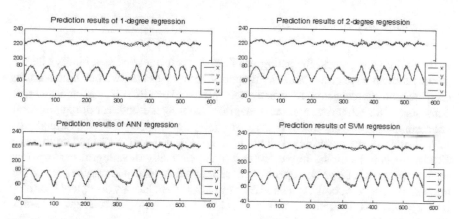

Fig. 10 Tracking results of four regression methods for patient 1. (x, y) are the ground truth 2D position of the tumor center, and (u, v) are the predicted results for (x, y)

Table 4 Tracking results for the four regression methods. $\bar{e}$ is the mean localization error, and e_{95} is the maximum localization error at a 95% confidence level. Pixel size is 0.486 mm for patients 2, 8 and 10, and 0.518 mm for the rest

Patient	Moving range (x, y) in pixels	One-degree linear regression $\bar{e}$, e_{95}	Two-degree linear regression $\bar{e}$, e_{95}	ANN regression $\bar{e}$, e_{95}	SVM regression $\bar{e}$, e_{95}
1	10, 25	1.7, 3.2	1.8, 3.9	1.9, 3.4	1.8, 3.6
2	7, 28	1.9, 3.7	1.9, 4.5	1.3, 2.9	1.7, 3.9
3	9, 29	2.4, 5.5	2.4, 7.2	2.3, 6.2	2.2, 5.8
4	25, 41	6.0, 12.9	6.1, 14.2	4.0, 6.5	6.9, 11.6
5	8, 28	1.4, 2.9	1.4, 3.4	1.7, 4.5	1.2, 2.5
6	11, 32	1.5, 3.2	1.2, 2.6	2.3, 4.5	0.9, 2.0
7	12, 37	1.6, 3.2	1.7, 3.9	1.8, 3.8	1.4, 3.0
8	10, 38	1.4, 2.8	1.6, 4.1	2.4, 5.7	1.5, 3.3
9	8, 24	1.5, 3.1	1.3, 2.6	1.3, 3.1	1.4, 2.7
10	11, 51	2.5, 6.8	2.6, 7.6	2.3, 5.8	2.8, 13.8
Average	11.1, 33.3	2.2, 4.7	2.2, 5.4	2.1, 4.6	2.2, 5.2

1.80 GHz CPU and 1.97 GB of RAM. The time required to find the estimated tumor position in a new acquired image is in the same order of magnitude as the time achieved by Moser et al. (2008) [21] of 6.4 ms, which is short enough for the purpose of real-time tracking.

5   Discussions

5.1   Summary of Our Work

In the tumor gating work, the gating problem was reformulated as a binary classification problem. Five dimensionality reduction techniques and two machine learning classification approaches were investigated. We found that PCA is in general superior compared to the other four nonlinear manifold learning methods for our application, suggesting that our data might lie in a (roughly) linear space. PCA combined with ANN leads to more accurate results in terms of CA, RR than SVM although TC is similar for both methods. In particular, for the clinically meaningful performance measure, we can achieve an upper 90% TC for most sequences in our data set. When combined with PCA, both ANN and SVM give a system latency acceptable for real-time applications. Therefore, for future real-time gated lung radiotherapy in clinics, we recommend PCA combined with ANN.

In the tumor tracking work, we have proposed a novel tracking algorithm without implanted fiducial markers. Commonly three surrogate ROIs are selected, and then the correlation between the tumor position and the surrogate representations can be captured by regression analysis techniques. Four regression methods were tested in this study: linear and two-degree polynomial regression, artificial neural network (ANN), and support vector machine (SVM). The experimental results based on fluoroscopic sequences of ten lung cancer patients demonstrate a mean tracking error of 2.1 pixels and a maximum error at a 95% confidence level of 4.6 pixels (pixel size is about 0.5 mm) for the proposed tracking algorithm. Experimental results demonstrated the feasibility of the proposed tracking algorithm, which can be clinically promising for respiratory gating or beam tracking in the future.

5.2 Limits of Our Work

For markerless tumor gating, to overcome the potential problems mentioned in the previous sections, we may need to resort to fluoroscopic images with implanted markers to get more accurate ground truth in the future. In some cases, using a smaller ROI may reduce the amount of interfering movements of other organs and increase classification accuracy. Some preprocessing such as low pass filtering may help reduce the effects of background noise. In general, the issue of shape and size changes in the tumor as well as irregular breathing patterns is more difficult to deal with. It is obvious that PCA is sensitive to these changes since it is an area-based approach and works directly with image intensity values. One solution is to investigate other feature extraction techniques or special-purpose image processing algorithms to overcome this problem.

As to the tumor tracking study, the results presented above indicate great promise for the development of algorithms that can track lung tumors in real time and in a non-invasive way with high accuracy. Nevertheless, the achievement of these goals requires a number of further improvements. First, the current work can be expanded to design regression functions capable of taking the smoothness of PCA trajectories (rather than single point locations) into account for the prediction of tumor positions. Second, surrogate ROIs should be selected automatically in an optimal way. Right now, we empirically selected three surrogate ROIs. There is no guarantee that the manually selected surrogates are the best ones for a particular patient, in terms of their predictive power with respect to the tumor position. Since the motion of surrogate features is used to predict tumor motion, the quality of tumor tracking is very likely to be improved if the ROIs are carefully selected.

There is also a need to determine the number of surrogates on which to base the prediction. We have used three ROIs in this work. There is, however, no reason to believe that this is the optimal number of surrogates. In contrast, as is well known in statistics, improved predictions can typically be obtained with recourse to the law of large numbers, by taking averages over large numbers of measurements. In the context of fluoroscopic image tracking, this advises the adoption of regression functions based on a large number of surrogate ROIs. However, the amount of training data required to estimate the regression function grows exponentially with the number of variables of the regression problem. This number is the product of the number of surrogate ROIs with the number of PCA coefficients per ROI. When too large a number of ROIs are used, the training requirements become practically infeasible. This implies that there is a trade-off between the prediction accuracy and dimensionality problem. Finding the optimal value for this trade-off requires a careful selection of both the number of surrogates and the number of coefficients per surrogate. We have, so far avoided dimensionality problems by resorting to three surrogates and three PCA coefficients. Once again, there is no reason to believe that those are optimal numbers which will lead to the best possible predictions. A better strategy is to rely on statistical learning techniques to determine which coefficients are most informative for the prediction, and limit the regression problem to these.

The technique presented here finds the regression between tumor and surrogate representation based on knowledge of the tumor position ground truth of the training set. The clinical implementation of this method has to be well thought in order to reduce treatment time. The regression could potentially be performed before the first treatment from a fluoroscopic sequence uniquely acquired for this purpose. However, PCA is sensitive to the tumor size and position, so if the tumor changes size or relative position with respect to the chosen surrogates, this regression needs to be re-calculated.

One may note that all the image sequences used in the tracking work are only from anterior Cposterior (AP) views. This is because tumors in images from other views, such as lateral view, are often much more difficult to identify even by expert observers. Thus for those images it is impossible to develop ground truth to test the developed algorithm.

Finally one should observe that due to the nature of fluoroscopic images, only 2D information of the tumor position can be extracted from them. Although superior Cinferior motion is normally the largest one among all directions of motions, the overlooking of other directions of motions will degrade the accuracy of radiotherapy. In order to achieve complete 3D tracking, either a good correlation between the third coordinate and the planar image is obtained, for example from a 4D-CT scan of the patient, or another imaging method is used for the third coordinate.

5.3   Follow-Up Work by Other Authors

The markerless gating and tracking methods described in this chapter were published in 2009 [19, 20]. Since then, many follow-up studies have been conducted in order to improve the accuracy and the running time; we review some significant advancements here since our publications.

Our work shows that the gating problem can be reformulated as a binary classification problem and using classifiers can generate marginally better results than template matching methods. In [16] Li et al. pointed out that classification-based methods usually require a training image set marked manually in each fluoroscopic template, which seems to be impractical to manually mark the tumor position in each image frame in a clinical setting. Thus Li et al. proposed a new and clinically more practical method based on template matching, where the templates are prepared from four-dimensional computed tomography (4DCT) at the stage of treatment planning. On the other hand, Li et al. also provided a new dimension reduction method to tumor gating called generalized linear discriminant analysis (GLDA), which explicitly takes the label information available in the training set into account [17].

Lewis et al. noticed several main challenges when applying our tracking method [15]. First, fluoroscopic image data should be acquired prior to treatment, and a clinician is needed to mark the tumor positions on the images for model training. Second, a training data set of fluoroscopic images must be acquired for each beam angle from which the tumor will be tracked. If the beam angle is changed, we need to prepare the new training data set for this specific beam angle. Third, tumors are often difficult to observe on fluoroscopic images, implying that purely dependence on fluoroscopic images might be clinically infeasible for some cases. To address these difficulties, Lewis et al. proposed an algorithm for direct tumor tracking in rotational cone-beam projections.

Rottmann et al. developed an algorithm that directly uses the on-board portal imaging device of the treatment machine for tracking lung tumors, which greatly reduce the additional dose exposed to the patients [30]. Interestingly he gave the following comments: "The classification approach lacks the ability to adapt to changes in the breathing pattern that cannot be described with the motion observed during the training session (extrapolation)". However, it works well for the application of gated treatment, where it is not necessary to know the precise location, but rather to decide whether the target is within a predefined region. To his comments we would like to mention that regression methods (rather than classification) are employed in our tracking system. We actually know little about the extrapolation capability of our tracking method when new motion patterns occur in the test data set rather than in the training set. But regression methods commonly have certain degrees of extrapolation capability to partially handle this scenario.

References

1. Adler, J.R., Murphy, M.J., Chang, S.D., Hancock, S.L.: Image-guided robotic radiosurgery. Neurosurgery **44**, 1299–1307 (1999)
2. Arslan, S, Yilmaz, A., Bayramgıleı, B., Uzman, O., et al.: CT-guided transthoracic fine needle aspiration of pulmonary lesions: accuracy and complications in 294 patients. Int. Med. J. Exp. Clin. Res. textbf8, CR493-497 (2002)
3. Balter, J.M., Wright, J.N., Newell, L.J., Friemel, B., et al.: Accuracy of a wireless localization system for radiotherapy. Int. J. Radiat. Oncol. Biol. Phys. **61**, 933–937 (2005)
4. Berbeco, R.I., Mostafavi, H., Sharp, G.C., Jiang, S.B.: Towards fluoroscopic respiratory gating for lung tumours without radiopaque markers. Phys. Med. Biol. **50**, 4481–4490 (2005)
5. Chang, C.C., Lin, C.J.: LIBSVM: a library for support vector machines. ACM Trans. Intell. Syst. Technol. **2**, 27 (2011)

6. Cui, Y., Dy, J.G., Sharp, G.C., Alexander, B., Jiang, S.B.: Robust fluoroscopic respiratory gating for lung cancer radiotherapy without implanted fiducial markers. Phys. Med. Biol. **52**, 741–755 (2007)
7. Cui, Y., Dy, J.G., Alexander, B., Jiang, S.B.: Fluoroscopic gating without implanted fiducial markers for lung cancer radiotherapy based on support vector machines. Phys. Med. Biol. **53**, N315–327 (2008)
8. Cui, Y., Dy, J.G., Sharp, G.C., Alexander, B., Jiang, S.B.: Multiple template-based fluoroscopic tracking of lung tumor mass without implanted fiducial markers. Phys. Med. Biol. **52**, 6229–6242 (2007)
9. Geraghty, P.R., Kee, S.T., McFarlane, G., Razavi, M.K., et al.: CT-guided transthoracic needle aspiration biopsy of pulmonary nodules: Needle size and pneumothorax rate. Radiology **229**, 475–481 (2003)
10. Haykin, S.: Neural Networks: A Comprehensive Foundation. Prentice-Hall International, Englewood Cliffs (1994)
11. Jiang, S.B.: Radiotherapy of mobile tumors. Semin. Radiat. Oncol. **16**, 239–248 (2006)
12. Jiang, S.B.: Technical aspects of image-guided respiration-gated radiation therapy. Med. Dosimetry **31**, 141–151 (2006)
13. Keall, P.J., Joshi, S., Vedam, S.S., Siebers, J.V., et al.: Four-dimensional radiotherapy planning for DMLC-based respiratory motion tracking. Med. Phys. **32**, 942–951 (2005)
14. Keall, P.J., Kini, V.R., Vedam, S.S., Mohan, R.: Motion adaptive x-ray therapy: a feasibility study. Phys. Med. Biol. **46**, 1–10 (2001)
15. Lewis, J.H., Li, R., Watkins, W.T., Lawson, J.D., et al.: Markerless lung tumor tracking and trajectory reconstruction using rotational cone-beam projections: a feasibility study. Phys. Med. Biol. **55**, 2505–2522 (2010)
16. Li, R., Lewis, J.H., Cervino, L.I., Jiang, S.B.: A feasibility study of markerless fluoroscopic gating for lung cancer radiotherapy using 4DCT templates. Phys. Med. Biol. **54**, N489–500 (2009)
17. Li, R., Lewis, J.H., Jiang, S.B.: Markerless fluoroscopic gating for lung cancer radiotherapy using generalized linear discriminant analysis. In: Fourth International Conference on Machine Learning and Applications, pp. 468–472 (2009)
18. Lin, T., Zha, H.: Riemannian manifold learning. IEEE Trans. Pattern Anal. Mach. Intell. **30**, 796–809 (2008)
19. Lin, T., Cervino, L.I., Tang, X., Vasconcelos, N., Jiang, S.B.: Fluoroscopic tumor tracking for image-guided lung cancer radiotherapy. Phys. Med. Biol. **54**, 981–992 (2009)
20. Lin, T., Li, R., Tang, X., Dy, J.G., Jiang, S.B.: Markerless gating for lung cancer radiotherapy based on machine learning techniques. Phys. Med. Biol. **54**, 1555–1563 (2009)
21. Moser, T., Biederer, J., Nill, S., Remmert, G., Bendl, R.: Detection of respiratory motion in fluoroscopic images for adaptive radiotherapy. Phys. Med. Biol. **53**, 3129–3145 (2008)
22. Murphy, M.J., Chang, S.D., Gibbs, I.C., Le, Q.T., et al.: Patterns of patient movement during frameless image-guided radiosurgery. Int. J. Radiat. Oncol. Biol. Phys. **55**, 1400–1408 (2003)
23. Murphy, M.J.: Tracking moving organs in real time. Semin. Radiat. Oncol. **14**, 91–100 (2004)
24. Neicu, T., Shirato, H., Seppenwoolde, Y., Jiang, S.B.: Synchronized moving aperture radiation therapy (smart): average tumour trajectory for lung patients. Phys. Med. Biol. **48**, 587–598 (2003)
25. Neicu, T., Berbeco, R., Wolfgang, J., Jiang, S.B.: Synchronized moving aperture radiation therapy (SMART): improvement of breathing pattern reproducibility using respiratory coaching. Phys. Med. Biol. **51**, 617–636 (2006)
26. Ozhasoglu, C., Murphy, M.J., Glosser, G., Bodduluri, M., et al.: Real-time tracking of the tumor volume in precision radiotherapy and body radiosurgery—a novel approach to compensate for respiratory motion. In: Computer Assisted Radiology and Surgery, pp. 691–696 (2000)
27. Papiez, L.: The leaf sweep algorithm for an immobile and moving target as an optimal control problem in radiotherapy delivery. Math. Comput. Model. **37**, 735–745 (2003)
28. Papiez, L., Rangaraj, D.: DMLC leaf-pair optimal control for mobile, deforming target. Med. Phys. **32**, 275–285 (2005)

29. Rangaraj, D., Papiez, L.: Synchronized delivery of DMLC intensity modulated radiation therapy for stationary and moving targets. Med. Phys. **32**, 1802–1817 (2005)
30. Rottmann, J., Aristophanous, M., Chen, A., Berbeco, R.: A multi-region algorithm for markerless beam's-eye view lung tumor tracking. Phys. Med. Biol. **55**, 5585–5598 (2010)
31. Roweis, S.T., Saul, L.K.: Nonlinear dimensionality reduction by locally linear embedding. Science **290**, 2323–2326 (2000)
32. Schweikard, A., Glosser, G., Bodduluri, M., Murphy, M.J., Adler, J.R.: Robotic motion compensation for respiratory movement during radiosurgery. Comput. Aided Surg. **5**, 263–277 (2000)
33. Shirato, H., Harada, T., Harabayashi, T., Hida, K., et al.: Feasibility of insertion/implantation of 2.0-mm-diameter gold internal fiducial markers for precise setup and real-time tumor tracking in radiotherapy. Int. J. Radiat. Oncol. Biol. Phys. **56**, 240–247 (2003)
34. Shirato, H., Shimizu, S., Kunieda, T., Kitamura, K., et al.: Physical aspects of a real-time tumor-tracking system for gated radiotherapy. Int. J. Radiat. Oncol. Biol. Phys. **48**, 1187–1195 (2000)
35. Suh, Y., Yi, B., Ahn, S., Kim, J., et al.: Aperture maneuver with compelled breath (AMC) for moving tumors: a feasibility study with a moving phantom. Med. Phys. **31**, 760–766 (2004)
36. Tang, X., Sharp, G.C., Jiang, S.B.: Fluoroscopic tracking of multiple implanted fiducial markers using multiple object tracking. Phys. Med. Biol. **52**, 4081–4098 (2007)
37. Tsao, A.: Lung Carcinoma: Tumors of the Lungs, Merck Manual Professional Edition (2007)
38. Trofimov, A., Rietzel, E., Lu, H.M., Martin, B., et al.: Temporo-spatial IMRT optimization: concepts, implementation and initial results. Phys. Med. Biol. **50**, 2779–2798 (2005)
39. Vapnik, V.N.: Statistical Learning Theory. Wiley (1998)
40. Webb, S.: The effect on IMRT conformality of elastic tissue movement and a practical suggestion for movement compensation via the modified dynamic multileaf collimator (dmlc) technique. Phys. Med. Biol. **50**, 1163–1190 (2005)
41. Webb, S.: Limitations of a simple technique for movement compensation via movement-modified fluence profiles. Phys. Med. Biol. **50**, N155–161 (2005)
42. Wijesooriya, K., Bartee, C., Siebers, J.V., Vedam, S.S., Keall, P.J.: Determination of maximum leaf velocity and acceleration of a dynamic multileaf collimator: implications for 4d radiotherapy. Med. Phys. **32**, 932–941 (2005)
43. Xu, Q., Hamilton, R.R., Alexander, B., Jiang, S.: Lung tumor tracking in fluoroscopic video based on optical flow. Med. Phys. **35**, 5351–5359 (2008)
44. Xu, Q., Hamilton, R.J., Schowengerdt, R.A., Jiang, S.B.: A deformable lung tumor tracking method in fluoroscopic video using active shape models: a feasibility study. Phys. Med. Biol. **52**, 5277–5293 (2007)

Image Guided and Robot Assisted Precision Surgery

Fang Chen, Jia Liu and Hongen Liao

Abstract Computer aided surgery (CAS) which integrates image guidance with surgical robot technologies is well accepted worldwide because of improved precision and small incisions. In this chapter, three key technologies in CAS will be introduced: (1) image processing based guidance, which involves analysis and integration of multimodality medical information; (2) 3D augmented reality based image guidance, which focuses on intuitive visualization of medical images; (3) various surgical robots that can be implemented precisely to complete complex tasks. Eventually, we discuss the future developments of image guidance and surgical robots in precise CAS.

1 Introduction

Traditional surgeries implement hand–eye coordination is limited in precision and efficiency due to inadequacies of human visualization and dexterity. Computer aided surgery (CAS) integrates image processing technology, computer technology, robot technology and clinical treatment technology. It is becoming more and more common worldwide compared with traditional surgeries [1]. CAS combines multiple medical image devices such as Computed Tomography (CT), Magnetic Resonance (MR), Positron Emission Tomography (PET), Digital Subtraction Angiography (DSA), and Ultrasound (US) and so on. By adding a positioning system, CAS can finish human anatomy display, preoperative planning and intra-operative localization [2]. CAS system improves surgical precision, reduces surgical invasiveness and overcomes many disadvantages of traditional surgeries [3].

Fang Chen and Jia Liu—equally contributed

F. Chen · J. Liu · H. Liao (✉)
Department of Biomedical Engineering, School of Medicine, Tsinghua University, Beijing 100084, People's Republic of China
e-mail: liao@tsinghua.edu.cn

© Springer International Publishing AG 2018
K. Suzuki and Y. Chen (eds.), *Artificial Intelligence in Decision Support Systems for Diagnosis in Medical Imaging*, Intelligent Systems Reference Library 140, https://doi.org/10.1007/978-3-319-68843-5_13

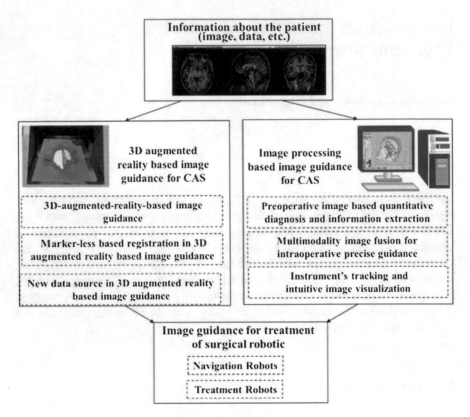

Fig. 1 Image guidance and surgical robot technologies in CAS

Figure 1 illustrates image processing, 3D augmented reality (AR) and surgical robot technologies in CAS. The input of CAS system derives from patient information, including medical images [CT, MR, PET, US, etc.], medical data [electroencephalograph (EEG), Electrocardiograph (ECG), etc.], lab test results, and so on. The next is image processing based guidance. It contains three contents: preoperative information is analyzed to achieve quantitative diagnosis; multimodality images are fused to guide intraoperative precise intervention; instruments are tracked and intuitive image visualization is applied. In addition to screen display based image guidance, the integrated information and images can be visualized intuitively through the 3D AR based image guidance. Based on image guidance, doctors and/or surgical robots can identify the targeted lesion accurately and perform the surgery precisely. In the following sections, we will introduce related technologies and application examples of image analysis, 3D AR and surgical robots in CAS.

2 Image Processing Based Guidance for CAS

Image analysis and guidance can enhance traditional diagnosis and treatment. Image analysis method contains multi-modality image fusion, image segmentation and surgical planning. Based on image guidance, doctors can perform minimally invasive therapy easier and safer. We will introduce related image processing techniques and applications of image guidance in CAS.

2.1 Overviews of Image Processing Based Guidance

Image analysis and guidance provide a solution to the blind area of observation caused by complex anatomical structures in operation. With the help of multi-modality medical images, such as MR, CT and US, more detail pathological information can be acquired [4]. Image-guided minimally invasive procedures reduce patient trauma, risk of complications and recovery time [5]. Image analysis and guidance can provide intuitive navigation information for doctors to assist interventional therapy and improve the accuracy of surgeries.

The rapid development of image processing and computing power makes it possible for the adoption of image guidance technology in clinical applications. A typical image-guided neurosurgery employs MR to identify critical brain tissues such as nerve fiber, tumor and so on. Intraoperative MR or US images are aligned with pre-operative data to correct brain shift, which often occurs during an operation [6]. During the spinal anesthesia surgery, real-time US image guidance is used to locate peripheral nerves and puncture needles. Traditional minimally invasive cardiovascular procedures rely on 2D X-ray angiography images to scan blood vessel and atherosclerotic plaque, simultaneously locate implantation stent. Therefore, image processing based guidance has increasingly played a significant role in addressing clinical problems.

Image processing based guidance is used in CAS in the following ways [4]. Firstly, by analyzing and reconstructing 2D cross-sectional images, the optimal path of surgical instrument can be decided to avoid damage to critical tissue. Secondly, the combination of multimodal images is acquired with various image registration and fusion methods to provide adequate information for surgeons. Thirdly, image based tracking method is used to locate the positions of anatomical structures and surgical tools. Finally, intuitive image visualization method is needed for surgeons to observe lesion and anatomical structures precisely.

To realize individualized treatment, image processing based pre-surgical planning is very important [7]. Pre-surgical planning involves modeling critical tissues and assessing trajectory of interventional devices (catheters, sheaths, guidewires, needles and so on). Sharifi et al. discussed the accuracy of surgery planning during orthognathic surgery [8]. Penkner et al. implemented soft tissue model to fabricate patient-specific auricular prostheses from CT images [9]. A virtual environment was produced to simulate the surgical procedure through 3D reconstructions of CT or MR images in liver surgery planning [10]. For maxillofacial surgical planning, automatic precise location method of the mid-facial plane was presented [11].

Besides modeling information from preoperative images, several researchers have proposed visualize intraoperative shape of critical structures by real-time US and MR images [12–14]. In neurosurgery, low field intraoperative MR image is fused with preoperative high field MR image to accommodate soft tissue deformation. Preoperative function MR and DT-MR images are non-rigidly aligned with intra-operative low field MR to enhance visualization and navigation in image-guided neurosurgery [12]. In addition, image guidance system incorporates pre-operative MR image with intraoperative 2D/3D US is used to estimate brain shift by deformable registration technologies. A rigid registration framework of US and CT images in the radiotherapy was proposed, which was based on a similarity measure that combined physical properties and artifacts in US image [13]. Intraoperative endoscopes are used through a small entry port, which can provide high-resolution real-time video images in a limited view of surgical site. So using ray-traced texture mapping, freehand endoscopic brain images were fused with 3D brain model of preoperative images by ray-traced texture mapping [14].

Accurate instruments tracking and intuitive navigation visualization are important components in CAS system. To acquire position of instruments relative to patient anatomy, optical tracking systems use optical markers and identify the markers in collected image sequence to estimate the pose and orientation of instruments [15]. The main problem of optical tracking systems is line-of-sight limitation. To avoid this limitation, the electromagnetic (EM) tracking system is presented which uses a motion-analysis-based tracking technology. Besides the tracking system based location method, intraoperative medical images can also localize instruments. During image-guided transcatheter aortic valve implantation surgery, the positions of valve and catheter are acquired by X-ray imaging [16]. For US-guided needle tracking, intraoperative US are widely used for localizing instruments [17].

Some commercial medical software platforms have been developed for realizing 3D modeling, tracking, registration, visualization and procedure training [18, 19]. An image guided neurosurgery system (Brainlab) involved surgical planning, CT/MR fusion, brain tissue segmentation [18]. Patient specific anatomical modeling and the alignment between preoperative and intraoperative image data were implemented in the neurosurgery navigator Medtronic StealthStation [19]. Coupled with upcoming image processing technologies, the CAS will create a paradigm change in patient treatment in the future.

We will introduce related techniques of image processing based guidance, including image analyzing and modeling, multi-modality information alignment, accurate instrument localization and intuitive visualization.

2.2 Related Techniques and Examples for Image Processing Based Guidance

Traditional surgeries rely on human eye to collect the information about lesion and tumor. However, they have limitations because of the inadequacies of human visualization. Image guidance uses medical image processing to guide surgeries. The related technologies of image processing shall be introduced here.

2.2.1 Preoperative Image Based Quantitative Diagnosis

To diagnose patient's disease precisely, different medical imaging modalities are used to detect lesions including tumor, plaque, and pulmonary abscess and so on. Various imaging modalities can provide different valuable structural and functional information about lesion but they have different limitations, such as image quality, time space resolution and field of view. Based on multi-modality preoperative medical imaging, surgeons can determine type and position of lesions to finish a surgery plan. However, manual image analysis lacks objectivity and is time-consuming. With the development of analytical algorithm and computing power, automatic quantitative image analysis is widely adopted. Several image analysis methods for overcoming manual subjectivity are introduced in the following text.

Noninvasive magnetic resonance angiography (MRA) is clinically popular to measure the pathological changes of vessels in cerebral aneurysm surgeries, cardiovascular interventional procedures and so on. Volumetric segmentation of blood vessels can achieve accurate assessment of plaque position and vessel wall measurement. To achieve automatic vessel segmentation, Gooya et al. proposed a unified segmentation framework R-FLUX, which integrated non-linear edge filter and geometric flux maximizing flow [20]. The main characteristics of the proposed method included three aspects: (1) the generalized definition of flux on Riemannian manifolds, which was suitable for vessel segmentation because of the oriented structures of vessels, (2) a new manifold metric method, (3) a function of vessel enhancing diffusion (VED) tensor. The R-FLUX method could effectively detect vessels in 3T MRA images and provide a variety of diagnostic information to clinicians without manual intervention.

In image guidance, preoperative images such as CT, MR and X-ray fluoroscopy are commonly used by registering with patient physical coordinate. Several registration methods such as point-based registration, surface-based registration and laser scan-based registration are implemented in the registration process. The deformation of tissue construct is an important factor affecting registration and navigation precision. Therefore, it is critical to study the displacement and physiological shift of tissue. An analysis method of carotid artery deformation in different head and neck positions was proposed for catheter navigation in oral cancer treatment [21]. In this study, the deformation of five branches from surrounding bones (such as the skull, jaw, cervical spine, etc.) was analyzed. Firstly, preoperative segmentation of two sets of CT angiography images was achieved to extract the carotid artery and the surrounding bones. Secondly, different data sets were aligned into a newly defined coordinate system to acquire the amount of deformation by iterative closest point registration method. The priori information of predicting shifts of carotid artery (CA) bifurcations can be used to improve the accuracy of patient-image registration process in image guided intervention.

Some software platforms have been developed for patient-specific preoperative image analysis and visualization. As open-source software, 3D slicer (see http://www.slicer.org/) supports various image file formats including DICOM, Raw, Standard Template Library (STL), etc. Basic modules have been integrated, including medical image segmentation, registration, modeling and 3D visualization. Some advanced modules and algorithms are also created including US calibration, fiber tracking, and visual endoscopy and so on. In addition, users can develop new image processing modules for specific applications on Slicer platform. Due to friendly interface, integrated image processing modulation and the support of re-development, Slicer has been more and more implemented in image processing based guidance. Figure 2 shows an example of segmenting and modeling brain tissue on 3D slicer platform. Another common used medical image software

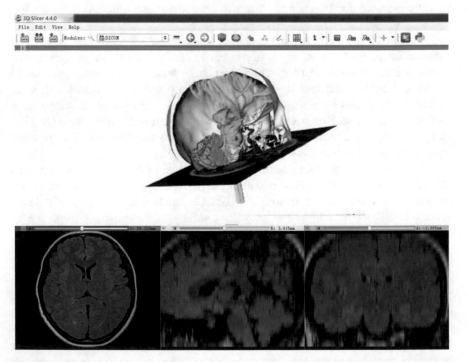

Fig. 2 The example of segmenting and modeling brain tissue for T1-weighted MR images on 3D slicer platform

platform is Mimics, which is an interactive medical image control system. Besides basic image modules such as segmentation, registration and visualization, the Mimics platform also integrates image measurement module and 3D re-meshing module. In addition, the Mimics platform has developed a convenient interface for data transmission with other software platform. For example, the FEA module in Mimics can process medical images and output corresponding files for finite element analysis. The Mimics platform has been used extensively in orthopedics operation, stent implantation operation, etc. These software platforms provide basic building blocks and components for CAS.

The goal of preoperative image processing is implementing automatic quantitative analysis to provide surgeons efficient and precision image information, and to reduce the influence of subjective factors.

2.2.2 Multimodality Image Fusion for Intraoperative Precise Guidance

Different image modalities are based on different imaging principles. Therefore, different image modalities have various image resolutions to provide various information of lesion. According to different classification criteria, image modalities can be divided into kinds of categories. Images modalities can be divided into preoperative and intraoperative images according to the image collection environment. Generally, preoperative images have high space resolution and intraoperative images have high time resolution. Besides, image modalities can be divided into global and local images according to the view of field. For example, global CT images can present whole abdomen, but endoscopic can only give local image because it has small field of view. Moreover, based on whether depicting the metabolism of anatomy, image modalities are divided into anatomical and functional images. Anatomical modalities include CT, US, MR, X-ray and so on. Functional modalities include PET, functional MR, fluorescence molecular images and so on. The information gained from multimodality images is usually of a complementary nature, so proper fusion of useful information from these images is often desired. Therefore, integration of multimodality images can guide intervention that is more precise. Three related multimodality images fusion techniques for intraoperative intervention shall be introduced in the following text.

Preoperative CT and intraoperative US fusion for vessel bifurcation localization in image-guided catheter intervention of oral cancers

Traditional 2D X-ray-fluoroscopy-guided catheter intervention of oral cancer lacks intuitive 3D images of the surrounding anatomy and causes repeated X-ray radiation. To solve this issue, an intraoperative fluoroscopy-free image navigation method was proposed by integrating preoperative 3D CT, intraoperative US and EM tracking information [22]. This navigation method combined catheter path information from EM tracking, preoperative 3D CT images and intraoperative

Doppler US images to localize target vessel bifurcations for image-guided catheter interventions.

There were three important coordinate systems, which need to be registered: EM tracker system coordinate, preoperative 3D CT image coordinate and intraoperative US image coordinate. To align EM tracker coordinate with preoperative 3D CT image coordinate, patients had to take CT scan with skin markers (fiducial points) around the head and neck. The centers of these markers were identified both in EM tracker coordinate with a stylus and in preoperative CT images. The transformation matrix from CT image to EM tracker coordinate was solved with iterative closest point method. Furthermore, the vessel centerline was extracted from freehand intraoperative Doppler US images by segmenting color pixels. The vessel center-lines in preoperative CT images were extracted on 3D Slicer platform by using least squares splines based curve fitting technologies. The vessel centerlines in US and CT images were registered. This registration between intraoperative US and pre-operative CT could compensate vessel deformation and accurately locate target vessel bifurcations. The proposed navigation method had been applied in a vivo image-guided catheter intervention experiment.

Fast mapping of local endoscopic image with global 3D US image for intrauterine fetal surgery

US image is commonly used in minimally invasive fetal surgery navigation to visualize 3D structure and shape of placenta. For visualization of placental vascular network, in twin-to-twin transfusion syndrome (TTTS), a fetoscope is used to collect real-time endoscopy video. However, it is difficult for surgeons to get all information of the placenta just based on endoscopic images because of small field of view. The fusion of global 3D US images and local endoscopic images can provide not only the structural information of whole placenta but also vascular connecting information. Liao et al. developed a system configuration for mapping endoscopic images with 3-D placenta model derived from US images to guide intrauterine fetal surgery [23] (see Fig. 3).

The proposed endoscopic and US image mapping system comprised three main steps. Firstly, endoscope calibration and tracking were used to calculate the transformation between endoscopic images coordinate and optical tracking system coordinate. The fish-eye lens in the camera produced a barrel-type spatial distortion, so the correction of endoscope images was needed by using camera's parameters from camera calibration. Secondly, another set of optical markers was mounted on US probe to track the poses of US probe. To acquire the poses of US images under US probe coordinate, a set of metal balls, which could be easily identified in US images, were used to calibrate the US probe. By integrating US probe's calibration and tracking results, the transformation between 3D US images coordinate and tracking system coordinate could be achieved. Thirdly, to map local endoscopic images onto the surface of placenta, a placenta model was generated from 3D US images. Finally, by using the transformation between 3D US images coordinate and tracking system coordinate, and transformation between endoscopic images

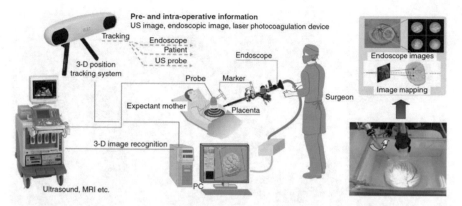

Fig. 3 System configuration for mapping endoscopic image mosaic with 3-D placenta model derived from US images (Liao et al. [23])

coordinate and tracking system coordinate, 3D US image coordinate and endoscopic image coordinate could be aligned to map endoscopic image onto placenta model.

The developed images mapping system for the treatment of TTTS can provide 3D large-scale images of placenta surface, which enables surgeons to observe vasculature system of twins without the need to memorize it.

Integrating anatomical MR images with functional fluorescence images for guiding laser ablation in precision neurosurgery

In tumor ablation surgery, surgeons need to identify the edges of tumor in order to perform a complete tumor resection and preserve normal tissues as much as possible. Nevertheless, it is difficult to distinguish tumor and normal tissues by using MR guidance alone although 3D MR images can provide 3D structure information. In contrast, functional fluorescence molecular imaging can illustrate brain tumor but cannot provide global structure of brain due to the limitation of imaging depth. For example, the 5-aminolevulinic acid (5-ALA)-induced protoporphyrin IX (PpIX) fluorescence can imaging tumor tissue. Therefore, Liao et al. developed an integrated diagnosis and therapeutic system using intraoperative 5-ALA-induced fluorescence guided robotic laser ablation for precision neurosurgery [24] (see Fig. 4).

During the integrated diagnosis and therapeutic system, 5-ALA-induced fluorescence measurement and analysis result were integrated into MR images to identify precisely the boundary of tumors, especially those of malignant tumors like glioma. The fluorescence detection was performed by a motor-driven fluorescence probe, and scanning probe was tracked under the tracking system. The collected fluorescence was guided into a spectrometer through an optical multi-mode fiber and then into a computer for spectral analysis. Based on spectral analysis results of the fluorescence, tissues could be divided into "tumor", "no-tumor" and "blended boundary". After accurate identification of tumor area, the micro ablation laser

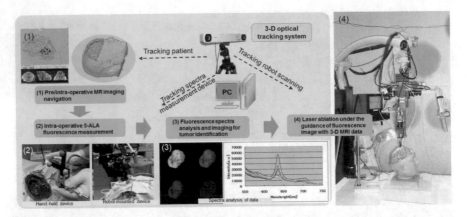

Fig. 4 System configuration of laser ablation treatment with guidance of 5-ALA-enhanced intra-operative navigation (Liao et al. [24])

ablated tumor area by automatic scanning. Therefore, the integration of high precision identification information of tumor contour from fluorescence images and entire brain construct information from MR images can obtain more precision tumor localization and navigate tumor ablation therapy.

2.2.3 Instrument's Tracking and Intuitive Image Visualization

Position information of surgical instruments is important in CAS. The instrument positioning methods can be divided into two categories: external tracking based and image based methods. Wang et al. proposed a catheter location method, which could accurately determine the pose and shape of catheter [25]. Two 5 degree of freedom (DOF) magnetic sensor coils were used to locate the tip of catheter unambiguously. The catheter shape between two sensors could be predicted using spline interpolation. However, external tracking systems have some limitations. For example, the accuracy of EM tracking is limited and optical tracking is complicated by line-of sight requirements. In image-based method, US and X-ray images are commonly used due to real-time imaging characteristics. An elegant framework was proposed for intraoperative instrument localization in minimally invasive fetoscopic surgery [26]. This framework used an US imaging system and a computation scheme without the requirement of external tracking system. In addition, intuitive image visualization is another essential component of image guidance. To obtain intuitive and continuous visual feedback, some studies about image visualization were proposed. A virtual endoscopy technique was adopted to generate virtual intravascular video as visual feedback to help surgeons place the stent precisely in oral cancer treatment [25].

In all, some studies have been made in the past decade about image processing based guidance, including more accurate image segmentation algorithms, more robust combinations of multimodality images and more precise tracking method of surgical tools, etc.

3 3D Augmented Reality Based Image Guidance in CAS

CAS is a new minimally invasive treatment method, which combines computer science, artificial intelligence, automatic control, image processing, 3D graphics, virtual reality and other clinical treatment technology. The multimodality images guidance will help doctors direct puncture surgical instruments into the body for local treatment. Besides, it can improve the quality of surgery and reduce surgical trauma. Although the image guidance technology plays a key role in CAS, conventional image guidance systems display the instrument and guidance image on a separate screen. In order to confirm the entrance of intervention and the position relationships between tools and targets, surgeons need to keep focus on the screen and patient. Thus, the accuracy and efficiency of operation are reduced significantly [27].

In CAS system, new technology is needed to address these issues. Augmented reality, which merges virtual computer-generated images into real surgical scene seamlessly and accurately, is a visualization technique [28]. Medical AR system can ensure the correspondence between real intervention environments and virtual images dynamically. AR visualization can facilitate hand-eye coordination, so that the physician can simultaneously observe real and virtual instruments.

3.1 Overview of 3D Augmented Reality

To achieve these goals, various techniques are applied to medical AR systems, such as 3D positioning technology, intra-operating imaging techniques and 3D visualization techniques [29]. Most AR system applied in surgical environment focus on the usage of augmented optics, head-mounted displays (HMD) and semi-transparent mirrors overlay systems [30].

Augmented optics is the method that operating microscope and binocular, can be inserted a semi-transparent mirror which reflects the virtual image into the optical path of real image. In 1985, Roberts et al. [31] presented the first augmented microscope, which showed a segmented tumor slice. However, this system used ultrasonic tracking which could not acquire real-time data. Augmented stereoscopic operating microscope for neurosurgical interventions was proposed by Edwards et al. [32] in 1995. However, this infrared tracking system limited the update rate to 1–2 Hz. In 2000, an augmented operating binocular was presented by Birkfellner et al. [33] for maxillofacial surgery. However, compared with other augmentation technology, the disadvantage of augmented optics was relative lag between the visualization of real and virtual images.

HMD is the method that combines real image and virtual image by a semi-transparent mirror. In 1992, Bajura et al. [34] proposed an augmented live video instead of optical image fusion using a magnetic tracking system. However, this system had poor image quality and was latency for the real view. In 2000, a video sees through system that allowed for a synchronized view of real and virtual images in real-time was developed by Sauer et al. [35]. Luo et al. [36] used HMD visualization to superimpose contour images. HMD system does not need the eye-to-display calibration, and just the camera-to-tracker transformation has to be calculated. However, this method produces the restriction of the position between eyes and eyepiece or screen.

Compared with the augmented optics and head-mounted displays, semi-transparent mirrors overlay systems can provide a larger viewing angle and a more comfortable visual perception for multiple observers. In 1995, a system with a semi-transparent mirror placed between the user and the object to be augmented was proposed by Masutani et al. [37]. This system used the virtual images, which were created by an auto-stereoscopic screen with integral photography technology. In 2001, Liao et al. [38] extended the integral photography technology to motion picture and proposed integral videography (IV) techniques. The medical AR system combines image overlay with IV techniques can display real 3D image on the geometry of space accurately, as shown in Fig. 5.

Through the IV techniques, doctors can get more complete and accurate patient information about organ morphology. Under the guidance of the naked eye 3D display of images, doctors can get flexible depth information to understand the hierarchy structure of tissues, organs and instruments.

Auto-stereoscopic image overlay is a good solution for AR in CAS, so this part focus most on the correlative methodology of image overlay.

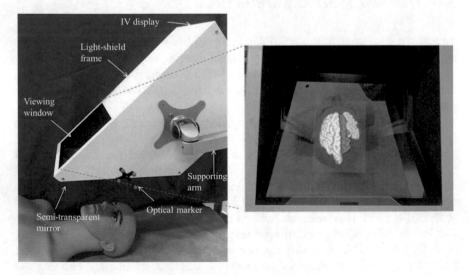

Fig. 5 IV image overlay device and IV images overlay of brain

3.2   Related Techniques and Examples of 3D AR Based Image Guidance

Image processing based guidance can provide doctors with 2D or 3D image of tissues on the computer screen, which requires surgeons with intensive hand-eye coordination to keep switching focus between the screen and patients. In comparison, 3D AR based image guidance can help surgeons obtain dynamic "see-through" scenes in CAS. The related technologies of 3D AR based image guidance and some research about marker-less based registration and high quality data source to improve the precision of the 3D AR based image guidance are presented in following text.

3.2.1   3D AR Based Image Guidance

3D AR based image guidance consists of an IV overlay device, a 3D data scanner, a position-tracking device and computers for image rendering and display. The IV overlay device is combined with an IV display aligned with a half-silvered mirror. Through the half-silvered mirror, surgeons can see the reflected IV image reflected in the corresponding location of surgical area. The tracking device is assembled on a robotic arm that can manipulate the overlay device to required position and posture. Working distance between the half-silvered mirror and surgical area can be adjusted by changing the distance between half-silvered mirror and IV display, as shown in Fig. 6.

The first part is the IV image generating and reconstruction. In order to create an IV image, every pixel on the background display needs to be computed. The calculation of elemental images can be achieved by two main IV rendering methods: volume rendering and surface rendering. To display 3D image of an object in real space, IV technique is a solution. The basis of IV comes from the principle of integral photography [39]. A micro lens array is placed in front of a high-density LCD display. Each pixel in the portion behind a micro lens emits a light ray in a unique direction that connects the pixel and the center of the lens. From a specific viewpoint, one can only see the set of light rays emitted from the pixels that lie on the straight lines connecting the viewpoint and the lenses. Consequently, different views of an IV image can be seen in various positions, just like a real 3D object in space. Data sources of IV images can be pre-operative, intra-operative medical images or computer-aided design models.

The second part is software system. The system includes two software modules, one is for navigation and the other is for IV image overlay. The preoperative segmented medical image data and the intraoperative spatial coordinate transformation matrix are required as navigation information, which is transmitted by transmission control protocol (TCP)/IP network to the image overlay device. The resulting IV images are displayed on the IV image overlay device. The 3D Slicer includes a GUI and a 2D/3D viewer, which uniquely integrates several medical

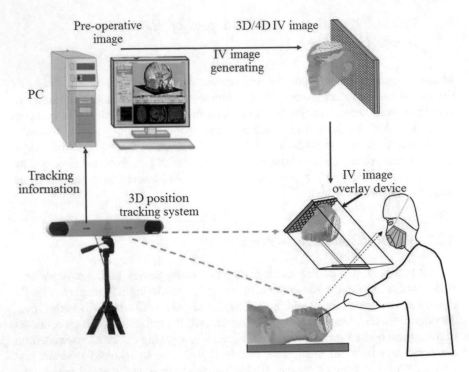

Fig. 6 Configuration of IV image overlay navigation system

image guidance modules into a single environment. The user interface of the IV image overlay navigation system is developed as an extended module based on 3D Slicer. Besides, 3D Slicer including volume-rendering algorithm and image segmentation model can be used as for navigation software development.

The third part is the registration between spatial 3D image and patient. Before the IV display, two important steps must be finished, pixel adjustment and image correction. Due to the errors between the width of the elemental image (corresponding to each lens) and the deformation of the IV image caused by the lens pitch, may significantly affect the perceived depth perception. A set of spatial test patterns can be used to calibrate the displayed IV image.

In image registration, a set of fiducial markers is used to track the position of the patient's body. These markers can be detected by MR, CT, US and other medical image acquisition devices. The registration process represents the relationship between the IV display and the coordinates of the reflected spatial IV image. It consists of the following three steps (Fig. 7): (a) IV image overlay device with IV image and reflected spatial image; (b) Using an optical probe to calibrate the spatial position of reflected IV images located in different planes; (c) Calibration of the position of the reflected spatial IV image. Thus, the relationship between the reflected spatial IV image and the patient can be determined.

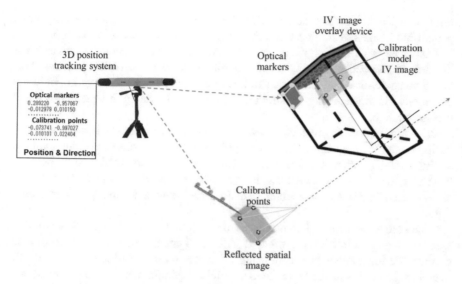

Fig. 7 Calibration of the position of the reflected spatial IV image

The 3D AR based image guidance is helpful in CAS that has been rapidly evolving since the last decade. There are some typical applications in CAS. Knee surgery is a type of minimally invasive surgery to treat the injured bone or the cartilage damage on knee. The positional precision of the tunnel is important, because it is closely related to the patient's rehabilitation. Although common navigation system can guide surgeons by the information displayed on the screen, it is not vivid and intuitive. Due to the limitations of unsatisfied hand-eye coordination and limited visual field, experienced surgeons are required to grasp the internal structure of knee joint. Liao et al. [40] presented a surgical navigation system for anterior cruciate ligament (ACL) reconstruction based on IV image overlay. This report was the first one that applied an IV image overlay system to ACL reconstruction surgery. Besides, by the means of 3D optical tracking system and semi-transparent mirror, the bone data obtained by CT could be reconstructed to 3D IV images and shown in the surgical view. The 3D reconstructed surgical navigation system could guide surgeons to see the structure of ACL and surgical tools inside the patient's body. Experiments testified that the average registration accuracy was about 1.16 mm and frame rate of IV image display was about 3 frames per second for organ, while 11 frames per second for surgical tools [41].

3.2.2 Marker-Less Based Registration in 3D AR Based Image Guidance

Although markers based methods in 3D AR work well in many applications, it is limited in some surgical environments, such as those operations performed within a limited space. Therefore, some researchers proposed some marker-less based patient-3D image registration techniques applied for AR navigation system.

Marmulla et al. [42] proposed an anatomical landmarks method to register the 3D data to the patient without using external fiducial markers. This method was based on anatomical landmarks on skull. However, anatomical landmarks could not be exactly identified during registration and surgery, therefore this method was not precise enough.

3D surface geometry matching is another approach of marker-less based registration method. For instance, Liao et al. [43] proposed a surface matching method. In this method, patient's image extracted from a 3D surface model could be matched to a 2D rendering surface model. Other methods of surface matching could also be used in 3D AR, like stereo-camera, laser surface scanning and structured light.

There are some new registration methods without markers in 3D AR navigation system. Wang et al. [41] presented AR navigation systems with automatic marker-free image registration by using IV image overlay and stereo tracking for dental surgery. This method overcame the main shortcomings in currently available technologies. Oral surgery was performed on the teeth and jaw in order to modify dentition. In most cases, operations were limited by the narrow space and surgical targets might be hidden in structures. Their proposed systems included a stereo camera tracker for tracking patients and instruments, an automatic real-time marker-free based patient-3D image registration method, an accurate IV image-camera registration method, and AR visualization using IV overlay. With the help of the 3D AR system, surgeons could obtain the depth perception, operate with both stereo, and motion parallaxes.

3.2.3 New Data Source in 3D AR Based Image Guidance

Pre-operative images such as MR and CT with high spatial resolution are often used for diagnosis and image guidance in surgeries such as orthopedics surgery, dental surgery and so on. In 3D AR based image guidance, these pre-operative images are commonly used as data source. However, preoperative images cannot reflect intraoperative soft-tissue deformation, which will influence the success rate of operation. To solve this problem, some research proposed to use the fused images of preoperative and intraoperative images as new data source of 3D AR navigation system.

Herlambang et al. proposed a 4D MR image visualization method that was generated from the registration between preoperative 3D MR image and intraoperative 4D US image [44]. The presented registration method integrated the inter-modality rigid registration between 3D MR image and 3D US image, and intra-modality non-rigid registration. Because IV rendering of 4D MR images is computationally costly, a flexible IV rendering pipeline with graphics processing unit (GPU) acceleration was significant. GPU provided a very effective way to perform interpolations through their naive texture accessing function, which solved the problem of time cost.

Intraoperative US image is commonly used for surgery guidance in liver surgery, fetal surgery and so on. Therefore, a real time 3D US surgical navigation system using IV technology was presented for minimally surgery [45]. To improve the image quality of 3D US IV images, a 3D median filter was implemented. Meanwhile, the IV rendering with the use of multi-threading made real-time visualization realized. Therefore, intraoperative image collection and IV rendering made online AR surgical navigation system developed. This system could overcome the drawbacks of traditional AR navigation system, which only used the preoperative medical images as data source.

3.3 Applications of 3D AR Based Image Guidance for Precise Surgery

To overcome the limitations of traditional spine surgery, 3D AR is used for spine revision cases and recommended in a preliminary report. Especially, when normal anatomic landmarks are difficult to identify during the surgery, the exact insertion of a cervical screw is needed. To improve the accuracy of screw placement in spine surgery, microscope, endoscope, navigation system and series of surgical instruments are used. Among these techniques, image-guide system is vital for successful access to the target area. During current spine surgery, image-guided system still suffers from the problem of hand-eye coordination as well as the lack of depth information. These drawbacks can be solved by 3D images, which can give depth information in the surgical region. Surgeons can have a better knowledge of the anatomic structure of lesion and position of surgical instruments through the 3D image guidance. 3D AR system is a promising solution that the virtual image in space is 3D with full parallax. Therefore, surgeons can see through the patient to know the relationship of internal structures. In this way, the accuracy and safety of the surgery will be increased.

Besides the applications in spine surgery, 3D AR has an extensive application in orthopedics surgery. Moreover, combined with the fluoroscopy, microscope and other therapy techniques, 3D AR can be used to show clear 3D vision of interested regions of the patient in minimally invasive orthopedics surgery.

We present several related technologies and analyze several clinical applications of 3D AR in CAS. By means of 3D AR, not only the problem about hand-eye coordination, but also the problem of hidden anatomical structure from the direct observation can be solved. IV image overlay systems provide auto-stereoscopic visualization of inner anatomical structure and surgical tools with correct depth information directly in the intraoperative scene. Furthermore, based on GPU accelerated algorithm, the data source of the IV images can contain pre-operative data as well as intraoperative data, such as MR/CT and US images. However, problems of IV image overlay still exist, such as the requirements of a suitable micro lens array and a display with high resolution. In the future, the method of seamless integration between the AR system and other operation instruments is worth investigating and clinical factors including efficiency and usability require further experiments and evaluations.

4   Image-Guided Surgical Robots

With the development of technologies, several new surgical robotic systems had been employed in various complex procedures. Through the application of surgical robot, the motions of surgeon's hand are replicated in the surgical field, while the hand tremors are filtered which leads to highly precision in surgery.

The surgical robotic systems can help surgeons to perform procedures with dexterity in areas not possible for bare hands. A surgeon sits on a console and performs procedure with the help of a robotic system in CAS. Robotics can be applied remotely to minimize X-ray exposure in needle placement surgery. For example, in acquired immunodeficiency syndrome (ADIS) treatment, the surgery is difficult because surgeons need to keep away from the infected blood and other biological samples. In the interventional radiology surgery supported by X-ray images, doctor is exposed to a large dose of radiation. The surgical robots can be employed in this situation. Surgical robots can be used in difficult procedures that require highly precise manipulations. It should be noted that instead of taking the place of a surgeon, robots would be operated by surgeons with improved accuracy, less time, and stability consistent motion control during a surgical procedure. Robots are used in conjunction with surgeons to reduce hand tremor and involuntary spasm.

4.1   Overview of Surgical Robots

A surgical robotic system generally contains a multiple DOF manipulation arm, which is coupled to a controller for controllably positioning the surgical tool. Furthermore, a safety monitoring processor can determine the relative positions between the surgical tool and a volumetric lesion model. The system further includes an optical tracking system. An output of the tracking system is coupled to the processor, which determines if the surgical tool is positioned outside of the volumetric model. A strain gage is contained in surgical robotic system for detecting slippage between an immobilized tissue and a reference point. The system also includes multiple safety features for suspending a motion of the surgical tool to prevent the tool from operating outside of the predetermined space.

The robot technology is integrated into minimally invasive surgery, so that it can better assist physicians to finish high quality surgery. Surgical robot has become a popular topic in medicine, machinery, automation, communications and other fields. In 1987, the first robotic surgery was completed in a laparoscopic chole-cystectomy on a woman [46]. Since then, there has been a steady increase in the research of robotic systems and technologies applied to critical surgical procedures. There were some representative surgical robots. One was EndoAssist system developed by Armstrong Project in 1993. The commercially available EndoAssist system was a robotic manipulator for minimally invasive thoracic and abdominal surgeries [47]. In 1996, Computer Motion Company in USA produced AESOP-2000 surgical robot, which achieved the voice recognition of the operating arm [48]. Based on the AESOP system, Computer Motion Company developed higher precision ZEUS surgical robotic system, which was the first generation of master-slave teleoperation surgical robots [49]. The main contribution of ZEUS system was to eliminate the shake of surgeons' hand, and make surgical procedure more accurate and stable. It had been successfully applied to valvular heart pros-thesis, total arterial coronary artery bypass grafting surgery, and so on. Intuitive Surgical Company in USA developed a new generation of minimally invasive surgical robotic system called da Vinci surgical robotic system [50] that was a telerobotic systems and equipped smart assistant tools such as 'hands-on' robots. The da Vinci system was the most famous example for telerobotic surgical robots, which used four arms. The da Vinci system consisted of two main components: a control console and the robotic apparatus with several manipulator arms. The development of surgical robotics is promising for improving the capabilities of surgeons when performing complex surgical procedures.

The development of medical image/information guided surgical robots also promotes the application of telesurgery. Telesurgery makes it possible for surgeons to diagnose, evaluate, consult and treat patients remotely [51]. The robots provide the possibility for developing master slave telesurgery systems for surgeries when surgeons and the patient are separated by a significant physical distance. Even now, the safety of the surgical robotic system is critical. Safety concerns are responsible for the cautious reception of autonomous robots. All surgical robots are designed to avoid injury within and outside the operational volume.

4.2 Classification of Surgical Robots

In accordance with the application of surgical robots, they can be divided into navigation robots and treatment robots. The task of navigation robots is to guide surgeons to operate properly surgical instruments and to determine the surgical site of lesion. The treatment behaviors shall still be completed by surgeons. In addition to the function of locating the lesion, treatment robots are also used to participate in specific treatment operations, such as bone cutting, laser ablation and anastomosis. Thus, more details about these two different surgical robots will be introduced.

4.2.1 Navigation Robots

Navigation robots can aid in precision targeting and act as a high-dexterity surgical tool to improve or enable new image-guided therapy options. A typical application of navigation robots is to use the preoperative images for surgical planning and execute the plan by using robot as a guidance tool. The application of navigation robots appeared earlier in the orthopedic therapies including osteotomy for total knee replacement and hip joint replacement [52, 53]. CT was used for surgical plan and actual osteotomy was carried out using robots. These orthopedic robots were placed in a CT scanner and were used in conjunction with imaging [54].

Preoperative images consist of MR and CT images. MR images can provide the most recent examination of a patient's anatomy to identify a target and critical surrounding tissue. Surgeons can use preoperative images to plan a trajectory to the target that avoids damage to critical anatomies. MR-compatible robots are particularly useful for guiding tools to the target following the planned trajectory and executing the treatment plan. From CT images, navigation robots offer the potential for automating instrument placement, alignment and insertion via a direct coupling to 3D positioning data. The first recorded surgical robotics application occurred in 1988 for CT-guided stereotactic brain surgery [54]. More recent examples included the Innomotion system (Innomedic Inc., Herxheim, Germany), which was mounted on a large frame that extended over the patient [55].

Besides these traditional image-guided robotic systems, 3D auto stereoscopic image overlay system integrated with a laser guidance device was a new image-guided robotic system, which improved the safety and accuracy of surgical treatments, especially those using linear surgical tools for puncturing and drilling [42].

Neurosurgery was one of the clinical applications of navigation robots. The entry and target points were planned on CT/MR images. The robot coordinate system was registered to the image coordinate system (typically with fiducials affixed to the patient's head). Registration was achieved by simultaneous tracking of the robot and fiducials attached to the patient's skull in the Neuromate system [56]. Special constraints of percutaneous access have led to the development of structures achieving remote center of motion (RCM) or fulcrum motion [57, 58]. In these systems, the RCM was positioned at the entry point, typically with an active Cartesian stage or a passive mechanical mechanism, and the robot set the needle direction and (sometimes) the depth.

Fetal surgery is different from general forms of surgery. Due to the fetus is fragile, the surgical instrument needs to be small and flexible enough not to hurt the fetus or the placenta. Liao et al. [59] designed a fetus-supporting flexible manipulator with balloon-type stabilizer for endoscopic intrauterine surgery (see Fig. 8). The flexible joint method enabled the stabilizer to reach the target sites within the confined space of the uterus under US image guidance. This navigation robotic system used US images to acquire real-time intraoperative information. After the stabilizer being inserted into the uterus through a small incision, the position of the fetus and the umbilical cord could be identified with the help of an endoscope.

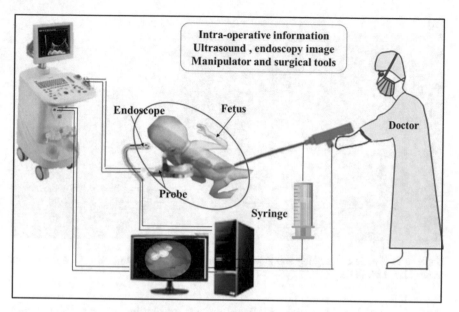

Fig. 8 Fetus support manipulator system for intrauterine surgery

4.2.2 Treatment Robots

The treatment robot as an extension of surgical navigation is used for the final execution of the surgical tasks. Both image-directed robots and surgical auxiliary robots are treatment robots [60]. The difference between an image-directed robot and a surgical auxiliary robot is the use of images. An example of an auxiliary robot is the da Vinci Surgical System (Intuitive Surgical, Inc.), which does not use preoperative or intraoperative images to guide the treatment device, but allows a physician to move surgical tools using robotic arms. An image-directed robot, like a surgical navigation system, performs preoperative planning by using preoperative images and drives the surgical device with a robotic arm according to the operative plan. An example of an image-directed robot is ROBODOC (with its software ORTHODOC, Curexo Technology Corporation) [61], which perform bone cutting precisely. A similar system, MAKO (Mako Surgical Corporation) has been used in total hip arthroplasty and total knee replacement surgery [62].

Complete removal of malignant gliomas is important for the prognosis in neurosurgery treatment. Currently, the challenge is how to detect any remaining tumors and remove them during the operation. Some researchers developed some laser ablation systems with accurate tumor analysis and image guidance for high-precision brain tumor resection during neurosurgery. Yamanaka et al. proposed a rigid endoscopic laser ablation system, and the diameter of the device was 7.0 mm [63]. The observation angle scope of this laser ablation system was constrained, which might lead to blind area in organs with sophisticated surface,

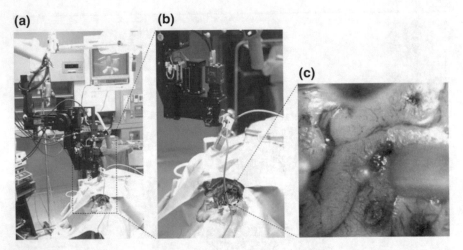

Fig. 9 **a** In vivo laser scanning and ablation experiment setup. **b** Surgical area. **c** Experiment scene (Liao et al. [24])

like colon. Patel et al. designed a laser scalpel employing a laser ablation unit produced by the New Scale Company, and the size of the scalpel was 17.0 mm [64]. Liao et al. studied automatic laser scanning ablation systems [65], especially a 5-ALA image guided laser scanning ablation system for high-precision treatment of brain tumors (Fig. 9). Though the proposed systems were integrated with imaging units for therapeutic operations, the sizes of the proposed systems were not appropriate for minimally invasive surgeries. Su et al. [66] proposed a laser ablation system whose distal module was a parallel four-bar mechanism combined with a micro CCD imaging sensor. The diameter of the distal module was 3.5 mm, which was very suitable for minimally invasive surgeries.

4.3   Application of Surgical Robots for Precise Surgery

High intensity focused ultrasound (HIFU) is a promising technique for cancer treatment owing to its minimal invasiveness and safety. MR-guided HIFU (MRgHIFU) and US-guided HIFU (USgHIFU) are two most common types of HIFU treatment systems.

The first MRgHIFU system built by GE Medical Systems (Milwaukee, WI) was tested by treating benign fibroadenomas in the breast at the Brigham and Women's Hospital [67]. In MRgHIFU, MR image guidance is expected to be a major advantage because both the tumor and its boundaries can be known during surgery. Thus, total ablation of the tumor can be accomplished. In addition, this noninvasive alternative to surgical lumpectomy requires no general anesthesia and leaves no surgical scar. However, the limitations of MRgHIFU still exist, including the oversize of the MR scanner, the complicated electronic control for HIFU focusing, the high manufacture and treatment cost. In contrast, USgHIFU has promising potentials in terms of its real-time imaging, compactness and low cost. Some robotic systems for HIFU treatment are also proposed to enable automatic and precise HIFU transducer positioning.

Yonetsuji et al. presented a novel HIFU robotic system for breast cancer treatment [68]. The robot had four rotational DOF with the workspace located in a water tank for HIFU beam imaging and ablation treatment. The HIFU transducer combined with a diagnostic 2D linear US probe was mounted on the robot end-effector, which was rotated around the HIFU focus while ablating the tumor. HIFU beams were visualized with the 2D probe by using beam imaging. The time cost could be significantly reduced, as there was no need to interrupt the ablation procedure for cooling the skin. In addition, these robot control strategies could avoid incomplete ablation.

5 Summary and Future Directions

This chapter presents several related technologies and applications examples about image guidance and surgical robots in CAS. With image analysis and guidance in CAS, surgeons can acquire adequate lesion information to achieve precision diagnosis and surgery planning. 3D AR provides surgeons perception that he is "seeing through" the anatomical structures and solves the problem of hand-eye coordination. Through intuitive guidance, surgeons can observe 3D images of lesion region directly. Furthermore, information driven surgical robots enable surgeons to treat individual patients with improved efficacy and reduced morbidity. Very significant researches have been made in three aspects: image processing algorithm, display resolution enhancement, auto-control way of surgical robotics. For 3D AR guidance, some researches focus on hard components development and the fusion of real and virtual images. In addition, under the guidance of intuitive medical images, some studies have developed more flexible robot to solve complex operations.

Future progress in CAS depends on the development of image analysis, 3D AR technology and surgery robot. New technologies of image analysis and guidance are being developed, which will produce more accurate target recognition, more quantitative lesion analysis, more intuitive navigation visualization and less treatment time. Novel diagnostic imaging techniques including specific fluorescence probe imaging and complex proteomics analysis, can improve the development of precise treatment. Popular deep learning will be implemented to realize precision classification of different levels of servility and provide quantitative diagnostic information. 3D AR is a promising means to achieve intuitive guidance, and will be applied in more types of surgery. Additionally, the surgery robot will be more flexible to achieve precise therapy. We foresee a significant future of CAS as it can improve safety and efficacy and reduce invasiveness compared with traditional surgeries.

References

1. Takakura, K., Iseki, H., Dohi, T.: Computer-Aided Aurgery. In: Computer-Assisted Neurosurgery, pp. 101–104. Springer, Japan (1998)
2. Berg, W.A., Gutierrez, L., NessAiver, M.S., Carter, W.B., Bhargavan, M., Lewis, R.S., Ioffe, O.B.: Diagnostic accuracy of mammography, clinical examination, US, and MR imaging in preoperative assessment of breast cancer 1. Radiology 233(3), 830–849 (2004)
3. Sati, M., De Guise, J.A., Drouin, G.: Computer assisted knee surgery: diagnostics and planning of knee surgery. Comput. Aided Surg. 2(2), 108–123 (1997)
4. Yaniv, Z., Cleary, K.: Image-guided procedures: a review. Comput. Aided Interv. Med. Robot. 3 (2006)
5. Fuchs, K.H.: Minimally invasive surgery. Endoscopy 34(2), 154–159 (2002)
6. Arbel, T., Arbel, T., Morandi, X., Comeau, R.M., Collins, D.L.: Automatic non-linear MRI-ultrasound registration for the correction of intra-operative brain deformations. Comput. Aided Surg. 9(4), 123–136 (2004)
7. Liao, H., Wong, K.K., Xue, Z.: Introduction to the special issue of image-guided surgical planning and therapy. Comput. Med. Imaging Graph. 34(1), 1–2 (2010)
8. Sharifi, A., Jones, R., Ayoub, A., Moos, K., Walker, F., Khambay, B., McHugh, S.: How accurate is model planning for orthognathic surgery. Int. J. Oral Maxillofac. Surg. 37(12), 1089–1093 (2008)
9. Penkner, K., Santler, G., Mayer, W., Pierer, G., Lorenzoni, M.: Fabricating auricular prostheses using three-dimensional soft tissue models. J. Prosthet. Dent. 82(4), 482–484 (1999)
10. Reitinger, B., Bornik, A., Beichel, R., Schmalstieg, D.: Liver surgery planning using virtual reality. IEEE Comput. Graph. Appl. 6, 36–47 (2006)
11. De Momi, E., Chapuis, J., Pappas, I., Ferrigno, G., Hallermann, W., Schramm, A., Caversaccio, M.: Automatic extraction of the mid-facial plane for cranio-maxillofacial surgery planning. Int. J. Oral Maxillofac. Surg. 35(7), 636–642 (2006)
12. Kuhnt, D., Bauer, M.H., Nimsky, C.: Brain shift compensation and neurosurgical image fusion using intraoperative MRI: current status and future challenges. Crit. Rev.™ Biomed. Eng. 40(3) (2012)
13. Wein, W., Röper, B., Navab, N.: Automatic registration and fusion of ultrasound with CT for radiotherapy. In: Medical Image Computing and Computer-Assisted Intervention–MICCAI 2005, pp. 303–311. Springer, Berlin (2005)
14. Dey, D., Gobbi, D.G., Slomka, P.J., Surry, K.J., Peters, T.M.: Automatic fusion of freehand endoscopic brain images to three-dimensional surfaces: creating stereoscopic panoramas. IEEE Trans. Med. Imaging 21(1), 23–30 (2002)
15. Khadem, R., Yeh, C.C., Sadeghi-Tehrani, M., Bax, M.R., Johnson, J.A., Welch, J.N., Shahidi, R.: Comparative tracking error analysis of five different optical tracking systems. Comput. Aided Surg. 5(2), 98–107 (2000)
16. Liu, Y., Liao, R., Lv, X.: Extended contrast detection on fluoroscopy and angiography for image-guided trans-catheter aortic valve implantations (TAVI). In: SPIE Medical Imaging, pp. 831618–831618. International Society for Optics and Photonics (2012)
17. Ungi, T., Abolmaesumi, P., Jalal, R., Welch, M., Ayukawa, I., Nagpal, S., Mousavi, P.: Spinal needle navigation by tracked ultrasound snapshots. IEEE Trans. Biomed. Eng. 59(10), 2766–2772 (2012)

18. BrainLab. Cranial navigation application. http://www.brainlab.com/art/2811/4/cranial-navigation-application
19. Medtronic. Image-guided surgery overview. http://wwwp.medtronic.com/
20. Gooya, A., Liao, H., Sakuma, I.: Generalization of geometrical flux maximizing flow on Riemannian manifolds for improved volumetric blood vessel segmentation. Comput. Med. Imaging Graph. **36**(6), 474–483 (2012)
21. Ohya, T., Iwai, T., Luan, K., Kato, T., Liao, H., Kobayashi, E., Tohnai, I.: Analysis of carotid artery deformation in different head and neck positions for maxillofacial catheter navigation in advanced oral cancer treatment. Biomed. Eng. Online **11**(1), 65 (2012)
22. Luan, K., Ohya, T., Liao, H., Kobayashi, E., Sakuma, I.: Vessel bifurcation localization based on intraoperative three-dimensional ultrasound and catheter path for image-guided catheter intervention of oral cancers. Comput. Med. Imaging Graph. **37**(2), 113–122 (2013)
23. Liao, H., Tsuzuki, M., Mochizuki, T., Kobayashi, E., Chiba, T., Sakuma, I.: Fast image mapping of endoscopic image mosaics with three-dimensional ultrasound image for intrauterine fetal surgery. Minim. Invasive Ther. Allied Technol. **18**(6), 332–340 (2009)
24. Liao, H., Noguchi, M., Maruyama, T., Muragaki, Y., Kobayashi, E., Iseki, H., Sakuma, I.: An integrated diagnosis and therapeutic system using intra-operative 5-aminolevulinic-acid-induced fluorescence guided robotic laser ablation for precision neurosurgery. Med. Image Anal. **16**(3), 754–766 (2012)
25. Wang, J., Ohya, T., Liao, H., Sakuma, I., Wang, T., Tohnai, I., Iwai, T.: Intravascular catheter navigation using path planning and virtual visual feedback for oral cancer treatment. Int. J. Med. Robot. Comput. Assist. Surg. **7**(2), 214–224 (2011)
26. Yang, L., Wang, J., Kobayashi, E., Liao, H., Yamashita, H., Sakuma, I., Chiba, T.: Ultrasound image-based endoscope localization for minimally invasive fetoscopic surgery. In: Engineering in Medicine and Biology Society (EMBC), 2013 35th Annual International Conference of the IEEE, pp. 1410–1413. IEEE (2013)
27. Peters, T., Cleary, K.: Image-Guided Interventions: Technology and Applications. Springer, Berlin (2008)
28. Liao, H., Edwards, P.J.: Introduction to the special issues of mixed reality guidance of therapy-Towards clinical implementation. Comput. Med. Imag. Gr. Off J. Comput. Med. Imaging Soc. **37**(2), 81 (2013)
29. Lamata, P., Ali, W., Cano, A., et al.: Augmented reality for minimally invasive surgery: overview and some recent advances. Augment Real 73–98 (2010)
30. Sauer, F., Vogt, S., Khamene, A.: Augmented reality. Image-Guided Interventions, pp. 81–119. Springer, US (2008)
31. Hatch, J.F.: Reference-display system for the integration of CT scanning and the operating microscope (1984)
32. Edwards, P.J., Hill, D.L., Hawkes, D.J., Spink, R., Colchester, A.C., Strong, M.A., Gleeson, M.M.: Neurosurgical guidance using the stereo microscope. In: Computer Vision, Virtual Reality and Robotics in Medicine, pp. 555–564. Springer, Berlin (1995)
33. Birkfellner, W., Figl, M., Huber, K., Watzinger, F., Wanschitz, F., Hummel, J., Bergmann, H.: A head-mounted operating binocular for augmented reality visualization in medicine-design and initial evaluation. IEEE Trans. Med. Imaging **21**(8), 991–997 (2002)
34. Bajura, M., Fuchs, H., Ohbuchi, R.: Merging virtual objects with the real world: Seeing ultrasound imagery within the patient. In: ACM SIGGRAPH Computer Graphics, vol. 26, no. 2, pp. 203–210. ACM (1992)
35. Sauer, F., Wenzel, F., Vogt, S., Tao, Y., Genc, Y., Bani-Hashemi, A.: Augmented workspace: Designing an AR testbed. In Augmented Reality. In: IEEE and ACM International Symposium on ISAR 2000. Proceedings, pp. 47–53. IEEE (2000)
36. Luo, G., Peli, E.: Use of an augmented-vision device for visual search by patients with tunnel vision. Invest. Ophthalmol. Vis. Sci. **47**(9), 4152 (2006)
37. Masutani, Y., Iwahara, M., Samuta, O., Nishi, Y., Suzuki, N., Suzuki, M., Takakura, K.: Development of integral photography-based enhanced reality visualization system for surgical support. In: Proceedings of ISCAS, vol. 95, pp. 16–17 (1995)

38. Liao, H., Nakajima, S., Iwahara, M., Kobayashi, E., Sakuma, I., Yahagi, N., Dohi, T.: Intra-operative real-time 3-D information display system based on integral videography. In: Medical Image Computing and Computer-Assisted Intervention—MICCAI 2001, pp. 392–400. Springer, Berlin (2001)

39. Lippmann, G.: Epreuves reversibles donnant la sensation du relief. J. Phys. Theor. Appl. 7(1), 821–825 (1908)

40. Liao, H., Nomura, K., Dohi, T.: Autostereoscopic integral photography imaging using pixel distribution of computer graphics generated image. In: ACM SIGGRAPH 2005 Posters, p. 73. ACM (2005)

41. Wang, J., Suenaga, H., Liao, H., Hoshi, K., Yang, L., Kobayashi, E., Sakuma, I.: Real-time computer-generated integral imaging and 3D image calibration for augmented reality surgical navigation. Comput. Med. Imaging Graph. 40, 147–159 (2015)

42. Marmulla, R., Hassfeld, S., Lüth, T., Mühling, J.: Laser-scan-based navigation in cranio-maxillofacial surgery. J. Cranio-Maxillofac. Surg. 31(5), 267–277 (2003)

43. Liao, H., Inomata, T., Hata, N., Dohi, T.: Integral videography overlay navigation system using mutual information-based registration. In: Medical Imaging and Augmented Reality, pp. 361–368. Springer, Berlin (2004)

44. Herlambang, N., Liao, H., Matsumiya, K., Masamune, K., Dohi, T.: Real-time autostereoscopic visualization of registration-generated 4D MR image of beating heart. In: Medical Imaging and Augmented Reality, pp. 349–358. Springer, Berlin (2008)

45. Herlambang, N., Yamashita, H., Liao, H., et al.: Real time integral videography auto-stereoscopic surgery navigation system using intra-operative 3D ultrasound: system design and in-vivo feasibility study. In: AMI-ARCS, vol. 61

46. Gatti, D.M., Shabalin, A.A., Lam, T.C., et al.: Fast map: fast eQTL mapping in homozygous populations. Bioinformatics 25(4), 482–489 (2009)

47. Halín, N., Loula, P., Aarnio, P.: Experiences of using the endo assist-robot in surgery. Stud. Health Technol. Inform. 125, 161–163 (2006)

48. Kraft, B.M., Jäger, C., Kraft, K., Leibl, B.J., Bittner, R.: The AESOP robot system in laparoscopic surgery: increased risk or advantage for surgeon and patient. Surg. Endosc. Other Interv. Tech. 18(8), 1216–1223 (2004)

49. Butner, S.E., Ghodoussi, M.: A real-time system for tele-surgery. In: ICDCS, p. 0236. IEEE (2001)

50. Miyamoto, S., Sugiura, M., Watanabe, S., Oyama, K.: Development of minimally invasive surgery systems. Hitachi Rev. 52(4), 189 (2003)

51. Zhao, D., Ma, L., Ma, C., Tang, J., Liao, H.: Floating autostereoscopic 3D display with multidimensional images for telesurgical visualization. Int. J. Comput. Assist. Radiol. Surg. 11, 207–215 (2016)

52. Taylor, R.H., Mittelstadt, B.D., Paul, H., Hanson, W., Kazanzides, P., Zuhars, J.F., Bargar, W.L.: An image-directed robotic system for precise orthopaedic surgery. IEEE Trans. Robot. Autom. 10(3), 261–275 (1994)

53. Kienzle, T.C., Stulberg, S.D., Peshkin, M., Quaid, A., Wu, C.: An integrated CAD-robotics system for total knee replacement surgery. In: Proceedings of IEEE International Conference on Robotics and Automation, Atlanta, pp. 899–894 (1993)

54. Kwoh, Y.S., Hou, J., Jonckheere, E., Hayati, S.: A robot with improved absolute positioning accuracy for CT guided stereotactic brain surgery. IEEE Trans. Biomed. Eng. 35(2), 153–160 (1988)

55. Melzer, A., Gutmann, B., Remmele, T., Wolf, R., Lukoscheck, A., Bock, M., Fischer, H.: Innomotion for percutaneous image-guided interventions. IEEE Eng. Med. Biol. Mag. 27(3), 66–73 (2008)

56. Li, Q.H., Zamorano, L., Pandya, A., Perez, R., Gong, J., Diaz, F.: The application accuracy of the NeuroMate robot—a quantitative comparison with frameless and frame-based surgical localization systems. Comput. Aided Surg. 7(2), 90–98 (2002)

57. Stoianovici, D., Whitcomb, L.L., Anderson, J.H., Taylor, R.H., Kavoussi, L.R.: A modular surgical robotic system for image guided percutaneous procedures. In: Medical Image

Computing and Computer-Assisted Intervention—MICCAI'98, pp. 404–410. Springer, Berlin (1998)

58. Taylor, R.H., Funda, J., Eldridge, B., Gomory, S., Gruben, K., LaRose, D., ..., Anderson, J.: A telerobotic assistant for laparoscopic surgery. IEEE Eng. Med. Biol. Mag. 14(3), 279–288 (1995)
59. Liao, H., Suzuki, H., Matsumiya, K., Masamune, K., Dohi, T., Chiba, T.: Fetus-supporting flexible manipulator with balloon-type stabilizer for endoscopic intrauterine surgery. Int. J. Med. Robot. Comput. Assist. Surg. 4(3), 214–223 (2008)
60. Dogangil, G., Davies, B. L., y Baena, F.R.: A review of medical robotics for minimally invasive soft tissue surgery. Proc. Inst. Mech. Eng. Part H: J. Eng. Med. 224(5), 653–679 (2010)
61. Taylor, R.H., Joskowicz, L., Williamson, B., Guéziec, A., Kalvin, A., Kazanzides, P., ..., Sahay, A.: Computer-integrated revision total hip replacement surgery: concept and preliminary results. Med. Image Anal. 3(3), 301–319 (1999)
62. Tarwala, R., Dorr, L.D.: Robotic assisted total hip arthroplasty using the MAKO platform. Curr. Rev. Musculoskelet. Med. 4(3), 151–156 (2011)
63. Yamashita, H., Matsumiya, K., Masamune, K., Liao, H., Chiba, T., Dohi, T.: Two-DOFs bending forceps manipulator of 3.5-mm diameter for intrauterine fetus surgery: feasibility evaluation. Int. J. Comput. Assist. Radiol. Surg. 1, 218 (2006)
64. Patel, S., Rajadhyaksha, M., Kirov, S., Li, Y., Toledo-Crow, R.: Endoscopic laser scalpel for head and neck cancer surgery. In: SPIE BiOS International Society for Optics and Photonics. p. 8207, 82071S–82071S (2012)
65. Liao, H., Noguchi, M., Maruyama, T., Muragaki, Y., Iseki, H., Kobayashi, E., Sakuma, I.: Automatic focusing and robotic scanning mechanism for precision laser ablation in neurosurgery. In: 2010 IEEE/RSJ International Conference on Intelligent Robots and Systems (IROS), pp. 325–330. IEEE (2010)
66. Su, B., Shi, Z., Liao, H.: Micro laser ablation system integrated with image sensor for minimally invasive surgery. In: 2014 IEEE/RSJ International Conference on Intelligent Robots and Systems (IROS 2014), pp. 2043–2048. IEEE (2014)
67. Hynynen, K., Pomeroy, O., Smith, D.N., Huber, P.E., McDannold, N.J., Kettenbach, J., ... Jolesz, F.A.: MR imaging-guided focused ultrasound surgery of fibroadenomas in the breast: a feasibility study 1. Radiology 219(1), 176–185 (2001)
68. Yonetsuji, T., Ando, T., Wang, J., Fujiwara, K., Itani, K., Azuma, T., Liao, H.: A novel high intensity focused ultrasound robotic system for breast cancer treatment. In: Medical Image Computing and Computer-Assisted Intervention—MICCAI 2013, pp. 388–395. Springer, Berlin (2013)